Psychedelic-Assisted EMDR Therapy

W0114821

Psychedelic-Assisted EMDR Therapy is a groundbreaking exploration of how eye movement desensitisation and reprocessing (EMDR) therapy can be harnessed to enhance the beneficial effects of psychedelic medications. EMDR is a clinically validated therapy that utilises bilateral stimulation of the brain to access and reconsolidate pathologically encoded memories. The protocolised methods outlined herein offer a practical roadmap for unlocking the full potential of EMDR within the context of psychedelic-assisted psychotherapies, paving the way for scalable psychedelic treatment options.

Drawing upon a rich tapestry of research, case material and clinical insight, this book provides readers with a comprehensive understanding of how EMDR's adaptive information processing (AIP) model conceptualises healing outcomes in psychedelic settings. Emphasising harm reduction, social justice and sustainability, this book systematically outlines a strong focus for the work, to ensure safer, more inclusive, equitable, environmentally conscious practices in psychedelic therapy delivery.

Authored by experts in the field, this is a compelling resource that expands the horizon of contemporary psychedelic psychotherapy, offering a novel perspective and a confident new voice in trauma-responsive healing.

Hannah Raine-Smith is an integrative psychotherapist and clinical supervisor working in private practice in the UK. She holds an MSc in EMDR and has studied postgraduate cognitive neuroscience at Cardiff University.

Jocelyn Rose is a psychotherapeutic counsellor, EMDR practitioner and clinical supervisor. She works as a psychedelic therapist on the DMT and 5-MeO-DMT clinical research trials. An educator and facilitator, Jocelyn also cofacilitates various community events.

"The insights and experiences shared here will challenge many preconceived notions and hopefully inspire new perspectives of fusing psychedelic therapy with EMDR. I think this book might serve as a beacon of innovation and knowledge and as a catalyst for positive developments in mental health treatment advancement."

David Nutt, professor of neuropsychopharmacology at Imperial College London and author of Psychedelics

"As someone who has explored a range of therapeutic modalities to integrate and heal the psychedelic-induced psychotic states I experienced in 1967, I found my EMDR sessions to be uniquely effective in revealing the roots of those terrifying experiences in early childhood trauma. I am deeply grateful for the healing that transpired during that work, and I applaud the timely publication of this comprehensive, groundbreaking volume."

Scott Hill, author of Confrontation with the Unconscious: Jungian Depth Psychology and Psychedelic Experience

"This is an original and compelling model of a trauma-focused psychedelic therapy with transformative potential for health care. This comprehensive book develops new protocols and models of best practice into a previously unexplored area of the psychedelic field."

Maria Papaspyrou and Tim Read, co-directors of the Institute of Psychedelic Therapy and co-authors of Psychedelics and Psychotherapy

Psychedelic-Assisted EMDR Therapy

A Memory-Consolidation Approach to Psychedelic Healing

Hannah Raine-Smith and Jocelyn Rose

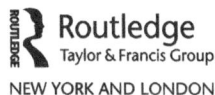

Routledge
Taylor & Francis Group

NEW YORK AND LONDON

Designed cover image: © Araminta Studio – Didier Kobi/Getty Images

First published 2025
by Routledge
605 Third Avenue, New York, NY 10158

and by Routledge
4 Park Square, Milton Park, Abingdon, Oxon, OX14 4RN

Routledge is an imprint of the Taylor & Francis Group, an informa business

ISBN: 978-1-032-55628-4 (hbk)
ISBN: 978-1-032-55627-7 (pbk)
ISBN: 978-1-003-43171-8 (ebk)

DOI: 10.4324/9781003431718

Typeset in Sabon
by codeMantra

This book is dedicated to the incredible humans, who, in pursuit of healing, have shared so much of themselves with us.

Contents

x *Contents*

Acknowledgements

The story that underpins this book first began in the Autumn of 2022. It was a post-pandemic world, and we both found ourselves in attendance at a very small psychedelic practitioners' event in London that had been organised by the Institute of Psychedelic Therapy (IPT). Upon first meeting, a spark was ignited, and we have been fanning these flames of enthusiasm ever since. There is strength in relationship, where ideas are cultivated, passions are validated and integrity is upheld. Each of us wants to acknowledge the tremendous impact that our relationship has had on the way that we work and on the quality of what we have been able to coproduce. We recognise that without one another, the material that we are about to share with you would never have come to fruition.

Moreover, our individual journeys to this point would not have been possible without the skills and wisdom gained through the rich tapestry of experiences that motherhood provides. Our wonderful children – Obi, Fred, Elizabeth, Jemima, Esther and Huey – have taught us more than we could ever have imagined possible and leave a heart-shaped imprint throughout our clinical practices and in all that we write. Alongside this, an endless list of unspeakable gratitude to Ben and Andy for their dedication to our homes and to our children as we birthed this project into existence. We really appreciate all that they did to make this possible. With loving thanks also to our parents, our wider families and our ancestors, each of whom cocreated these systemic conditions and who will continue to make this work so meaningful to us.

We wish to deliver a special mention of thanks to Maria and Tim and the wonderful community of practitioners who make up the IPT. Our IPT family have become an infinite resource of community support, expertise and love. In you, we have found our tribe. To dear Scott, a million thanks for allowing us to be a small part of your continuing journey, and as this is the acknowledgements section, you can't ask the editors to remove this celebration of all that you have done to normalise psychotraumatology in the field of psychedelics. You model vulnerability with such refreshing humility. Scott, you are an absolute legend! We are also especially grateful to Jono for the long days and sleepless nights, for his dedication to precision thinking and for his unwavering support of this project. Thanks to JP, who served as a constant reminder of the bigger picture and the importance of re-politicising mental health. Thanks to Ben who championed our leadership and whose passion for sustainability has so deeply influenced our thinking. And thanks too to Martin, Graham and Silvia for their expertise, sage advice, tireless reviews and endless generosity with their time. Each of you has broadened our perspectives and significantly contributed to the overall quality of the piece. Your marks are undeniably etched into every chapter.

Extending thanks to Julie for her feedback on the developing protocol despite being so unwell. At the time of writing, there were very few people who knew both EMDR and psychedelic therapy well enough to have offered this gift to us. Julie's parting words of encouragement to us were of her hope that "life isn't getting in the way of the brilliant work you are doing." Words that continue to resonate so deeply and remind us of the preciousness of our 'life(s) work.'

With thanks to Gabriella Cook for her beautiful artwork, whose ink is dotted throughout these pages. Each diagram required tireless patience through countless revisions as we slowly developed our theoretical frameworks and adopted ever more sophisticated models for our ideas. Gabriella works as a tattoo artist, and her exquisite body art can be found on Instagram: @gabriellafrancestattoo.

As we embrace all that the future has to offer, we also want to acknowledge the role that technological innovation has played in what we have been able to share with our audiences. The artificial intelligence of Chat-GPT, QuillBot and basic spellchecking software has helped us to pull our ideas together and has somehow managed to coordinate these two dyslexic scattered brains of ours into a coherent product that we hope you will enjoy. Throughout our practice, we see that innovation cannot be ignored as we move towards better education and healthcare outcomes for all.

With thanks to our editor, Anna Moore, and the team at Routledge for tying up the loose ends and for helping us to publish material positioned at the forefront of clinical advancement. Despite the social stigmas that still surround the use of psychedelics, their work has contributed to our confidence in bringing our ideas and expertise out into the public domain.

Forever in gratitude of Francine Shapiro, whose contribution to evidence-based trauma-focused practice sculpted the foundations upon which our work is based. We acknowledge the contributions of the many advocates and enthusiasts who have trailblazed the way in getting the psychedelic movement going again after many years of scientific censorship. And thanks to the countless underground and shamanic practitioners who kept the healing arts of natural rhythms, plant and animal medicine work alive, despite generations of persecutory practices.

Finally, we give thanks to the lands upon which we live. The beauty of the natural world serves as a constant reminder that our lives are interconnected and that our communal healing journey is shared with all that coexists on this, our shared planet.

About the authors

Hannah is a psychotherapist, clinical supervisor and trainer working in private practice. She has a long-standing special interest in trauma and psychedelics. During her BSc in psychotherapeutic counselling, she developed a specialism in complex PTSD early on through work in a number of domestic violence charities. During this time, she began researching the use of psychedelics to facilitate the integration of trauma. She went on to study postgraduate cognitive neuroscience at the Cardiff University Brain Research Imaging Centre in Wales. Here she discovered EMDR, and through reviewing the literature, she noticed similarities between the underlying neurobiological mechanisms of altered states of consciousness elicited by psychedelics and EMDR reprocessing and went on to train under Professor Derek Farrell on the EMDR master's programme in the UK. Hannah has been using EMDR to facilitate the integration of difficult psychedelic experiences in her private practice since 2018 and has been adapting the eight phases of EMDR to treat PTSD caused by psychedelics. Her extensive training in attachment, trauma, neuroscience and the AIP model informs her research into psychedelic-assisted EMDR. More information can be found on her website: www.traumatology.co.uk

Jocelyn is a psychodynamic psychotherapeutic counsellor, EMDR practitioner and clinical supervisor working in private practice. She co-facilitates the Brighton Psychedelic Integration Circle and Brighton Psychedelics events. She holds a two-year diploma in psychedelic-assisted therapy and has worked in clinical research since 2021, first as a psychedelic therapist on the DMT for treatment-resistant depression clinical research trial and now also as a lead therapist on several 5-MeO-DMT clinical trials. Jocelyn is an educator. For over a decade, she worked with adults and young people as a qualified teacher and lecturer in psychology and developmental neuroscience. She was involved in educational research and had a special interest in teaching psychopathology. Jocelyn continues her work as an independent researcher in various contexts. More information about Jocelyn and how she works can be found on her website: www.jocelynclairerose.co.uk.

Both women are members of the Drug Science psychedelic therapies working group and cohost the psychedelic-assisted EMDR international working group. They also facilitate an EMDR special interest group (SIG) at the IPT.

Until Hannah and Jocelyn met, both of them had been independently enthusing about the potential of EMDR as a psychedelic therapy to anyone who would listen. Then, in 2022, their paths finally crossed at an in-person event at the IPT in London, and they have been nerding out about the synergistic benefits of combining EMDR and psychedelics ever since. Their shared passion has taken them on a journey of discovery. Drawing on their extensive experiences in private practice and their learning from various practitioner trainings and from their involvement in clinical research, their expertise has since been further enriched through self-experimentation in legal retreat settings abroad. The information shared herein is based on a diverse blend of these varied skill sets. The process of writing has also helped to cultivate, sculpt and further refine their thinking. Within a few months of meeting, they had co-written and published two articles for EMDR UK's online magazine. The psychedelic-assisted EMDR therapy protocol emerged as a consequence of their collaboration and this developing expertise. Fuelled on by their enthusiasm and inspired by the results that they were getting in their clinical work, their ideas soon evolved to include EMDR as a psychedelic-assisted therapy across the preparation, dosing and integration phases of delivery. They facilitate a variety of harm-reduction and training initiatives, utilising the AIP framework (Shapiro, 2001) to support individuals, practitioners and healthcare settings to adopt a trauma-focused approach to psychedelic healing.

Both women run their own businesses and are industriously busy working parents. Their analytic drive and determination have come about as a consequence of their own resilience-building life experiences. Despite their expertise, intellectual curiosity and extensive training, both recognise that their real work is, and will continue to be, the deep inner work that they do on themselves.

Foreword by Professor David Nutt

The field of psychotherapy now stands at a crossroads, where traditional approaches meet innovative paradigms, offering new pathways to healing and personal growth. This book marks the beginning of a journey of exploration and discovery at the intersection of two remarkable healing modalities: eye movement desensitisation and reprocessing (EMDR) and psychedelic-assisted therapy. This groundbreaking book ventures into uncharted territories, guided by some of the practitioners who are reshaping the landscape of psychedelic therapy.

As a professor of neuropsychopharmacology and an advocate for evidence-based drug policy reform, I have long been intrigued by the transformative potential of psychedelic drugs and the potential synergistic benefits of using them in conjunction with established psychotherapeutic modalities. Eventually, I expect a cohesive evidence base to emerge that will help to orchestrate which treatments become most widely available, and of course, any therapy that can be demonstrated to enhance the effects and safety of these medicines will become the most clinically useful and therefore the most likely to be used.

EMDR has already gained widespread recognition and a compelling evidence base demonstrating its effectiveness in treating trauma-related disorders. Its adaptive information processing model, coupled with bilateral stimulation techniques, has already revolutionised trauma-focused therapy. Now, imagine merging this scientifically validated methodology with the healing benefits of expanded states of consciousness, facilitated by psychedelic substances.

At first glance, the idea of combining EMDR with psychedelics may seem audacious or even controversial. Yet, as we delve deeper into the science and therapeutic potential, we uncover a wealth of possibilities. Psychedelics, when used judiciously and within a supportive therapeutic framework, such as those outlined in the PsyA-EMDR protocols, can catalyse profound shifts in perception, cognition and emotional processing. These methods offer a unique window into the subconscious mind, opening doors into adaptive insights, enhanced clinical malleability and healing outcomes that may otherwise remain blocked.

In this book, pioneers in the field share their knowledge, experiences and innovative approaches to integrating EMDR with psychedelic-assisted therapy. Through detailed case studies, clinical insights and theoretical frameworks, they illuminate the transformative potential of adopting this synergistic approach.

This book also delves into the neurobiological underpinnings of EMDR and psychedelics, exploring how these modalities interact at the level of brain function and neural structure. It examines the therapeutic mechanisms at play and the nuances of guiding individuals through psychedelic experiences, all laid out within a trauma-informed context.

One of the most intriguing aspects of this emerging field is its potential to address complex psychological conditions. EMDR frameworks are already well versed in dealing with psychological complexity, and this book maps out what adaptations might be needed to bring these clinical cohorts into psychedelic treatment settings. The ethics of accessibility, working within diversity and inclusive practice, is also addressed, illustrating a justification for adopting the PsyA-EMDR therapy approach.

As we navigate this frontier, it is essential to maintain a balance between innovation and evidence-based practice. Rigorous research, ethical guidelines and professional standards form the bedrock of responsible psychedelic therapy. The insights shared in this book reflect a commitment to advancing the field with integrity and compassion and act as a guide for those who will, in time, build the emergent evidence base where it becomes possible and when it becomes necessary.

To the readers embarking on this journey, I encourage you to approach these pages with an open mind and a spirit of analytical enquiry. The insights and experiences shared here may challenge preconceived notions, inspire new perspectives and ignite curiosity. May this book serve as a beacon of innovation and knowledge as well as a catalyst for positive change in the evolving landscape of mental health advancement.

David Nutt is a professor of neuropsychopharmacology at Imperial College London and author of *Psychedelics* (published by Yellow Kite Press).

Acronyms and abbreviations

5-HT	serotonin
5-HT1A	serotonin 21A receptor
5-HT2A	serotonin 2A receptor
ACT	acceptance and commitment therapy
ACE	accept, embody, connect model
ACEs	adverse childhood experiences
AIP	adaptive information processing
BLS	bilateral stimulation of the brain
CBT	cognitive behavioural therapy
cPTSD	complex post-traumatic stress disorder
DMT	dimethyl tryptamine
DEA	Drug Enforcement Administration
EMDR	eye movement desensitisation and reprocessing
GAD-7	general anxiety disorder questionnaire
HPPD	hallucinogen persisting perceptive disorder
LSD	lysergic acid diethylamide
MAPS	Multidisciplinary Association for Psychedelic Studies
MDMA	3,4-Methylenedioxymethamphetamine
NC	negative cognition
PAP	psychedelic-assisted psychotherapy
PC	positive cognition
PHQ-9	patient health questionnaire (depression scale)
PTSD	post-traumatic stress disorder
REBUS	relaxed beliefs under psychedelics
SSRI	selective serotonin reuptake inhibitor
SUD	subjective unit of distress scale
TRD	treatment-resistant depression
VOC	validity of cognition scale

Disclaimer

Nothing contained herein is intended to encourage or support illegal behaviour. However, as the therapeutic use of psychedelics is being legalised incrementally across the globe, access to these substances is becoming more widespread; therefore, this material has been prepared with the core aim of harm reduction in this rapidly changing climate.

This book contains information obtained from authentic and highly regarded sources. While all reasonable efforts have been made to publish reliable data and information, neither the authors nor the publisher can accept any legal responsibility or liability for any errors or omissions that may be made. The publishers wish to make clear that any views or opinions expressed in this book by individual editors, authors or contributors are personal to them and do not necessarily reflect the views/opinions of the publishers. The information or guidance contained in this book is intended for use by medical, scientific or healthcare professionals and is provided strictly as a supplement to the medical or other professional's own judgement, their knowledge of the patient's medical history, relevant manufacturer's instructions and the appropriate best practice guidelines. Because of the rapid advances in medical science, any information or advice on dosages, procedures or diagnoses should be independently verified.

The reader is strongly urged to consult the relevant national drug formulary and the drug companies' and device or material manufacturers' printed instructions, and their websites, before administering or utilising any of the drugs, devices or materials mentioned in this book. This book does not indicate whether a particular treatment is appropriate or suitable for a particular individual. Ultimately, it is the sole responsibility of the medical professional to make his or her own professional judgements so as to advise and treat patients appropriately.

Romanesco traumatology

The structure of the Romanesco cauliflower on the front cover showcases a natural example of the mathematical beauty and complexity of fractals. When you look closely, you'll notice that each bud is made up of smaller buds, which in turn are made up of even smaller buds. This self-similarity across scales is a hallmark of fractal geometry.

The fractal nature of the Romanesco arises from its growth pattern. The unique structure is made from flowers that fail to bloom. These buds then produce shoots that produce new flowers that also fail, and this process is repeated time and time again. In response to their trauma, they harden and move closer to the light, edging towards self-actualisation. The post-traumatic growth creates a spectacular fractal form that encapsulates the ancient tension between light and darkness.

1 Introduction

Serotonin
5-hydroxytryptamine ($C_{10}H_{12}N_2O$)

DOI: 10.4324/9781003431718-1

The neurotransmitter serotonin (5-HT) was discovered in blood in the late 1800s. Later, scientist Dilworth Woolley PhD located the structure of serotonin in LSD and realised that it could be used as a tool to study the role of serotonin in mental illness (Woolley & Shaw, 1954). Since then, it has been shown to impact mood, cognition, appetite, memory, as well as numerous physiological processes such as vomiting and vasoconstriction (Sanders-Bush & Nichols, 2012). Serotonin is synthesised from L-tryptophan, an amino acid that occurs naturally in many foods. It was first discovered in the digestive tract in 1937 (Erspamer & Vialli, 1937). Indeed, over 90% of the body's serotonin is synthesised by enterochromaffin cells in the gut. However, 1–2% of serotonin is produced in the central nervous system, where it serves a wide variety of functions:

- **Mood Regulation:** The 5-HTP system is closely associated with mood regulation, and alterations in serotonin levels are linked to mood disorders such as depression and anxiety.
- **Sleep:** Serotonin plays a role in regulating sleep patterns and the sleep-wake cycle.
- **Appetite and Weight Regulation:** Serotonin influences appetite and satiety and is involved in the control of food intake.
- **Pain Perception:** The serotonin system can modulate pain perception and sensitivity.
- **Cognition:** Serotonin contributes to cognitive functions such as learning and memory.

Serotonergic systems have long been the target of psychopharmaceutical interventions for psychiatric conditions. Selective serotonin reuptake inhibitors (SSRIs) were developed to block the reuptake of serotonin at the presynaptic cell, in an attempt to rectify a hypothesised 'chemical imbalance' in mood and anxiety-related disorders. However, initial success rates of SSRIs have waned, and the long-term efficacy of such treatments is being called into question (Hare, 2018). With a relaxation in the legislative restrictions for pharmaceutical testing of Schedule I (Class A) drugs, interest has now turned to look at this category of serotonergic compounds. Serotonergic psychedelics, also referred to as serotonergic hallucinogens, include psilocybin, LSD, ketamine and mescaline. These drugs moderate the effect of serotonin, its receptor sites and reuptake mechanisms (Tófoli & de Araujo, 2016). Whilst MDMA is not a classic psychedelic, it also influences the serotonin system, causing excess serotonin release, resulting in mood-elevating effects. This new class of medications could be used to ease the ever-increasing prevalence of mental illness, which is increasingly recognised as stemming from multitudinous contemporary economic, social and environmental adversities.

The climate emergency is a health emergency (NHS England, 2022). Tackling climate change through reducing harmful carbon emissions will improve health and save lives, which is why 50 countries committed to develop climate-resilient and low-carbon health systems at COP26, the UN Climate Change Conference.

Sustainable healthcare happens when we meet economic, social and environmental agendas. Mental disorders increasingly contribute to the global burden of disease, with huge costs across all three areas (Whiteford et al., 2013). The climate emergency calls for a paradigm shift in our approach to mental health, where we need to implement sustainable models of care at scale. The four principles of sustainable healthcare, in order of importance, have been outlined by Mortimer (2010):

1 Prevention
2 Patient empowerment/supported self-care
3 Lean service pathways
4 Low-carbon treatment alternatives

These principles will be revisited in Chapter 4, 'Ethics,' to consider their place in relation to the interventions outlined in this book.

As things stand, the prevalence of mental disorders is rising, whilst the rate of developing novel treatments is in decline. Shortcomings in the current diagnostics and explanations for mental disorders generate intense debate, which is further fuelled by the stalling of innovative treatments to tackle these conditions. This constitutes a paradigmatic crisis (Schengberg, 2018). It has been proposed that a psychiatric paradigm shift is required to address how we conceptualise, diagnose and treat mental health issues. Shifting away from traditional models that categorize mental illness as discrete disorders, towards an approach which embraces descriptions of mental injury, recognizing a multidimensional spectrum of conditions and emphasizing individualised formulations. Until now, commissioned treatments have tended to be medically orientated; a paradigm shift would require a transition to a more holistic treatment approach (Schengberg, 2018).

Psychedelic-assisted psychotherapy (PAP) offers a novel panacea. Evidence from contemporary clinical research indicates that PAP can be used transdiagnostically to treat a spectrum of conditions, including but not limited to alcoholism (Garcia-Romeu et al., 2019), end-of-life anxiety (Rosenbaum et al., 2019), addiction (Garcia-Romeu et al., 2020), anorexia (Springs, 2021), OCD (Moreno et al., 2006), fibromyalgia (Bornemann, 2021), anxiety (King, 2021), treatment-resistant depression (Palhano-Fontes et al., 2018) and post-traumatic stress disorder (PTSD) (Mitchell et al., 2021). The pace of psychedelic advancement is fast and attempts to capture contemporary findings are quickly superseded by evermore recent advances. A more exhaustive overview of psychedelic research would be quickly outdated, and so it is not explored in any depth herein.

Psychedelics have been implicated in the modulation of serotonin (Aghajanian & Marek, 1999), the default mode network (DMN, Gattuso et al., 2022), serotonin 5-HT receptor subtypes (Lopez-Gimenes & Gonzalez-Maeso, 2018), neuroplasticity (de Vos et al., 2021), increased connectivity (Avram et al., 2021), synaptogenesis (Ly et al., 2018), gene expression and inflammation (Nichols, 2003). In this book, a selection of key compounds from psychedelic neuroscience are outlined at the start of each chapter.

The pharmaceutical value of such compounds has led to a psychedelic gold rush (Pollan, 2018). In what has been described as a renaissance in the healing potential of psychedelics, some have been keen to emphasise the value of the therapeutic interaction as the crucial moderator of clinical efficacy (Cavarra, 2022), whilst some have suggested that repeated dosing is necessary for prolonged therapeutic effects (Strong & Kabbaj, 2018). To date, the impact of such therapeutic interventions has not been formally assessed for its place in treatment outcomes.

Trauma-informed practice has already revolutionised the efficacy of contemporary therapy practice, leading to innovative psychotherapeutic interventions (Van Der Kolk, 1989; Seigel, 1999; Shapiro, 2001; Levine, 2015). Eye movement desensitisation and reprocessing (EMDR) therapy has emerged in this field as an efficacious trauma-focussed intervention that has been empirically validated to treat a wide variety of mental health presentations (de Jongh et al., 2024). Previously the authors have theorised a clinical basis for using EMDR as a PAP, in their previous publication of the proposed psychedelic-assisted (PsyA)-EMDR protocol (Raine-Smith & Rose, 2023). This book is an evolution of these concepts and focuses on the application and delivery of PsyA-EMDR therapy and its potential to enhance the therapeutic value of PAP. A comprehensive overview of EMDR therapy can be found in other resources, and exploring standard protocol EMDR therapy in any level of detail goes beyond the remit of this book. A foundational knowledge in EMDR therapy will therefore be assumed. However, the book is presented in a way that is accessible to a wider, non-EMDR readership, with the rationale for developing the PsyA-EMDR therapy framework and illustrative case examples separated out from the PsyA-EMDR protocol and troubleshooting sections. We therefore recommend that readers who are not qualified in basic EMDR training (Parts 1–4) skip the PsyA-EMDR protocol in Chapter 3. The value of each chapter will depend on the audience and the layout supports readers to pick and choose the sections that are most relevant to them. It is the authors' intention that all audiences will get something from the ideas presented herein.

A systematic appraisal of existing psychedelic-assisted psychotherapies

Psychedelic-assisted therapeutic protocols have been developed to help integrate insights gained through the administration of psychedelic compounds and facilitate sustained positive change (Mithoefer et al., 2019; Watts & Luoma, 2020; Wolff et al., 2020; Brennan & Belser, 2022; Raine-Smith & Rose, 2023). To date, PAP has largely been based on pre-existing therapeutic frameworks. Modifications and adjustments have been made to these frameworks to enhance their suitability to work with psychedelic content. In (loosely) chronological order, this next section uses the Socratic method to define, appraise and question a number of these models in their use as a PAP. Although an extensive analysis of these therapeutic paradigms goes beyond the remit of this publication, this review demonstrates that the current psychotherapeutic approaches do not always provide the best starting point in terms of safety and efficacy in psychedelic treatments.

Indigenous Practices

Indigenous practices encompass traditional rituals and healing methods rooted in the cultural heritage of indigenous communities. Archaeological and anthropological evidence suggests that psychedelics have been used for thousands of years (Miller, 2019). Generally offered in ritualistic settings, and accompanied by the society's religious worldviews, the psychedelic space is commonly held by a religious leader (Miller, 2019), involving the use, for example, of songs (icaros), dancing, burning of incense, prayer, fasting and rites of passage rituals, to name but a few. The rationale for the use of indigenous practice in the therapeutic setting is that some of these ancient rituals may have been honed over many generations, optimising and complimenting the effects of that specific plant medicine. Proponents of indigenous practices to support psychedelic healing suggest that we ignore these practices at our peril and that such practices could benefit participants and patients in contemporary healthcare settings (Dufrene & Coleman, 1992; King, 2008; Gone, 2010; Trimble, 2010; George et al., 2020). Indigenous practices and contexts should be studied and preserved; however, using these practices within clinical settings is problematic, for several reasons.

Key limitations

- Indigenous practices have not been empirically scrutinised in clinical settings; thus, their safety and effectiveness when working with individuals from westernised backgrounds is unknown.

- Indigenous practices held outside of the milieu of that cultural setting may be problematic.
- Cultural misappropriation and decontextualising practices become both problematic (and offensive) if transplanted into a secular health-care setting.
- Pairing with tribal elders and overseers raises moral concerns because of power differentials that exist and the potential to profit from adopting indigenous practices into economically driven healthcare settings.

Psychodynamic approaches

In the late 19th and early 20th centuries, Sigmund Freud, an Austrian neurologist and founder of psychoanalysis, introduced a therapeutic approach, aimed at exploring unconscious mental processes and conflicts, to understand and treat psychological disorders (Grosskurth, 1991). Based on these early Freudian foundations, psychodynamic theory emphasises the impact of the psychological forces underlying human behaviour and how these forces might relate to early experiences. Psychedelics reveal primary processes (unconscious functioning) that can be interpreted by a psychoanalyst, contributing to a shared understanding eliciting an emotional expression, and this 'corrective emotional experience' (Alexander & French, 1946) elicits behavioural change. In the 1950s and 1960s, psychoanalysis was the predominant therapeutic modality, widely influencing a range of psychological theories and treatment approaches during that era, and dominated the theoretical and practical foundations of early psychedelic research. Jung was the first of the early proponents of psychodynamic theory to briefly mention the use of psychedelics (Jaffe, 2015). For those working in early research, "observations from LSD psychotherapy could be considered laboratory proof of the basic Freudian premises" (Grof, 1982, p. 64). The value of the psychodynamic perspective continues to be promoted by many clinicians and contemporary researchers in the field (Carhart-Harris et al., 2014). Contemporary psychodynamic frameworks conceptualise psychopathology in developmental, cultural and temporal contexts, whereby the 'persistent personality' operates alongside psychological processes which defend against emotional pain (Paulhus et al., 1997).

Key limitations

- Whilst psychodynamic approaches provide a flexible and intuitive way of working, they fail to keep pace with the falsifiable requirements of empirical research.
- Psychodynamic approaches are largely separate from scientific scrutiny and have been used as an example of an unfalsifiable form of pseudoscience (Popper, 1983).

- Thorough psychodynamic psychedelic integration is a slow and nuanced process. For many, this raises issues of affordability and accessibility.
- At the foundation of this approach sits the therapeutic relationship. Broad application of which raises issues of replicability, objectivity and reliability.
- In cases where a relational alliance is not possible, clinical application of this approach has little or no foundation.

Transpersonal approaches

The transpersonal approach is defined as "experiences in which the sense of identity or self extends beyond the individual or personal to encompass wider aspects of humankind, life, psyche or cosmos" (Walsh, 1993, p. 22). Transpersonal approaches recognise the value of spiritual or transcendent aspects of the human experience. In PAP, the most prominent transpersonal framework is promoted in the work of Stanislav Grof, with theoretical roots in psychoanalysis (depth psychology), and claims that the acute subjective effects of psychedelic substances can be understood as a figurative (and perhaps literal) memory of being born (Grof, 2000). This 'peri-natal theory' of psychedelic experience came to inform his preferred psychotherapeutic framing of psychedelic treatments. See Chapter 11 'Transpersonal Healing' for an expanded view of his conceptual framework.

Key limitations

- Like many criticisms of the psychodynamic approach, transpersonal approaches fail to keep pace with the falsifiable requirements of empirical research and clinical practice.
- Abstract and symbolic content can be difficult to translate into emotional resolution or behavioural modification.
- Without the support of other therapeutic frameworks, emergent emotional and somatic content may be left unintegrated.

New-age spirituality approaches

The most high-profile research into psychedelics conducted during the 1960s was by Professors Timothy Leary and Richard Alpert at Harvard University (Baumeister & Placidi, 1983). Their findings, and later publicity, facilitated the process of psychedelics becoming mainstream. Psychedelics were then adopted by various sub-cultures, including those incorporating new-age spiritual practices. Mixing new-age spiritual ideals with a therapeutic context was hoped to enhance the therapeutic effects of psychedelics (Lattin, 2010). Emerging evidence suggests that spiritual insight might be a spontaneous psychedelic effect (Yaden et al., 2017; Griffiths et al., 2019;

Davis et al., 2020) and that encountering material within a spiritual frame-work reduces the likelihood of adverse experiences. Indeed, it may enhance the value of the emergent psychological material.

Key limitations

- Spiritual bypassing, the act of using spiritual beliefs or practices to avoid facing or dealing with unresolved psychological or emotional issues, can lead to the neglect of personal growth and authentic healing.
- It is unclear the extent to which psychedelic-induced spiritual insights are culturally constructed experiences, innate cognitive systems or spiritually intrinsic effects.
- Adopting a spiritually orientated therapeutic frame is without an evidence base and thus presents unknown risks (Johnson, 2020).
- As with many other ontological assumptions, metaphysical assumptions of spirituality are problematic.

Underground (illegal) therapy approaches

Initially, even after licensing and legislative change, it is unlikely that psychedelic treatment will be made ubiquitously available. As access to psychedelic therapy is rolled out, individuals without a formal diagnosis of an approved condition, those with more complex needs and higher levels of risk or for those who do not otherwise meet the inclusion criteria, there are no alternatives to accessing psychedelic treatments other than to travel abroad or turn to illegal underground settings. Often, this forces the most vulnerable individuals to look for unlicensed, entirely unregulated alternatives. There is no standardisation in the therapeutic interventions used, and many settings do not posit a theoretical orientation for their work; albeit both transpersonal methodologies and new-age spiritual approaches have been influential in underground psychedelic contexts. Ethical controversy from the increasing numbers of people participating in underground settings is already emerging (Brennan et al., 2021). Underground treatments present many practical and ethical issues.

Key limitations

- There are no formalised/standardised ethical standards in underground settings.
- Working without a theoretical orientation means that bridging the gaps that inevitably emerge during an intervention has no practical or intellectual foundation. Whilst offering space for creativity and new ideas, these methods rely on emergent 'practice-based evidence.'

- Standard ethical considerations such as staying within one's scope of competency go entirely unchecked.
- Opportunities for clinical supervision and reflective practice are limited, in part because this work cannot be insured.
- Most interventions are not trauma-informed which can lead to enactments and further traumatisation, bringing the therapeutic use of psychedelics into disrepute.
- A lack of continued professional development (CPD) training opportunities for PAP clinicians is pushing some to seek illegal alternatives.

Risk reduction and psychoeducational approaches

The harm-reduction perspective is based on adopting a compassionate stance and focuses on reducing the risks associated with substance use (Marlatt, 1996; Marlatt et al., 2011). Gorman et al. (2021, p. 1) outline one such approach, detailing "Psychedelic Harm Reduction and Integration (PHRI) [as] a transtheoretical and transdiagnostic clinical approach to working with patients who are using or considering using psychedelics in any context." PHRI is designed for trained therapists to use in both brief and ongoing psychotherapeutic interactions. Incorporating principles of harm reduction, psychoeducation, mindfulness-based modalities and psychodynamic therapy, it provides a non-directive framework for examining and working with psychedelic experiences from both recreational and clinical care settings. Mindfulness-based relaxation exercises create a framework for supporting those with more complex presentations and those who have been destabilised by their experiences.

Key limitations

- Managing and working therapeutically with adverse reactions is still problematic.
- This is a non-directive, unfolding process with undefined parameters for the integration of psychedelic content.
- Outside of festival and event-based harm-reduction initiatives, there is a lack of suitable training opportunities in risk reduction and psychoeducation techniques.

Community-based approaches

Moved by the moral and ethical imperative to offer some form of ongoing support, community-based psychedelic integration circles have emerged and are now becoming a popular therapeutic tool in their own right. Little research exists on the value of psychedelic integration communities, group work or horizontal models of care in PAP. The efficacy of horizontal care structures has been previously verified both in substance misuse (Donovan et al., 2013) and in brain injury patients (Reistetter & Abreu, 2005). The community integration group is an emerging clinical tool and may hold untapped potential for amplifying the effects of PAP. The question posed in an academic thesis on the subject asked some important questions. "Can 21st century psychotherapy incorporate group therapy with the use of psychedelics to produce a reorganization of consciousness necessary for true healing?" And "Is thorough integration a collaborative and group process?" (Gross, 2021). Either way, community-based psychedelic integration circles offer an adjunctive wraparound to assist the therapeutic process, whereby the group process provides opportunities for content to be further explored and healed. There is very limited research into psychedelic-assisted group therapy (PAGP), and currently, only a handful of empirical studies on group therapy with psychedelics have been conducted (Anderson et al., 2020; Oehen & Gasser, 2022; Schmid et al., 2021).

Key limitations

- Funding for community groups is often problematic leading to inconsistent provision.
- Accessibility is based on geographical location.
- There is a lack of therapeutic consistency as each group is unique.
- Community groups often lack the wider care structures to hold more complex needs.
- There are risks associated with inadequate therapeutic input.

Cognitive-Behavioural Therapy (CBT) approaches

Traditional CBT interventions begin with a systematic assessment of thoughts and behaviour, then intentional actions are taught to enable adaptive thinking and enhanced behavioural response. Sessions are structured to promote efficacy; an initial check-in is followed by setting an agenda for the session. The agenda is then completed and summarised into setting a plan of action (McGinn & Sanderson, 2001). Developing a collaborative therapeutic alliance, establishing treatment goals, providing psychoeducation, self-monitoring, skills training, developing alternatives to struggling and avoidance, connecting with values, core beliefs/unhelpful thoughts, cognitive restructuring, relaxation techniques, mindfulness skills, emotional regulation skills, distress tolerance skills, assigning homework (behavioural experiments) and monitoring progress all form part of the CBT approach to PAP (Yaden et al., 2022).

Key limitations

- CBT focuses on management of symptoms.
- Control or avoidance of dysfunctional thinking or difficult emotions may contribute to suffering.
- Frameworks to support the integration of unconscious material and mystical experiences do not feature in cognitive-behavioural interventions.
- Cognitive-behavioural approaches are often rigidly manualised which limits the individualisation of care.
- Harm may be done when clients lose ownership of their meaning making.

Acceptance Commitment Therapy (ACT)/Accept, Connect and Embody (ACE) model

Traditional CBT has given way to third-wave CBT interventions such as dialectic behavioural therapy (DBT) and ACT. To illustrate, ACT is founded on six core processes; diffusion, acceptance, present moment, self-as-content, values and committed action. ACT is underpinned by the 'cognitive flexibility model' (Hayes, 2004). Using qualitative and quantitative data from clinical trials, ACT has been adapted for psychedelic-assisted therapy, to create ACE (Watts & Luoma, 2020). Like traditional CBT, in ACE, there is an emphasis on developing an awareness of thoughts, feelings and sensations. However, the ACE model cultivates an acceptance of difficult emotions and bodily sensations, encouraging people to connect to the meaning behind these feelings. The ACE model is flexible and non-prescriptive and employs a series of interventions to develop and enhance acceptance, connection and embodiment. It is the embodiment phase of ACE that deviates most from traditional ACT frameworks. Embodiment is practised during preparation with a guided visualisation and a body scan where participants are encouraged to 'let go and dive into (their) bodies'. The diving metaphor encourages participants to go towards difficult emotions and identify the 'pearls of wisdom' that the difficult emotion elicits. An intention for dosing is then based on this (Watts & Luoma, 2020). Psychedelic content is then worked with therapeutically using the ACT core processes.

Key limitations

- Embodiment visualisation is not comparable to the strong somatic responses that can emerge during a psychedelic treatment and does not serve as adequate preparation.
- Acceptance is not the same as working through and integrating the root cause of a psychological issue.

- Managing adverse reactions using this framework is still problematic.
- Exclusion criteria have meant that this approach has not been tested in those with underlying sensitivities or more complex presentations.

EMBARK approach

EMBARK is described as an evidence-based therapy, formed from an acronym that gives the approach its name: existential-spiritual, mindfulness, body-aware, affective-cognitive, relational and keeping momentum. EMBARK has already been adopted as a therapeutic framework by several of the PAP clinical research trials (Brennan, 2022). EMBARK's six clinical domains are flexibly employed by the therapist to individualise treatment. Therapists have clearly defined tasks and guidelines which operationalise the process, whilst drawing on their existing therapeutic skill set. Like many PAPs, EMBARK describes three phases of treatment, preparation, medicine and integration. The six clinical domains can be applied in any of these three phases. In addition, EMBARK rests on its own ethical framework, described as the four pillars of ethical care; trauma-informed care, culturally competent care, ethically rigorous care and collective care.

Key limitations

- It is an integrative approach, resting on a previously gained therapeutic training. Each clinician will bring their own modality making clinical consistency difficult to achieve.
- Tools for addressing the underlying trauma are not outlined in the intervention.
- Identifying and responding to trauma can be difficult, as much is unconscious process, and enactments are difficult to spot.
- Insufficient containment for those with undiagnosed sensitivities.

Pharmaceutical company specific approaches

When testing a new compound in medicines research, technically, any variables that are not the effect of the drug are considered to be expectancy effects (Butler et al., 2022). This is problematic in PAP research trials because the role of therapy is not a drug effect and yet is (probably) integral to the benefits of the PAP. The data gleaned from psychedelic research can be confounded by the impact of the therapeutic intervention as well as the difficulty blinding subjects in randomised controlled PAP trials. The sponsors of clinical research are developing their own approaches to working therapeutically with these compounds. Generally, there are non-disclosure agreements in place to ensure that the therapy used remains the intellectual property of the pharmaceutical sponsor. These therapies are continuously refined and updated in the study protocols and so would be quickly outdated in any publication. As new pharmaceutical companies emerge, so do new methods of working to optimise the efficacy of these drugs. Any such appraisal is limited by these constraints.

One example that has been shared in the public domain is the MAPS psilocybin therapy protocol. It will be outlined here as an illustrative example. This protocol offers a two-therapist model using a non-directive approach with what is described as 'integrative psychotherapy'. Preparatory and integration sessions are offered either side of the dosing session. Participant goals, desires, spiritual beliefs and psychoeducation around the study procedures all form part of the preparatory therapy. In integration, any thoughts, feelings or experiences that arose during the psilocybin session are explored, with the broad intention to integrate this material into everyday life loosely framing the agenda (MAPS, 2008).

Key limitations

- Intellectual property limitations mean that the efficacy of these interventions cannot be scrutinised.
- Samples are not representative and those with complex presentations are screened out.
- Pharmaceutical companies are limiting access to the interventions by ensuring that the licence for the drug is granted based on their own model of therapy. This may affect the price and therefore accessibility.
- Adverse events are managed using medical interventions and as such, the psychological value of adverse events may be overlooked.
- There is a conflict between the interests of pharmaceutical companies and the (lack of) disclosure of adverse events.
- The need to measure overall efficacy of the drug with the therapy makes it difficult for researchers to optimise therapy, as standardisation is needed to produce results which stand up to scientific scrutiny.

Basic support models

Many clinical trials are offering limited therapeutic support before, during or after drug administration. Some ketamine clinics also follow this model, offering therapeutic input (if any) as an optional upgrade. Some provide sitters to hold the psychedelic space, with the rationale that treatment benefit depends on an 'inner healing intelligence' that resides within the patient and is facilitated by psychedelic administration (Grof, 2000; Clare, 2018; Gorman et al., 2021). The adoption of an inward attentional focus then guides the participant/patient to healing. Many such sitters are not psychologically trained.

Key limitations

- Risks associated when working without a theoretical orientation.
- Lack of skilful evidence-based interventions may lead to suboptimal outcomes.
- Introduces a significant source of variability.
- Unprepared for challenging clinical situations that might arise.
- Unprepared for appearance of trauma and boundary testing.

Socratic questioning of current viewpoints and perspectives

The authors recognise that all therapies should be seen as potential candidates for working with psychedelic material and that no one treatment should be assumed the default; adopting a dialectic stance is necessary until the evidence base suggests otherwise. From a transtheoretical perspective, deductive inferences lead us to question what has been omitted from the current PAP axiom:

- Given that those who are most prone to adverse reactions tend to be those with complex trauma histories, how might trauma-informed and trauma-focused practice be rigorously applied in PAP?
- How might clinical populations with complex PTSD and those with undiagnosed sensitivities be accommodated?
- How do we systematically, objectively and quantifiably assess successful integration of psychedelic content?
- How do we support, respond to, reduce or eliminate somatic responses skilfully and ethically?
- How do we work therapeutically with all emergent material, including underwhelming/disappointing experiences?
- How do we improve the reliability of PAP delivery to ensure therapeutic consistency?
- How do we work psychologically with destabilised individuals, rather than signposting them to medicalised interventions?
- How do we more fully integrate the psychological themes that emerge (past, present and future)? Working with memory network/schema/COEX as psychological frameworks?
- How do we work ethically with substances that appear to create a suggestable state (Carhart-Harris et al., 2015) and could put participants/patients in a vulnerable position (Johnson, 2020)?
- How do we work with ethical concerns that emerge around a therapist/shaman/medicalised setting imposing their worldview (Johnson, 2020) on a participant or patient?

In developing PsyA-EMDR therapy, our goal is to develop a PAP that can:

- Widen inclusivity.
- Adequately prepare people for the psychedelic medication phase.
- Develop strategies to manage strong affect and uncomfortable emotions safely and ethically.
- Develop cohesive protocols.
- Facilitate the integration of cognitive, somatic and emotional material that may arise.
- Stabilise participants who experience adverse reactions.
- Provide a cohesive theoretical framework that underpins the transdiagnostic use of psychedelics.
- Be used alongside harm reduction, psychoeducation and community-based integration practices.
- Develop a more effective and therefore more sustainable PAP.

References

Aghajananian, G. K., & Marek, G. J. (1999). Serotonin and hallucinogens. *Neuropsychopharmacology, 21*(2 Suppl 1), 16S–23S. https://doi.org/10.1016/S0893-133X(98)00135-3

Alexander, F., & French, T. M. (1946). *Psychoanalytic therapy: Principles and application.* New York: Ronald Press.

Anderson, B. T., Danforth, A., Daroff, P. R., Stauffer, C., Ekman, E., Agin-Liebes, G., Trope, A., Boden, M. T., Dilley, P. J., Mitchell, J., & Woolley, J. (2020, Sep 24). Psilocybin-assisted group therapy for demoralized older long-term AIDS survivor men: An open-label safety and feasibility pilot study. *E Clinical Medicine, 27,* 100538. https://doi.org/10.1016/j.eclinm.2020.100538

Avram, M., Rogg, H., Korda, A., Andreou, C., Muller, F., & Borgwardt, S. (2021). Bridging the gap? Altered thalamocortical connectivity in psychotic and psychedelic states. *Frontiers in Psychiatry: Sec. Psychopathology, 12,* 706017. https://doi.org/10.3389/fpsyt.2021.706017

Baumeister, R. F., & Placidi, K. S. (1983). A social history and analysis of the LSD controversy. *Journal of Humanist Psychology, 23,* 25–58. https://psycnet.apa.org/doi/10.1177/0022167883234003

Bornemann, J., Close, J., Spriggs, M., Carhart-Harris, R., & Roseman, L. (2021). Self-medication for chronic pain using classic psychedelics: A qualitative investigation to inform future research. *Frontiers in Psychiatry: Sec. Psychological Therapies, 12,* 735427. https://doi.org/10.3389/fpsyt.2021.735427

Brennan, W., Jackson, M., Maclean, K., & Ponterotto, J. (2021). A qualitative exploration or relational ethical challenges and practices in psychedelic healing. *Journal of Humanistic Psychology.* http://dx.doi.org/10.1177/00221678211045265

Brennan, W., & Belser, A. B. (2022). Models of psychedelic-assisted psychotherapy: A contemporary assessment and an introduction to EMBARK, a transdiagnosis, trans-drug model. *Frontiers in Psychology: Sec. Psychology for Clinical Settings,* *13,* 866018. https://doi.org/10.3389/fpsyg.2022.866018

Butler, M., Jelen, L., & Rucker, J. (2022). Expectancy in placebo – controlled trials of psychedelics: If so, so what? *Psychopharmacology, 239*(10), 3047–3055. https://doi.org/10.1007/s00213-022-06221-6.

Carhart-Harris, R. L., Leech, R., Hellyer, P. J., Shanahan, M., Feilding, A., Tagliazucchi, E., Chialvo, D. R., & Nutt, D. (2014). The entropic brain: A theory of conscious states informed by neuroimaging research with psychedelic drugs. *Frontiers in Human Neuroscience, 8,* 20. https://doi.org/10.3389%2Ffnhum.2014.00020

Carhart-Harris, R. L., Kaelen, M., Whalley, M. G., Bolstridge, M., Feilding, A., & Nutt, D. J. (2015). LSD enhances suggestibility in healthy volunteers. *Psychopharmacology, 232*(4), 785–794. https://doi.org/10.1007/s00213-014-3714-z

Cavarra, M., Falzone, A., Ramaekers, J., Kuypers, K., & Mento, C. (2022). Psychedelic-assisted psychotherapy – A systematic review of associated psychological interventions. *Frontiers in Psychology: Sec. Psychology for Clinical Settings,* *13,* 887255. https://doi.org/10.3389/fpsyg.2022.887255

Clare, S. (2018). Cultivating inner growth: The inner healing intelligence in MDMA-assisted psychotherapy. *MAPS Bull, 28,* 30–33.

Davis, A. K., Barrett, F. S., May, D. G., Cosimano, M. P., Sepeda, N. D., Johnson, M. W., Finan, P. H., & Griffiths, R. R. (2021). Effects of psilocybin-assisted therapy on major depressive disorder: A randomized clinical trial. *JAMA Psychiatry, 78*(5), 481-489. https://doi.org/10.1001/jamapsychiatry.2020.3285; Erratum in: Effects of psilocybin-assisted therapy on major depressive disorder. *JAMA Psychiatry, 78*(5), 569. https://doi.org/10.1001/jamapsychiatry.2020.4714

Davis, A. K., Clifton, J. M., Weaver, E. G., Hurwitz, E. S., Johnson, M. W., & Griffiths, R. R. (2020). Survey of entity encounter experiences occasioned by inhaled N, N-dimethyltryptamine: Phenomenology, interpretation, and enduring effects. *Journal of Psychopharmacology, 34,* 1008–1020. https://doi.org/10.1177/0269881120916143

de Jongh, A., de Roos, C., & El-Leithy, S. (2024). State of the science: Eye movement desensitization and reprocessing (EMDR) therapy. *Journal of Traumatic Stress,* 37(2), 205–216. https://doi.org/10.1002/jts.23012

de Vos, C. M. H., Mason, N., & Kuypers, K. (2021). Psychedelics and neuroplasticity: A systematic review unravelling the biological underpinnings of psychedelics. *Frontiers in Psychiatry: Sec Psychopathology,* 12, 724606. https://doi.org/10.3389/fpsyt.2021.724606

Donovan, D., Ingalsbe, M., Benbow, J., & Daley, D. (2013). 12-Step interventions and mutual support programs for substance use disorders: an overview. *Social Work Public Health,* 28 (0), 313–332. https://doi.org/10.1080/19371918.2013.774663

Dufrene, P., & Coleman, V. (1992). Counselling native Americans: Guidelines for group process. *The Journal for Specialists in Group Work, 17*(4), 229–234. https://doi.org/10.1080/01933929208414354

Erspamer, V., & Vialli, M. (1937). Ricerche sul secreto delle cellule enterocromaffini. *Boll d Soc Med-chir Pavia, 51,* 357–363. https://doi.org/10.1007/BF00391792

Garcia-Romeu, A., Davis, A., Ewowid, F., Erowid, F., Griffiths, R., & Johnson, M. (2019). Cessation and reduction in alcohol consumption and misuse after psychedelic use. *Journal of Psychopharmacology, 33*(9),1088–1101. https://doi.org/10.1177/0269881119845793

Garcia-Romeu, A., Davis, A., Ewowid, F., Erowid, F., Griffiths, R., & Johnson, M. (2020). Persisting reductions in cannabis, opioid, and stimulant misuse after naturalistic psychedelic use: An online survey. *Frontiers in Psychiatry: Sec. Psychopharmacology,*10, 955. https://doi.org/10.3389%2Ffpsyt.2019.00955

Gattuso, J., Perkins, D., Ruffell, S., Lawrence, A., Hoyer, D., Jacobson, L., Timmermann, C., Castle, D., Rossell, S., Downey, L., Pagni, B., Galvao-Coelho, N., Nutt, D., & Sarris, J. (2022). Default mode network modulation by psychedelics: A systematic review. *International Journal of Neuropsychopharmacology, 26*(3), 155–188. https://doi.org/10.1093%2Fijnp%2Fpyac074

George, J. R., Michaels, T. I., Sevelius, J., & Williams, M. T. (2020). The psychedelic renaissance and the limitations of a White-dominant medical framework: A call for indigenous and ethnic minority inclusion. *Journal of Psychedelic Studies, 4*(1), 4–15. https://doi.org/10.1556/2054.2019.015

Gone, J. P. (2010). Psychotherapy and traditional healing for American Indians: Exploring the prospects for therapeutic integration. *The Counselling Psychologist, 38*(2), 166–235. https://doi.org/10.1177/0011000008330831

Griffiths, R. R., Hurwitz, E. S., Davis, A. K., Johnson, M. W., & Jesse, R. (2019). Survey of subjective "God encounter experiences": Comparisons among naturally occurring experiences and those occasioned by the classic psychedelics psilocybin, LSD, ayahuasca, or DMT. *PLOS ONE, 14*(4), e0214377. https://doi.org/10.1371/journal.pone.0214377

Grof, S. (1982). Realms of the unconscious: The enchanted frontier. *Journal of Transpersonal Psychology, 14*, 186–188.

Grof, S. (2000). *Psychology of the Future. Lessons from modern consciousness research.* Albany: State University of New York Press.

Gross, B. (2021). Communal psychedelic integration: How group therapy is integral to wholeness. Master of arts in counselling psychology pacifica graduate institute. Found at https://www.proquest.com/openview/fd4490c8c1e4446cc5bff729743ec6e9/1?pq-origsite=gscholar&cbl=18750&diss=y

Gorman, I., Nielson, E., Molinar, A., Cassidy, K., & Sabbagh, J. (2021). Psychedelic harm reduction and integration: A transtheoretical model fir clinical practice. *Frontiers in Psychology, 12*, 645246. https://doi.org/10.3389%2Ffpsyg.2021.645246

Grosskurth, P. (1991). *The Secret Ring: Freud's Inner Circle and the Politics of Psychoanalysis.* London: Jonathan Cape Ltd.

Hare, J. (2018). *Lost connections.* London: Bloomsbury Publishing.

Hayes, S. C., Strosahl, K. D., & Wilson, K. G. (2004). *Acceptance and Commitment Therapy: An Experiential Approach To Behavior Change.* Guilford Press.

Jaffe, A. (2015). Letters of CG Jung. Vol 2, (pp. 1951–1961). London: Routledge.

Johnson, M. W. (2020). Consciousness, religion, and gurus: Pitfalls of psychedelic medicine. *ACS Pharmacology Translational Science, 4*(2), 578–581. https://doi.org/10.1021/acsptsci.0c00198

King, J. (2008). Psychotherapy within an American Indian perspective, In M. Gallardo and B. McNeill (Eds.), *Multicultural Counselling* (pp. 113–136). Mahwah, NJ: Erlbaum.

King, F., 4th & Hammond, R. (2021). Psychedelics as remerging treatments for anxiety disorders: Possibilities and challenges in a nascent field. *Focus: The Journal of Lifelong Learning in Psychiatry, 19*(2), 190–196. https://doi.org/10.1176/appi.focus.2020047

Lattin, D. (2010). *The Harvard Psychedelic Club: How Timothy Leary, Ram Dass, Huston Smith, and Andrew Weil killed the fifties and ushered in a new age for America.* New York: Harper One/HarperCollins.

López-Giménez, J. F., & González-Maeso, J. (2018). Hallucinogens and serotonin 5-HT2A receptor-mediated signaling pathways. *Current Topics in Behavioral Neurosciences, 36*, 45-73. https://doi.org/10.1007/7854_2017_478

Ly, C., Greb, A., Cameron, L., Wong, J., Barragan, E., Wilson, P., Burbach, K., Zarandi, S., Sood, A., Paddy, M., Duim, W., Dennis, M., McAllister, K., Ori-McKenney, O., Gray, J., & Olson, D. (2018). Psychedelics promote structural and functional neural plasticity. *Cell Reports, 23*(11), 3170–3182. https://doi.org/10.1016%2Fj.celrep.2018.05.022

Levine, P. (2015). *Trauma and memory: Brain and body in a search for the living past: A practical guide for understanding and working with traumatic memory.* Berkeley, CA: North Atlantic Books.

Multidisciplinary Association for Psychedelic Studies (MAPS).(2008). Psilocybin-assisted psychotherapy in the management of anxiety associated with stage IV melanoma. Found at https://maps.org/research-archive/cluster/psilo-lsd/pca1protocol.pdf.

Marlatt, G. A. (1996). Harm reduction: Come as you are. *Addictive Behaviours, 21*(6), 779–788. https://doi.org/10.1016/0306-4603(96)00042-1

Marlatt, G. A., Larimer, M. E., & Witkiewitz, K. (2011). *Harm reduction: Pragmatic strategies for managing high-risk behaviours.* New York: Guilford Press.

McGinn, L. K., & Sanderson, W. C. (2001). What allows cognitive behavioural therapy to be brief: Overview, efficacy, and crucial factors facilitating brief treatment. *Clinical Psychology: Science and Practice, 8*(1), 23–37. https://doi.org/10.1093/clipsy.8.1.23

Miller, M. (2019). Chemical hints of ayahuasca use in pre-Columbian shamanic rituals. *Proceedings of the National Academy Sciences U.S.A, 116*, 11079-11081.

Mitchell, J., Bogenschutz, M., Liliensteinr, A., Harrison, C., Kleinman, S., Parker-Guilbert, K., Ot'alora, M., Garas, W., Paleos, W., Gorman, I., Nicholas, C., Mithoefer, M. Calin, S., Poulter, B.,Mithoefer, A., Quevedo, S., Wells, G., Klare, S., Van Der Kolk, B., Tzarfaty, K., Amiaz, R.,Worthy, R., Shannon, S., Woolley, J. D., Matra, C., Gelfand, Y., Hapkem E., Amar, S., Wallach, Y., Brown, R., Hamilton, S., Wang, J., Coker, A., Matthews, R., De Boer, A., Yazar-Klosinski, B., Emerson, A., & Doblin, R. (2021). MDMA-assisted therapy for severe PTSE: A randomised, double-blind, placebo-controlled phase 3 study. *Nature, 27*(6), 1025–1033. https://doi.org/10.1038/s41591-021-01336-3

Mithoefer, M. C., Feduccia, A. A., Jerome, L., Mithoefer, A., Wagner, M., Walsh, Z., Hamilton, S., Yazar-Klosinski, B., Emerson, A., & Doblin, R. (2019). MDMA-assisted psychotherapy for treatment of PTSD: Study design and rationale for phase 3 trials based on pooled analysis of six phase 2 randomized controlled trials. *Psychopharmacology (Berl), 236*(9), 2735–2745. https://doi.org/10.1007/s00213-019-05249-5 Erratum: MDMA-assisted psychotherapy for treatment of PTSD. *Psychopharmacology (Berl), 241*(11), 2405. https://doi.org/10.1007/s00213-024-06666-x

Moreno, F. A., Weigand, C. B., Taitano, E. K., & Delgado, P. L. (2006). Safety, tolerability, and efficacy of psilocybin in 9 patients with obsessive-compulsive disorder. *Journal of Clinical Psychiatry, 67*(11), 1735–1740. https://doi.org/10.4088/jcp.v67n1110

Mortimer, F. (2010). The sustainable physician. *Clinical Medicine, 10*(1), 110–111. https://doi.org/10.7861/clinmedicine.10-2-110

National Health Service (NHS) England. (2022). National commitments for a greener NHS. Found at https://www.england.nhs.uk/greenernhs/national-ambition/national-commitments/

Nichols, C. D., Garcia, E. E., & Sanders-Bush, E. (2003). Dynamic changes in prefrontal cortex gene expression following lysergic acid diethylamide administration. *Molecular Brain Research, 111*(1–2), 182–188. https://doi.org/10.1016/s0169-328x(03)00029-9

Oehen, P., & Gasser, P., (2022). Using a MDMA- and LSD-group therapy model in clinical practice in Switzerland and highlighting the treatment of trauma-related disorders. *Frontiers in Psychiatry, 13*, 863552. https://doi.org/10.3389/fpsyt.2022.863552

Paulhus, D. L., Fridhandler, B., & Hayes, S. (1997). Psychological defence: contemporary theory and research. In R. Hogan, J. Johnson, and S. Briggs (Eds.), *Handbook of Personality Psychology* (pp. 543–579). Boston, MA: Academic Press.

Popper, K. R. (1983). *Realism and the aim of science.* London: Hutchinson.

Palhano-Fontes, F., Barreto, D., Onias, H., Andrade K. C., Novaes, M., Pessoa, J. A., Mota-Rolim, S., Osório, F. L., Sanches, R., Santos, R. G., Tófoli, F. L., Silveira, G. O., Yonamine, M., Riba, J.,Santos, F., Silva-Junior, A., Alchieri, J.C., Galvão-Coelho, N. L., Lobão-Soares, B., Hallak, J.,Arcoverde, E., Maia-de-Oliveira, J. P., & Araújo, D. B. (2018). Rapid antidepressant effects of the psychedelic ayahuasca in treatment-resistant depression: A randomized placebo-controlled trial. *Psychological Medicine. 49*(4), 655–663. https://doi.org/10.1017%2FS0033291718001356

Pollan, M. (2018). *How to change your mind. The new science of psychedelics.* New York: Allen Lane.

Raine-Smith, H., & Rose, J. (2023). Psychedelic-assisted EMDR therapy (PsyA-EMDR): A memory consolidation approach to psychedelic healing. *EMDR Therapy Quarterly, 4*, 1. http://dx.doi.org/10.13140/RG.2.2.24683.35366

Reistetter, T., & Abreu, B. (2005). Appraising evidence on community integration following brain injury: A systematic review. *Occupational Therapy International, 12*(4), 196–217. https://doi.org/10.1002/oti.8

Rosenbaum, D., Boyle, A. B., Rosenblum, A. M., Ziai, S., Chasen, M. R., & Med, M. P. (2019). Psychedelics for psychological and existential distress in palliative and cancer care. *Current Oncology, 26*(4), 225-226. https://doi.org/10.3747/co.26.5009

Sanders-Bush, E., & Nichols, C. D. (2012) Chapter 17 – Serotonin receptors and neurotransmission. In D. Robertson, et al., (Eds.), *Primer on the Autonomic Nervous System* (3rd ed., pp. 83–86). San Diego: Academic Press.

Schmid, Y., Gasser, P., Oehen, P., & Liechti, M. E. (2021, Apr). Acute subjective effects in LSD- and MDMA-assisted psychotherapy. *Journal of Psychopharmacology, 35*(4), 362–374. https://doi.org/10.1177/0269881120959604

Seigel, D. (1999). *The developing mind: How relationships and the brain interact to shape who we are.* New York: Guilford Press.

Schengberg, E. (2018). Psychedelic-assisted psychotherapy: A paradigm shift in psychiatric research development. *Frontiers in Pharmacology, 9*, 733. https://doi.org/10.3389/fphar.2018.00733

Shapiro, F. (2001). *Eye movement desensitization and reprocessing: Basic principles, protocols and procedures* (2nd ed.). New York: Guilford Press.

Springs, M., Douglass, H., Park, R., Read, T., Danby, J., Magalhaes, F., Alderton, K., Williams, T.,Blemings, A., Lafrance, A., Nicholls, D., Erritzoe, D., Nutt, D., & Carhart-Harris, R. (2021). Study protocol for psilocybin as a treatment for anorexia nervosa: A pilot study. *Frontiers in Psychiatry: Sec. Psychological Therapies, 12*, 735523. https://doi.org/10.3389/fpsyt.2021.735523

Strong, G. E., & Kabbaj, M. (2018). On the safety of repeated ketamine infusions for the treatment ofd epression: Effects of sex and developmental periods. *Neurobiology of Stress, 9*, 166–175. https://doi.org/10.1016/j.ynstr.2018.09.001.

Trimble, J. E. (2010). The virtues of cultural resonance, competence and relational collaboration with native American Indian communities: A synthesis of the counselling and psychotherapy literature. *Counsel Psychology, 38*, 243–256. https://doi.org/10.1177/0011000009344348

Tófoli, L. F., & de Araujo, D. B. (2016). Treating addiction: Perspectives from EEG and imaging studies on psychedelics. *International Review of Neurobiology, 129*, 157–185. https://doi.org/10.1016/bs.irn.2016.06.005

Van Der Kolk, B., & Ducey, C. P. (1989). The psychological processing of traumatic experience: Rorschach patterns in PTSD. *Journal of Traumatic Stress, 2*(3), 259–274. https://doi.org/10.1002/jts.2490020303

Walsh, R., & Vaughan, F. (1993). On transpersonal definitions. *Journal of Transpersonal Psychology, 25*(2), 125–182.

Watts, R., & Luoma, J. B. (2020). The use of the psychological flexibility model to support psychedelic-assisted therapy. *Journal of Contextual Behavioral Science, 15*, 92-102. https://doi.org/10.1016/j.jcbs.2019.12.004

Whiteford, H.A., Degenhardt, L., Rehm, J., Baxter, A. J., Ferrari, A. J., Erskine, H. E., Charlson, F. J., Norman, R E., Flaxman, A. D., Johns, N., Burstein, R., Murray, C. J., & Vos T. (2013, Nov 9). Global burden of disease attributable to mental and substance use disorders: Findings from the global burden of disease study 2010. *Lancet.* 382(9904), 1575–1586. https://doi.org/10.1016/s0140-6736(13)61611-6

Wolff, M., Evens, R., Mertens, L. J., Koslowski, M., Betzler, F., Gründer, G., & Jungaberle, H. (2020). Learning to let go: A cognitive-behavioral model of how psychedelic therapy promotes acceptance. *Frontiers in Psychiatry, 11*, 5. https://doi.org/10.3389/fpsyt.2020.00005

Woolley, D. W., & Shaw, E. A. (1954). Biochemical and pharmacological suggestion about certain mental disorders. *Proceedings of the National Academy of Sciences of the United States of America, 40*(4), 228-231. https://doi.org/10.1073/pnas.40.4.228

Yaden, D., Earp, D., Graziosi, M., Friedman-Wheeler, D., & Johnson, M. (2022). Psychedelics and psychotherapy: Cognitive-behavioural approaches as default. *Frontiers in Psychology, 13*, 873279. https://doi.org/10.3389/fpsyg.2022.873279

Yaden, D. B., Haidt, J., Hood, R. W., Jr., Vago, D. R., & Newberg, A. B. (2017). The varieties of self-transcendent experience. *Review of General Psychology, 21*(2), 143–160. https://doi.org/10.1037/gpr0000102

2   An AIP model of the psychedelic space

Psilocybin
4-phosphoryloxy-N, N-dimethyltryptamine ($C_{12}H_{17}N_2O_4P$)

DOI: 10.4324/9781003431718-2

Psilocybin and psilocin are naturally occurring classic psychedelic compounds, found in over 200 species of the *Psilocybe* genus of mushroom. Psilocybin mushrooms, often referred to as 'magic mushrooms,' have a long history of use in various spiritual and cultural practices but were only unearthed by modern science in the late 1950s (Hoffman et al., 1958).

Chemically, psilocybin is a tryptamine alkaloid prodrug, meaning that when mixed with acid in the stomach, it is metabolised into its active form, psilocin. The active metabolite, psilocin, primarily interacts as an agonist with the serotonin 5-hydroxytryptamine type 2A (5-HT2A) receptor, leading to altered perception, changes in mood and shifts in consciousness (Halberstad & Geyer, 2011). Findings suggest that these changes could be associated with a temporary state of increased plasticity and decreased connectivity in certain brain regions (Brouwer & Carhart-Harris, 2021) and could be responsible for the mystical-type experiences reported (Griffiths et al., 2006). While the modulation of the serotonin system is hypothesised to play a role in the antidepressant and anxiolytic effects observed, the experience induced by psilocybin is not merely pharmacological; set and setting, as well as the psychological state of the individual, contribute significantly to its therapeutic effects.

As the scientific community continues to explore the multifaceted effects of psilocybin, there is increasing optimism regarding its role in mediating improved mental health outcomes. Research on psilocybin has surged in recent years, with studies exploring its impact on conditions such as depression (Carhart-Harris et al. 2021), PTSD (Khan et al. 2022), chronic pain (Whelan & Johnson, 2018), traumatic brain injury (Khan et al., 2021), Alzheimer's disease (Jones & O'Kelly, 2020), end-of-life anxiety (Grob et al., 2011), obsessive-compulsive disorder (Moreno et al., 2006), anorexia nervosa (Knatz Peck et al., 2023), alcohol dependence (Bogenschutz et al., 2015), along with a potential for performance enhancement effects (Mason et al., 2021).

Historically, psilocybin research has faced regulatory challenges, but a growing body of evidence indicating the drug's therapeutic potential has caused some jurisdictions to re-evaluate its legal status. In 2023, Australia was the first country to officially recognise psilocybin as a medicine.

Since the inception of EMDR therapy in the late 1980s, the adaptive information processing (AIP) framework has developed alongside this ground-breaking modality to conceptualise the pathogenesis of psychological issues and subsequent adaptive change (Shapiro, 2017). Over the past 30 years, the application of EMDR therapy has progressed from the treatment of single-event trauma to treat a wide range of psychological presentations; evidence of its efficacy has been reported in randomised controlled trials for the treatment of bipolar disorder (Novo et al., 2014; Moreno-Alcázar et al., 2015), pain management (Tesarz et al., 2014), fibromyalgia (Zat Çiftçi et al., 2023), depression (Hase et al., 2015), alcohol dependency (Perez-Dandieu & Tapia, 2014), psychosis (Varese et al., 2024) and panic disorder (Faretta, 2012). An extensive systematic review of 208 meta-analyses by the International Society for Traumatic Stress Studies (ISTSS) strongly recommends EMDR for the treatment of adults with PTSD (ISTSS, 2018). Now, in what has been coined the 'psychedelic renaissance,' the eight phases of EMDR therapy are being adapted to work alongside the therapeutic application of psychedelics (Raine-Smith & Rose, 2023). This chapter summarises current theories about the underlying mechanisms of EMDR and psychedelic therapy to give a picture of how these two powerful healing modalities can work synergistically alongside each other.

The AIP model

Research suggests that experience can be 'dissociated' from conscious awareness as a psychological defence against emotional flooding of the nervous system (Janet, 1901; Schore, 2015). Here we make a clear distinction between the subjective phenomenon of 'dissociation' and the resulting dysfunctionally encoded memory that is 'dissociated' from the main adaptive network in non-declarative memory. This compartmentalised sensory information can then be reactivated in the present by internal and external stressors that disrupt general functioning (Bourne et al., 2013). The AIP model postulates that a significant proportion of psychopathology is the result of these reactivations triggering a stress response in the present. Furthermore, chronic activation of the nervous system has been linked to many physical and mental health issues including IBS and autoimmune issues, as well as higher risk of a variety of health problems across the lifespan (Felitti et al., 1998). Considering these outcomes, it is important to refine treatments for psychological trauma, and psychedelics have the potential to optimise trauma-focussed modalities such as EMDR.

The AIP model hypothesises that impairments to the information processing systems of the brain under stress cause memories to be stored in an unprocessed, state-specific form that is not connected to adaptive information that is necessary to calm the nervous system, such as a sense of safety in the present (Van der Kolk & Van der Hart, 1989; Hase et al., 2017). If left unprocessed, this maladaptively stored sensory information (thoughts, images, emotions and somatic sensations) becomes the basis of the symptoms of PTSD. Chronic maladaptive encoding is conceptualised as being responsible for a plethora of presenting psychopathologies because of the way the brain processes stored information to navigate the world (Van der Kolk & Fishler, 1995; Dere et al., 2010). The AIP model posits that if traumatic memories are sufficiently reprocessed (reconsolidated) and integrated, the dysfunctional symptoms in the present can be eliminated. This view of psychopathology is gaining traction, and many neuroscientists are discussing the impact of pathogenic memories on implicit learning and the role this plays in mental disorders (e.g. Centonze et al., 2005).

Reprocessing in EMDR therapy "involves the accessing of dysfunctionally stored memories (which contain negative emotions, physical sensations, and beliefs) and forging their subsequent connection to more adaptive networks" (Shapiro, 2007, p. 73). In EMDR, adaptive memory networks are described as information that is sufficiently processed and stored in long-term memory. This information no longer holds its original emotional charge and is stored in the thematically appropriate pre-existing neural memory networks (Schore, 2015). EMDR's procedures have been developed to access dysfunctionally stored information and stimulate the brain's innate processing system, allowing it to transmute the information to an adaptive resolution (Stickgold, 2002).

Current EMDR theory

There are a number of theories about the underlying neurobiological mechanisms of EMDR with an array of contradictory evidence in the existing literature. Arguably, the most controversial component of EMDR therapy – and the intervention that sets it apart from traditional talking therapies – is the use of BLS, which is commonly elicited with horizontal saccadic eye movements, tactile (e.g. the 'butterfly hug,' Artigas & Jarero, 2014) and auditory BLS, or any combination of the three can be used. But to date, visual BLS has been shown to be the most efficacious at trauma memory reprocessing and fear extinction (Lee & Cuipers, 2013).

Comparisons have been made between the EMs in BLS and the saccades observed during rapid eye movement (REM) sleep. This is because sleep appears to be critical in memory-related processes and it is likely that it is necessary for resolution of emotional arousal whilst awake (Stickgold, 2008). It was initially proposed that lateral EMs in EMDR induce a neurological state characteristic of REM sleep, during which we are thought to consolidate memories. However, there is a lack of direct evidence to support this. REM sleep is associated with theta brain waves (3.5 to 7.5 Hz) and it has been hypothesised that BLS can entrain this frequency and moderate the flow of information that can be processed (Boyce et al., 2016; Huang, & Charyton, 2008). Sleep-like, delta wave oscillations (1.5 Hz) have been shown to be induced by EMDR in several EEG studies which is thought to depotentiate the 'fear memory' α-amino-3-hydroxy-5-methyl-4-isoxazolepropionic acid (AMPA) synapses in the amygdala and fronto-polar regions (Rasolkhani-Kalhorn & Harper, 2006; Pagani, et al., 2017). The depotentiation of AMPA receptors has been observed at a cellular level in animals (Lin et al., 2003) and is thought to be a biomarker of the fear extinction process (Hong et al., 2009).

The slow wave sleep (SWS) theory of EMDR posits that reprocessing with BLS modulates a naturally occurring low-frequency rhythm in the brain, similar to SWS (Pagani, et al., 2017). The BLS elicited during EMDR sessions is approximately 1–2 Hz, and Pagani et al. (2017) suggest that moving between reprocessing with BLS and engaging in cognitive thinking (SUDs, PC, VOC) mimics the cycle between REM and SWS, as waking memory is processed in a dialogue between the hippocampus and neocortex. During this process, newly encoded memories are reactivated during SWS and are moved from the short-term store (hippocampus) into the long-term store (neocortex). It is thought that REM sleep plays a role in the consolidation of these memories and is responsible for the wake-like EEG activity observed during this stage of sleep. This cycle between REM and SWS happens three to five times a night (Rasch & Born, 2013), which may account for the volume of memory reconsolidation achieved in EMDR because this cycle is repeated many times in one reprocessing session.

It is widely accepted that nested electrophysiological brain oscillations involving the neocortex, thalamus and the hippocampus form the basis of memory consolidation (Cohen, 2008). This phenomenon, whereby the amplitude of a faster rhythm is coupled to the phase of a slower rhythm, is also implicated in sleep (Steriade, 2006), and it has been proposed that nested theta and gamma oscillations are also linked to working memory (WM) capacity. Lisman and Idiart (1995) even suggest that the seven gamma cycles that approximately fit into a theta cycle correspond with the seven (±2) items that can be stored in the WM of the average person (Miller, 1956).

The WM model of EMDR posits that taxing WM resources reduces the vividness and emotionality of negative memories (Engelhard et al., 2010) and WM has been shown to be anti-correlated with the default mode network (DMN) during sustained cognitive processing in a nuanced, load-dependent manner (Cole et al., 2014). The dual-attention task of EMs and visual imagery is hypothesised to draw on the limited capacity of the WM resources, resulting in a reduction in vividness of disturbing images.

Tip! Sleep theory informed BLS

Aim: to mimic the cycle between REM and SWS seen during memory reconsolidation in sleep, whereby the memory is activated in the hippocampus and kicked up into the neocortex to be assimilated.

1 Use a combination of concurrent auditory and visual BLS.
2 To get the delta frequency (SWS, 1- 3Hz = approx. 2 beats per second) oscillating across the brain, the client can start by doing a short set of EMs before closing their eyes and reactivating (retrieving) the target memory.
3 When they have connected with the memory, open their eyes and do a set of eye movements.
4 Then, with the BLS still running, ask them to close their eyes again and re-assess the memory.
5 At this point they can either stop and check-in with the therapist or carry on the cycle (repeating this cycle entrains the brain waves and keeps them going to optimise reprocessing).

Warning: This technique is not part of the standard protocol. It is therefore advisable to assess a person's tolerance for EMDR prior to using this technique. Long sets of BLS can lead to chaining and overwhelm for some clients and therefore need to be monitored closely by an experienced clinician.

It has been suggested that the EMs in EMDR impair the visual imagery in conscious awareness, and research of this hypothesis has revealed that EMs in particular have the greatest treatment effect (de Jong et al., 2013). The main criticism of this model is that the partial explanations that are demonstrated in clinical research are based on protocols that do not fully reflect a standard EMDR session. The eight phases of EMDR consist of a number of interventions that have been developed to target a range of areas impacted by traumatic stress and therefore it is likely that there are a number of mechanisms of action.

Another theory about the underlying neurobiological mechanisms of EMDR is that the interhemispheric connectivity elicited by BLS appears to increase neuronal activity and facilitate access to and processing of information (Christman et al., 2003; Parker et al., 2008). It is thought that the sustained symptoms of psychological trauma are due to a fault in the information processing system and that BLS facilitates the integration of this information by synchronising interhemispheric functions

(Bergmann, 2008). Miller et al. (2018) go further and posit that reprocessing with BLS facilitates the repair and integration of somatosensory, memorial and cognitive integration by restoring the 40 Hz (gamma band) frequency to the thalamo-cortical system through a process they call 'stochastic resonance.' This term refers to the additional random neuronal 'noise' created by dual attention and BLS that facilitates the 'gating' of sensory information through the thalamus. This mechanism is often impaired in PTSD and stochastic resonance is posited to facilitate the return to functional memory encoding (Bergmann, 2008).

This neurobiological model is being further elucidated by the integration of the core principles of the AIP model with the predictive processing model (PPM) from cognitive neuroscience (Gregory, 1968), which posits that changes in automatic inferences in the brain's processing systems underlie PTSD symptoms as well as EMDR's treatment effects (Chamberlin, 2019; Vanderschoot & Van Dessel, 2022). The model refers to the prediction-based nature of memory, where psychopathology is conceptualised as the result of what the AIP model refers to as dysfunctionally stored memories. The PPM links the 'past' domain of the AIP model (maladaptively encoded memories) with the impact that these memories have on the brain's predictions in the 'present' of the 'future,' supporting the use of the 'three-pronged approach' in EMDR.

Chamberlain (2019) proposes that Friston's (2010) prediction error model explains the updating of beliefs when a traumatic memory is retrieved and reconsolidated in a reprocessing session. They highlight research that shows how saccadic EMs play a crucial role in synchronising the flow of incoming information through the brain's processing systems, namely the hippocampus and prefrontal cortex (Jutras et al., 2013). They also reference research showing that the theta rhythm plays a vital role in the flow of information during the encoding and retrieval of episodic memory (Hasselmo & Stern, 2014). Chamberlain acknowledges the complexity of EMDR as a therapy by highlighting that different elements of the EMDR standard protocol target different networks in the brain. For example, assessing the target is designed to reactivate the trauma memory and is posited to activate the default mode and salience networks. The dual-attention task of BLS during reprocessing is thought to activate the central executive network, therefore restoring balance to the nervous system. This allows the individual to take in information from the external world, orient to the safety of the present and update the prior-held beliefs accordingly (Chamberlain, 2019). Chamberlain proposes that the PPM of EMDR provides an integrative framework that explains what Francine Shapiro referred to as the 'inherent system' that enables the spontaneous reprocessing of maladaptively stored memories (Shapiro, 2002). This development in EMDR theory is an interesting progression because it aligns with the 'Entropic Brain' theory of psychedelics, which is also informed by the PPM (Carhart-Harris et al., 2014).

Altered states of consciousness

Robin Carhart-Harris, who headed the psilocybin trials at Imperial College London, and his research group have developed a theory of conscious states that weaves together recent data from neuroimaging with Freud's psychoanalytic concepts and Darwin's theory of evolution. The theory alludes to the once radical hypothesis that psychedelics could be the missing link that accounts for the shift in consciousness between primates and humans. They expand on Freud's concepts of primary and secondary consciousness:

Primary: Psychedelic states, REM sleep, psychosis and temporal lobe epilepsy. Described as a pre-ego style of cognition, based wholly in the present with no concept of past or future.

Secondary: Waking conscious awareness that has evolved with the ego as a mechanism to process our environment by exerting control over our experience. This includes our sense of self, metacognition, self-reflective awareness and abstract thinking.

Freud categorised non-ordinary states such as dreaming and psychosis as a primitive style of cognition and recognised that certain functions, that are normally present during ordinary waking consciousness, are deactivated. He postulated that these functions are the job of the ego and a core function of this system is to minimise 'free energy' in the mind (Freud, 1923). In a continuation of the research of the mid-20th century, altered states elicited by psychedelics have been studied to further elucidate Freud's theories of human consciousness (Freud, 1915).

Notice that REM sleep is in the primary consciousness group alongside psychedelic states. This link between psychedelic states and sleep could be relevant to EMDR because of the parallels drawn between the brain oscillations elicited during reprocessing with BLS and the oscillations observed during memory reconsolidation in sleep.

Entropic brain theory and EMDR

Entropy – Lack of order or predictability; gradual decline into disorder.

Early psilocybin trials showed less blood flow in the DMN, the system in the brain proposed to be involved in the separate sense of self and associated cognitive processes (Lanius et al., 2020). Carhart-Harris hypothesised that this was demonstrating a dissipation of blood flow across the brain and came upon the term 'entropy' (Carhart-Harris, 2021). Entropic brain theory posits that the 'entropy of spontaneous brain activity indexes the richness (i.e., the diversity and vividness) of subjective experience' and that psychedelics dramatically increase this (Carhartt-Harris & Friston, 2019, p. 317). Fundamentally, entropy is a dimensionless measure of 'uncertainty,' i.e. an increase in 'disorder' that can be measured by applying statistical analysis to neuroimaging data to quantify the uncertainty of fluctuation in activations across the brain. The neuroimaging data of individuals who have been administered psychedelics shows unpredictable neurological activity. Qualitative reports of psychedelic experience consistently indicate a heightened richness of experience; combining the objective neurological scanning data with such reports suggests that psychedelic-induced entropic brain states coincide with this reported "richness of experience" (Carhart-Harris et al., 2014).

The evidence base for entropic brain theory is a combination of empirical data from neuroimaging studies combined with subjective and behavioural data and it informs the Relaxed Beliefs Under Psychedelics (REBUS) model that was developed alongside the psilocybin trials (Carhartt-Harris & Friston, 2019). A core tenet of this model is the 'free energy' principle, a Bayesian model of the brain, whereby the brain minimises free energy by adapting the way it samples the environment or changes its expectations in a bid to maintain homeostasis (Friston, 2010). The REBUS model uses the principle that the brain predicts the world as a way of maintaining stability whereas psychedelics remove all prior assumptions, allowing for dramatic shifts in behaviour and perception. Under the influence of psychedelics, one's sense of self, referred to as 'ego' by Freud (1923), is removed and any basis of who we think we are dissolves (Feduccia & Mithoefer, 2018). Traumatic memories are theorised to maintain homeostasis and avoid flooding the nervous system (Vermetten et al., 2007). Neuroimaging studies have shown that psychedelics follow many pathways of the brain, creating connectivity that mimics that of an infant (Carhartt-Harris et al., 2016). From an AIP perspective, psychedelics appear to facilitate the integration of dissociated memory networks as well as the maladaptively stored sensory material encoded within them, which would account for the positive (and negative) side effects of psychedelics. Whilst under the influence of psychedelics, subconscious psychological barriers are removed, enabling an individual to connect with – and ideally reconsolidate or integrate – the aforementioned sensory information (Carhart-Harris et al., 2014). This is why trauma and attachment history, as well as affect regulation capacity of participants, must be taken into account for harm-reduction purposes.

Troubleshooting – Learning from the complex PTSD population

The neural 'interconnectedness' observed during psychedelic therapy flags up a warning for people with complex trauma histories or individual sensitivities that have not been addressed in therapy prior to the administration of psychedelics. This is because compartmentalisation of trauma is a mechanism that maintains homeostasis and avoids flooding of the nervous system (Maldonado & Spiegel, 1991). If dissociative barriers are suddenly removed in psychedelic therapy, there is a risk that individuals can become overwhelmed by the sudden reconnection with traumatic material and this can cause lasting side effects such as severe dissociation or heighten anxiety levels (Hoper et al., 2007; Halpern et al., 2018).

The term 'hallucinogen persisting perception disorder' (HPPD, American Psychological Association, 2013) has been used to describe a non-psychotic disorder where an individual experiences visual hallucinations that persist after the use of any drug, including psychedelics. From an AIP perspective, this could be conceptualised as a type of PTSD where the psychedelics have reactivated a maladaptively encoded memory network. The persisting visual and somatic responses often have thematic links, not only to the recent psychedelic experience but also to traumatic experiences in early childhood.

There has been a notable increase in individuals presenting with this condition in both private practice and acute care settings, driven by the growing publicity and interest surrounding psychedelics. Many of these clients experience persistent dysregulation following psychedelic treatments and often have complex trauma histories involving early childhood adversity and the development of coping mechanisms such as dissociation, which have become deeply ingrained over time.

In the following chapters, we discuss the adaption of the stabilisation and preparation phases of EMDR to specifically support complex trauma populations, including the use of EMDR reprocessing as a screening tool for psychedelic therapy.

DMN and 'high-level beliefs'

The DMN is a large-scale cortical network located along the brain's mid-line that is thought to be involved in high-level processing of sensory information (Raichle, 2015). Memories are encoded in hippocampal-cortical networks within the DMN, and it is involved in autobiographical memory processing as well as self-related cognition (Lanius et al., 2020). The brain is an inference machine (von Helmholtz, 1866; Rao & Ballard, 1998) and uses hierarchical models to predict its sensory input in an attempt to reduce prediction error. The brain tries to minimise prediction error in an attempt to reduce free energy and conserve energy and maintain homeostasis. Therefore, prediction error is a quantifiable measurement of free energy and is routinely used to model data (Friston, 2009). It has been proposed that the DMN is the neurobiological substrate of the Freudian concept of the 'ego' whose main function is to minimise free energy by repressing endogenous excitation (Carhart-Harris & Friston, 2010).

Our model of the world is proposed to be encoded in a hierarchy of brain regions (Huang & Rao, 2011). Low-level brain regions such as primary somatosensory, visual and the auditory cortex process sensory information, and the DMN is involved in the high-level processing of global sensory input and constructs an abstract belief system in response to this. The DMN has the ability to modulate activity in the lower regions in the system through prior-held beliefs based on previous experience. For example, it is proposed that the perception of physical pain is an inferential process whereby prior beliefs about pain are combined with incoming sensory data to give rise to pain perception. This Bayesian model of pain proposes that chronic pain emerges when prior beliefs have a bias towards inferring pain from sensory data that would otherwise be perceived as harmless (Eckert et al., 2022). This model has also been applied to psychological pain whereby current pain perception is based on prior experience (Feldmann et al., 2023). Pain protocols in EMDR will often target the client's prior-held beliefs about pain, by targeting their emotional reaction to the pain, as well as targets based on environmental stressors around the time it began (Zat Çiftçi et al., 2023).

Trauma can disrupt the normal functioning of the DMN, resulting in feelings of fragmentation, dissociation and distorted self-perception. Furthermore, alterations to the connectivity in the DMN can lead to impaired self-referential processing, compromised autobiographical memory retrieval and challenges with social cognition (Lanius et al., 2020). Such changes are argued to contribute to a distorted self-concept, including negative beliefs about oneself. The fragmentation of the self, caused by trauma, can result in difficulty delineating the past, present and future, leading to a sense of disorientation (Schore, 2015; Lanius et al., 2020).

Serotonergic psychedelics preferentially bind to the serotonin 2A (5-HT2A) receptors in the DMN (Hahn, 2012; Nichols, 2016), stimulating the receptors by binding to them, mimicking the action of serotonin. The key outcome is an increase in excitability of the hosting neuron, resulting in an increase in entropy (instability) across the DMN (Carhart-Harris et al., 2014). Carhart-Harris and Friston (2019) have revealed an inverse link between brain entropy on psychedelics and confidence in prior-held beliefs; when entropy is increased, there is less confidence in a prior-held belief. They state that "the general (entropic) action of psychedelics is to render the brain/mind's (variational free) energy landscape flattened or opened up" (Carhartt-Harris & Friston, 2019, p. 319). The free energy principle that informs the REBUS model is based on the concept that living systems monitor their internal environment through interoception and adapt accordingly to maintain homeostasis through a predictive process of allostasis (Zsoldos & Ebmeier, 2016). Here entropic brain theory is combined with the hierarchical predictive coding hypothesis that 'high-level priors or beliefs' have a constraining influence on the lower level components and can exert and inhibit their influence. The theory is that the relaxation of prior-held beliefs caused by brain entropy on psychedelics can then be harnessed by good-quality therapeutic interventions to facilitate sustained positive change.

Memory networks, COEXs and complexes

The concept of prior-held beliefs is a familiar one in the field of EMDR; defining such beliefs forms a core part of the case conceptualisation process. The AIP model refers to working within different 'memory networks' that are delineated by the cognitive (negative self-referencing belief/ negative cognition/schema), emotional and somatic responses that are assigned to it. In the assessment phase, this information is used to group memories together into networks (themes), for them to be cross-referenced with the client's presenting symptoms to create a case conceptualisation based on the AIP model.

This theory of associative memory networks is clearly demonstrated by the somatic bridge intervention in EMDR whereby a somatic response to a stressor in the present (combined with the negative cognition and emotion) is used to access earlier material in a specific memory network. See Chapter 8, 'Bridging to the Matrix.' Through an AIP lens, we conceptualise that emergent material in the psychedelic space often represents material from biographical memory networks that have been encoded maladaptively. These networks form a matrix and converge at points where trauma occurs. Emotionally salient material is given the opportunity to emerge during the transient hyperplastic state, in an attempt to integrate it adaptively in an innate move towards wholeness. Reprocessing with BLS can then be used as an adjunct therapy to facilitate the integration of psychedelic material during psychedelic dosing (psycholytic therapy) or post-dose (psychedelic therapy).

The AIP model and its conceptualisation of memory networks mirrors that of Carl Jung's concept of 'complexes' (Jung, 1960) and Stanislav Grof's 'systems of condensed experience (COEX) theory' (Grof, 2019) – two influential concepts in psychedelic-assisted psychotherapy (PAP). The main difference being that Grof's COEX systems expand the networks further to perinatal stages and even transgenerational or ancestral trauma. There is the potential to combine these theories to conceptualise PsyA-EMDR through a transpersonal lens, for example, when bridging somatically to abstract material that has no obvious reference point in their biographical history. Intergenerational and attachment informed (AI) EMDR protocols can be adapted to work with perinatal and transpersonal material. See Chapter 11, 'Multidimensional healing,' for an expanded view.

An AIP model of holotropic states

Stanislav Grof MD, an eminent researcher of the clinical applications of psychedelics since the 1960s, coined the term 'holotropic state' to describe a non-ordinary state of consciousness, experienced on psychedelics or during meditation or breathwork (Grof & Grof, 2023). The term holotropic is derived from Greek and means 'moving in the direction of wholeness.' When we consider that the most notable neurophysiological signature of psychedelics is increased spontaneous global neural activity, the concept of moving towards wholeness is demonstrated in the neuroimaging data. A core principle in EMDR is the brain's innate ability to heal itself under the right conditions. BLS is used to create the optimum conditions for the brain to reconsolidate dissociated trauma memories and integrate them with the main adaptive memory networks.

There is a distinct similarity between the holotropic states elicited by psychedelics and the reprocessing phase of EMDR therapy because they are both altered states of consciousness that seem to allow access to the subconscious. During reprocessing with BLS, subconscious information emerges from the memory network being targeted, and somatic releases and insights are experienced as the information is processed. It is possible that bilateral activation of the brain is partly responsible for this, and the WM taxation model of EMDR goes some way to account for the brain gaining access to emotionally salient material during reprocessing (van den Hout et al., 2011, 2014; Matthijssen et al., 2017). The stochastic resonance theory that reprocessing in EMDR adds extra noise to the neural circuits (Miller et al., 2018) echoes the increased entropy observed in neuroimaging of the effects of psychedelics.

It is thought that the degree to which functional brain networks are divided into subnetworks, known as 'modularity,' could be a biomarker of psychopathology because it constrains the flow of information across the brain (Bassett & Bullmore, 2009; Rubinov & Sporns, 2010). On the psilocybin for depression trials, a link has been demonstrated between decreased brain network modularity and sustained psychotherapeutic effects (Daws et al., 2022). The innate move towards wholeness is captured in these imaging studies showing that the greater the decrease in modularity on psychedelics, the greater the decrease in depression and that a sustained decrease in modularity correlates with improvements in symptom severity one-month post-high-dose psilocybin (Carhart-Harris et al., 2017; Daws et al., 2022). From an AIP perspective, perhaps the levels of modularity are a biomarker for maladaptively encoded information in the brain and the fragmentation of larger networks represents the compartmentalisation of sensory information in an attempt to maintain homeostasis.

Psychedelic integration with EMDR

The concept of integration varies dramatically across psychotherapeutic modalities, and psychedelic-assisted therapy is no exception. Here psychedelic integration is defined in terms of memory consolidation theory and the AIP model. It is proposed that the integration of psychological and somatic material that has emerged in response to the administration of psychedelics can be achieved through EMDR reprocessing. Material is considered sufficiently integrated when the subjective unit of distress is 0 or 1 (out of 10) when the target is held in close psychological proximity. See Chapter 8, 'Integration.'

A key reason for the combination of therapeutic interventions such as EMDR therapy with psychedelic treatments is the neuroplasticity that psychedelics promote (Ly et al., 2018; Aleksandrova & Philips, 2021). Classic 'serotonergic' psychedelics (e.g. psilocybin, DMT and LSD) have been shown to have an affinity for the 5-H2A receptor in the cerebral cortex, an area responsible for association (Beliveau et al., 2017). Serotonin 2A receptor agonism has been shown to promote a broad range of plasticity in the brain including promoting synapse growth, learning rate and cognitive flexibility. From an AIP perspective, these neuroplastogenic effects could enhance the effects of EMDR therapy by facilitating the reprocessing and integration of emotionally salient material that is dysfunctionally stored in memory networks (Vollenweider & Preller, 2020).

The term 'transient hyperplastic state' has been applied to describe the mechanism of action for psychological transformation caused by psychedelics (Brouwer & Carhart-Harris, 2021). A similar 'pivotal mental state' is also seen in response to stress, which has been shown to upregulate the 5-HTP system (Brouwer & Carhartt-Harris, 2021). It has been proposed that the 5-HT2A system has evolved to facilitate an adaptive response to adversity and perhaps accounts for the unique adaptability that we see in humans (Carhart-Harris & Nutt, 2017). It is hypothesised that the 5-HT2A receptors developed as a mechanism to attenuate acute or chronic stress which has been demonstrated in animal models (Takao et al., 1995). Chronic stress has been shown to prime the serotonin receptor system and upregulate the release of the natural chemical or ligand (serotonin) that stimulates the primed system. Deprivation states such as hyperthermia (Janssen et al., 2016) and fasting are thought to also activate this system. During reprocessing in EMDR, traumatic memories are reactivated and the noradrenergic activation could theoretically stimulate a primed 5-HTP system, causing an increase in neuroplasticity that facilitates memory reconsolidation.

The REBUS model, which is rooted in third-wave CBT notions of behavioural change, uses the term 'canalisation,' derived from the entrenchment of the canal to describe the entrenchment of pathological ways of thinking, feeling and behaving (Carhart-Harris et al., 2022). This model, along with all the PAPs based on acceptance and commitment therapy (ACT), focus on facilitating behavioural change by harnessing the neuroplastogenic effect of psychedelics with future-focussed goal-oriented behavioural interventions. We propose that this fails to directly address any past trauma and therefore old behaviours often return. From an AIP perspective, this framework fails to adequately address the impact of past trauma and maladaptive attachment dynamics on present functioning.

The predictive processing model and free energy principle that inform entropic brain theory further elucidate the spontaneous shifts in neuroplasticity in response to traumatic stress. If the system becomes overwhelmed by incoming sensory information, the brain is required to take drastic measures to re-stabilise the system. It is proposed that a primed 5-HTP system is triggered by traumatic stress (Murnane, 2019) and it is feasible that the resulting transient hyperplastic state is a means for the brain to separate the emotionally salient information from the main memory network in an attempt to stabilise the system through dissociation (Spiegel, 2012). The PPM of reprocessing in EMDR (Chamberlin, 2019) illustrates this concept: restoration of balance across networks elicited by interhemispheric activation with BLS creates the physiological conditions required for optimal processing of memory to be re-established. The resulting excess in free energy in the brain facilitates the re-establishment of prediction error minimisation of the traumatic memory, and saccadic EMs have been hypothesised to modulate this process. This results in the reconsolidation of memory and its re-integration with the main (adaptive) memory network.

The reconsolidation of traumatic memories in EMDR using bilateral stimulation can potentially be enhanced by the neuroplasticity elicited by serotonergic psychedelics. This is already being done in private practices in different parts of the world, where clients are receiving legal psychedelic treatments whilst engaged in EMDR therapy. Another way to harness the effects of these compounds is to pair them with interventions based on the therapeutic goal. For example, utilising the effects of the 'empathogen' 3,4-methylenedioxymethamphetamine (MDMA) by pairing it with the preparation phase of EMDR could augment the adaptive information formed in the memory networks through the embodied sense of safety and connectedness elicited by this compound. This could be particularly beneficial for clients who have suffered chronic childhood abuse and/or neglect.

Summary

Francine Shapiro discussed the 'inherent system' within the brain that has developed to process and integrate information and naturally move towards a state of balance and mental health. The AIP model proposes that in order to achieve this, maladaptively stored information needs to be reprocessed and integrated. This trauma-informed view of psychopathology is validated by a plethora of research showing the link between psychological trauma and general health, conversely, as well as positive outcomes following EMDR. The Groffian term 'holotropic' also alludes to this innate system that 'moves towards wellness,' and interhemispheric activation (BLS) in EMDR or entropy caused by psychedelics seem to both play a key role in this process.

The adaption of EMDR therapy to work alongside psychedelics feels like a natural progression in the evolution of trauma-informed PAP because the phases of EMDR have been developed over the past 40 years with the specific aims of stabilisation and harm reduction during trauma integration. The AIP model can be used as a transtheoretical case conceptualisation tool that can be applied across PAP settings and integrates neatly with the frameworks of key theorists in the field of psychedelic therapy, such as Freud, Jung, Grof and Carhart-Harris.

It is apparent that EMDR therapy has a number of underlying mechanisms of action, but it is evident that the BLS is what sets it apart from other therapies. It is likely that there are similarities between the neurological state elicited by EMDR and the holotropic state elicited by psychedelics, partly because they both act on the processing systems of the brain, allowing the integration of information. The dreamlike state elicited by BLS in EMDR allows access to the subconscious and firmly aligns it with psychedelic therapy, and it is possible that the research coming from this burgeoning field can further solidify the AIP model's foundations.

References

Aleksandrova, L. R., & Phillips, A. G. (2021). Neuroplasticity as a convergent mechanism of ketamine and classical psychedelics. *Trends in Pharmacological Sciences*, 42(11), 929–942. https://doi.org/10.1016/j.tips.2021.08.003

American Psychiatric Association. (2013). *Diagnostic and statistical manual of mental disorders* (5th ed.). Arlington, VA: American Psychiatric Association. https://doi.org/10.1176/appi.books.9780890425596

Artigas, L., & Jarero, I. (2014). *The butterfly hug. Implementing EMDR early mental health interventions for man-made and natural disasters* (pp. 127–130). New York: Springer. https://doi.org/10.1891/9780826122452.0001

Bassett, D. S., & Bullmore, E. T. (2009). Human brain networks in health and disease. *Current opinion in neurology, 22*(4), 340-347. https://doi.org/ 10.1097/ WCO.0b013e32832d93dd

Beliveau, V., Ganz, M., Feng, L., Ozenne, B., Højgaard, L., Fisher, P. M., Svarer, C., Greve, D. N., & Knudsen, G. M. (2017). A high-resolution in vivo atlas of the human brain's serotonin system. *The Journal of Neuroscience, 37*(1), 120–128. https://doi.org/10.1523/jneurosci.2830-16.2016

Bergmann, U. (2008). The neurobiology of EMDR: Exploring the thalamus and neural integration. *Journal of EMDR Practice and Research, 2*(4), 300–314. http://dx.doi.org/10.1891/1933-3196.2.4.300

Bogenschutz, M. P., Forcehimes, A. A., Pommy, J. A., Wilcox, C. E., Barbosa P. C. R., & Strassman, R. J. (2015). Psilocybin-assisted treatment for alcohol dependence: A proof-of-concept study. *Journal of Psychopharmacology, 29*(3), 289–299. https://doi.org/10.1177/0269881114565144

Bourne, C., Mackay, C. E., & Holmes, E. A. (2013). The neural basis of flash-back formation: The impact of viewing trauma. *Psychological Medicine, 43*(7), 1521–1532. https://doi.org/10.1017/s0033291712002358

Boyce, R., Glasgow, S. D., Williams, S., & Adamantidis, A. (2016). Causal evidence for the role of REM sleep theta rhythm in contextual memory consolidation. *Science, 352*(6287), 812–816. https://doi.org/10.1126/science.aad5252

Brouwer, A., & Carhart-Harris, R. L. (2021). Pivotal mental states. *Journal of Psychopharmacology, 35*(4), 319–352. https://doi.org/10.1177/0269881120959637

Carhartt-Harris, R. L. (2021). PT245 – Robin Carhart-Harris – Psychedelics, entropy, and plasticity. Found at https://www.youtube.com/watch?v=IOAiJc78Qmg. Accessed 5.9.23

Carhart-Harris, R. L., & Friston, K. J. (2010). The default-mode, ego-functions and free-energy: A neurobiological account of Freudian ideas. *Brain, 133*(4), 1265–1283. https://doi.org/10.1093/brain/awq010

Carhart-Harris, R. L., & Friston, K. J. (2019). REBUS and the anarchic brain: Toward a unified model of the brain action of psychedelics. *Pharmacological Reviews, 71*(3), 316–344. https://doi.org/10.1124/pr.118.017160

Carhart-Harris, R. L., & Nutt, D. J. (2017). Serotonin and brain function: A tale of two receptors. *Journal of Psychopharmacology, 31*(9), 1091–1120. https://doi.org/10.1177/0269881117725915

Carhart-Harris, R., Giribaldi, B., Watts, R., Baker-Jones, M., Murphy-Beiner, A., Murphy, R., Martell, J., Blemings, A., Erritzoe, D., & Nutt, D. J. (2021). Trial of psilocybin versus escitalopram for depression. *New England Journal of Medicine, 384*(15), 1402–1411. https://doi.org/10.1056/nejmoa2032994

Carhart-Harris, R. L., Chandaria, S., Erritzoe, D. E., Gazzaley, A., Girn, M., Kettner, H., Mediano, P. A. M., Nutt, D. J., Rosas, F.E., Roseman, L., & Timmermann, C. (2022). Canalization and plasticity in psychopathology. *Neuropharmacology, 226*, 109398. https://doi.org/10.1016/j.neuropharm.2022.109398

Carhart-Harris, R. L., Leech, R., Hellyer, P. J., Shanahan, M., Feilding, A., Tagliazucchi, E., Chialvo, D. R., & Nutt, D. (2014). The entropic brain: A theory of conscious states informed by neuroimaging research with psychedelic drugs. *Frontiers in Human Neuroscience, 8,* 20. https://doi.org/10.3389/fnhum.2014.00020

Carhart-Harris, R. L., Muthukumaraswamy, S., Roseman, L., Kaelen, M., Droog, W., Murphy, K., Tagliazucchi, E., Schenberg, E. E., Nest, T., Orban, C., & Leech, R. (2016). Neural correlates of the LSD experience revealed by multimodal neuroimaging. *Proceedings of the National Academy of Sciences USA, 113*(17), 4853–4858. https://doi.org/10.1073/pnas.1518377113

Centonze, D., Siracusane, A., Calabresi, P., & Bernardi, G. (2005). Removing pathogenic memories. *Molecular Neurobiology, 32*(2), 123–132. https://doi.org/10.1385/mn:32:2:123

Chamberlin, D. E. (2019). The predictive processing model of EMDR. *Frontiers in psychology, 10,* 2267. https://doi.org/10.3389/fpsyg.2019.02267

Christman, S. D., Garvey, K. J., Propper, R. E., & Phaneuf, K. A. (2003). Bilateral eye movements enhance the retrieval of episodic memories. *Neuropsychology, 17*(2), 221–229. https://doi.org/10.1037/0894-4105.17.2.221

Cohen, M. (2008). Assessing transient cross-frequency coupling in EEG data. *Journal of Neuroscience Methods, 168*(2), 494–499. https://doi.org/10.1016/j.jneumeth.2007.10.012

Cole, M., Bassett, D., Power, J., Braver, T., & Petersen, S. (2014). Intrinsic and task-evoked network architectures of the human brain. *Neuron, 83*(1), 238–251. https://doi.org/10.1016/j.neuron.2014.05.014

Daws, R., Timmermann, C., Giribaldi, B., Sexton, J. D., Wall, M. B., Erritzoe, D., Roseman, L., Nutt, D., & Carhart-Harris, R. (2022). Increased global integration in the brain after psilocybin therapy for depression. *Nature Medicine, 28*(4), 844–851. https://doi.org/10.1038/s41591-022-01744-z

de Jongh, A., Ernst, R., Marques, L., & Hornsveld, H. (2013). The impact of eye movements and tones on disturbing memories involving PTSD and other mental disorders. *Journal of Behavior Therapy and Experimental Psychiatry, 44*(4), 477–483. https://doi.org/10.1016/j.jbtep.2013.07.002

Dere, E., Pause, B. M., & Pietrowsky, R. (2010). Emotion and episodic memory in neuropsychiatric disorders. *Behavioural Brain Research, 215*(2), 162–171. https://doi.org/10.1016/j.bbr.2010.03.017

Eckert, A. L., Pabst, K., & Endres, D. M. (2022). A Bayesian model for chronic pain. *Frontiers in Pain Research, 3,* 966034. https://doi.org/10.3389/fpain.2022.966034

Engelhard, I. M., van den Hout, M. A., Janssen, W. C., & van der Beek, J. (2010). Eye movements reduce vividness and emotionality of "flashforwards". *Behaviour Research and Therapy, 48*(5), 442–447. https://doi.org/10.1016/j.brat.2010.01.003

Faretta, E. (2012). EMDR and cognitive-behavioural therapy in the treatment of panic disorder: A comparison. *Rivista di Psichiatria, 47*(2 Suppl), 19–25. https://doi.org/10.1708/1071.11735

Feduccia, A. A., & Mithoefer, M. C. (2018). MDMA-assisted psychotherapy for PTSD: Are memory reconsolidation and fear extinction underlying mechanisms? *Progress in neuro-psychopharmacology and biological psychiatry, 84*(Pt A), 221–228. https://doi.org/10.1016/j.pnpbp.2018.03.003

Feldmann, M., Kube, T., Rief, W., & Brakemeier, E. L. (2023). Testing Bayesian models of belief updating in the context of depressive symptomatology. *International Journal of Methods in Psychiatric Research, 32*(2), e1946. https://doi.org/10.1002/mpr.1946

Felitti, V. J., Anda, R. F., Nordenberg, D., Williamson, D. F., Spitz, A. M., Edwards, V., & Marks, J. S. (1998). Relationship of childhood abuse and household dysfunction to many of the leading causes of death in adults: The adverse childhood experiences (ACE) study. *American Journal of Preventive Medicine, 14*(4), 245–258. https://doi.org/10.1016/S0749-3797(98)00017-8

Freud, S. (1915). The Unconscious. *James Strachey, translator*. London: Hogarth Press.

Freud, S. (1923). The ego and the id. In J. Strachey (Ed.), *The standard edition of the complete psychological works of Sigmund Freud* (vol. 19). London: Hogarth Press.

Friston, K. (2009). The free-energy principle: A rough guide to the brain? *Trends in cognitive sciences, 13*(7), 293–301. https://doi.org/10.1016/j.tics.2009.04.005

Friston, K. (2010). The free-energy principle: A unified brain theory? *Nature Reviews Neuroscience, 11*, 127–138. https://doi.org/10.1038/nrn2787

Gregory, R. (1968). Perceptual illusions and brain models. *Proceedings of the Royal Society London B, 171*, 179–296. https://doi.org/10.1098/rspb.1968.0071

Griffiths, R. R., Richards, W. A., & McCann, U. (2006). Psilocybin can occasion mystical-type experiences having substantial and sustained personal meaning and spiritual significance. *Psychopharmacology, 187*, 268–283. https://doi.org/10.1007/s00213-006-0457-5

Grob, C. S., Danforth, A. L., Chopra, G. S., Hagerty, M., McKay, C. R., Halberstadt, A. L., & Greer, G. R., (2011). Pilot study of psilocybin treatment for anxiety in patients with advanced-stage cancer. *Archives of General Psychiatry, 68*, 71–78. https://doi.org/10.1001/archgenpsychiatry.2010.116

Grof, S. (2019). *Psychology of the future: Lessons from modern consciousness research*. Albany: State University of New York Press. https://doi.org/10.1515/9780791492383

Grof, S., & Grof, C. (2023). *Holotropic breathwork: A new approach to self-exploration and therapy*. Albany: State University of New York Press.

Hahn, A., Wadsak, W., Windischberger, C., Baldinger, P., Höflich, A. S., Losak, J., Nics, L., Philippe, C., Kranz, G. S., Kraus, C., & Mitterhauser, M. (2012). Differential modulation of the default mode network via serotonin-1A receptors. *Proceedings of the National Academy of Sciences, 109*(7), 2619–2624. https://doi.org/10.1073/pnas.1117104109

Halberstadt, A. L., & Geyer, M. A. (2011). Multiple receptors contribute to the behavioral effects of indoleamine hallucinogens. *Neuropharmacology, 61*(3), 364–381. https://doi.org/10.1016/j.neuropharm.2011.01.017

Halpern, J. H., Lerner, A. G., & Passie, T. (2018). A review of hallucinogen persisting perception disorder (HPPD) and an exploratory study of subjects claiming symptoms of HPPD. *Behavioral Neurobiology of Psychedelic Drugs, 36*, 333–360. https://doi.org/10.1007/7854_2016_457

Hase, M., Balmaceda, U. M., Hase, A., Lehnung, M., Tumani, V., & Huchzermeier, C. (2015). Eye movement desensitization and reprocessing (EMDR) therapy in the treatment of depression: a matched pairs study in an inpatient setting. *Brain Behavior, 5*(6), e00342. https://doi.org/10.1002/brb3.342

Hase, M., Balmaceda, U. M., Ostacoli, L., Liebermann, P., & Hofmann, A. (2017). The AIP model of EMDR therapy and pathogenic memories. *Frontiers in Psychology, 8*, 1578. https://doi.org/10.3389/fpsyg.2017.01578

Hasselmo, M. E., & Stern, C. E. (2014). Theta rhythm and the encoding and retrieval of space and time. *Neuroimage, 85*(Pt 2), 656–666. https://doi.org/10.1016/j.neuroimage.2013.06.022

Hofmann, A., Heim, R., Brack, A., & Kobel, H. (1958). Psilocybin, a psychotropic substance from the Mexican mushroom Psilicybe mexicana Heim. *Experientia, 14*(3), 107-109. https://doi.org/10.1007/BF02159243

Hong, I., Song, B., Lee, S., Kim, J., Kim, J., & Choi, S. (2009). Extinction of cued fear memory involves a distinct form of depotentiation at cortical input synapses onto the lateral amygdala. *European Journal of Neuroscience, 30*, 2089–2099. https://doi.org/10.1111/j.1460-9568.2009.07004.x

Huang, T. L., & Charyton, C. (2008). A comprehensive review of the psychological effects of brainwave entrainment. In Database of Abstracts of Reviews of Effects (DARE), *Quality-assessed Reviews*. UK: Centre for Reviews and Dissemination.

Huang, Y., & Rao, R. P. (2011). Predictive coding. *Wiley Interdisciplinary Reviews: Cognitive Science, 2*(5), 580–593. https://doi.org/10.1002/wcs.142

International Society of Traumatic Stress Studies (ISTSS). (2018). New ISTSS prevention and treatment guidelines. Found at https://istss.org/clinical-resources/treating-trauma/new-istss-prevention-and-treatment-guidelines. Accessed 12.04.2023

Janet, P. (1901). *The mental state of hystericals: A study of mental stigmata and mental accidents*. New York: GP Putnam's sons. https://doi.org/10.1037/10597-000

Janssen, C. W., Lowry, C. A., & Mehl, M. R. (2016). Whole-body hyperthermia for the treatment of major depressive disorder: A randomized clinical trial. *JAMA Psychiatry, 73*, 789–795. https://doi.org/10.1001/jamapsychiatry.2016.1031

Jones, S. A.V., & O'Kelly, A. (2020). Psychedelics as a treatments for Alzheimer's disease dementia. *Frontiers in Synaptic Neuroscience, 12*, 34. https://doi.org/10.3389/fnsyn.2020.00034

Jung, C. G. (1960). *A Review of the Complex Theory. Collected Works, (Vol. 8). Bollingen Series XX*. Princeton, NJ: Princeton University Press.

Jutras, M. J., Fries, P., & Buffalo, E. A. (2013). Oscillatory activity in the monkey hippocampus during visual exploration and memory formation. *Proceedings of the National Academy of Sciences USA, 110*(32), 13144–13149. https://doi.org/10.1073/pnas.1302351110

Khan, A. J., Bradley, E., O'Donovan, A., & Woolley, J. (2022). Psilocybin for trauma-related disorders. *Current Topics in Behavioural Neuroscience, 56*, 319–332. https://doi.org/10.1007/7854_2022_366

Khan, S. M., Carter, G. T., Aggarwal, S. K., & Holland, J. (2021). Psychedelics for brain injury: A mini-review. *Frontiers in Neurology: Sec. Neurorehabilitation, 12*, 685085. https://doi.org/10.3389/fneur.2021.685085

Knatz Peck, S., Shao, S., Gruen, T., Yang, K., Babakanian, A., Trim, J., Finn, D., & Kaye, W. (2023). Psilocybin therapy for females with anorexia nervosa: A phase 1, open-label feasibility study. *Nature Medicine, 29*, 1947–1953. https://doi.org/10.1038/s41591-023-02455-9

Lanius, R. A., Terpou, B. A., & McKinnon, M. C. (2020). The sense of self in the aftermath of trauma: Lessons from the default mode network in posttraumatic stress disorder. *European Journal of Psychotraumatology, 11*(1), 1807703. https://doi.org/10.1080/20008198.2020.1807703

Lee, C. W., & Cuijpers, P. (2013). A meta-analysis of the contribution of eye movements in processing emotional memories. *Journal of Behavior Therapy Experimental Psychiatry, 44*, 231–239. https://doi.org/10.1016/j.jbtep.2012.11.001

Lin, C. H., Lee, C. C., & Gean, P. W. (2003). Involvement of a calcineurin cascade in amygdala depotentiation and quenching of fear memory. *Molecular Pharmacology, 63*(1), 44–52. https://doi.org/10.1124/mol.63.1.44

Lisman, J. E., & Idiart, M. A. (1995). Storage of 7±2 short-term memories in oscillatory subcycles. *Science, 267*(5203), 1512–1515. https://doi.org/10.1126/science.7878473

Ly, C., Greb, A. C., Cameron, L. P., Wong, J. M., Barragan, E.V., & Wilson, P. C.(2008). Psychedelics promote structural and functional neural plasticity. *Cell Reports, 23*, 3170–82. https://doi.org/10.1016/j.celrep.2018.05.022

Maldonado, J., & Spiegel, D. (1991). Dissociative Disorders. In A. Tasman and S. M. Goldfinger (Eds.), *Release of Psychiatry*, Vol. 10. (pp. 145–160). Washington, DC: American Psychiatric Press.

Mason, N. L., Kuypers, K. P. C., Reckweg, J. T., Muller, F., Da Rios, B., Toennes, S. W., Stiers, P., Feilding, A., & Ramaekers, J. G. (2021). Spontaneous and deliberate creative cognition during and after psilocybin exposure. *Translational Psychiatry, 11*, 209. https://doi.org/10.1038/s41398-021-01335-5

Matthijssen, S. J., Verhoeven, L. C., Van den Hout, M. A., & Heitland, I. (2017). Auditory and visual memories in PTSD patients targeted with eye movements and counting: The effect of modality- specific loading of working memory. *Frontiers in Psychology, 8*, 1937. https://doi.org/10.3389/fpsyg.2017.01937

Miller, G. (1956). The magical number seven, plus or minus two: Some limits on our capacity for processing information. *Psychological Review, 63*(2), 81–97. https://doi.org/10.1037/h0043158

Miller, P. W., McGowan, I. W., Bergmann, U., Farrell, D., & McLaughlin, D. F. (2018). Stochastic resonance as a proposed neurobiological model for Eye Movement Desensitization and Reprocessing (EMDR) therapy. *Medical Hypotheses, 121*, 106–111. https://doi.org/10.1016/j.mehy.2018.09.010

Moreno-Alcázar, A., Radua, J., Landín-Romero, R., Blanco, L., Madre, M., & Reinares, M. (2015). The EMDR therapy protocol for bipolar disorder, In M. Luber (Ed.), *Eye movement desensitization and reprocessing (EMDR) therapy scripted protocols and summary sheets: Treating anxiety, obsessive-compulsive, and mood-related conditions.* New York: Springer Publishing Co. https://doi.org/10.4088/JCP.v67n1110

Moreno, F., Wiegand, C., Keolani Taitano, E., & Degado, P. (2006). Safety, tolerability, and efficacy of psilocybin in 9 patients with OCD. *Journal of Clinical Psychiatry, 67*, 1735–1740. https://doi.org/10.4088/JCP.v67n1110

Murnane, K. S. (2019). Serotonin 2A receptors are a stress response system: Implications for post-traumatic stress disorder. *Behavioural pharmacology, 30*(2 and 3-Spec Issue), 151–162. https://doi.org/10.1097/FBP.0000000000000459

Nichols, D. E. (2016). Psychedelics. *Pharmacological reviews, 68*(2), 264–355. https://doi.org/10.1124/pr.115.011478

Novo, P., Landin-Romero, R., Radua, J., Vicens, V., Fernandez, I., & Garcia, F. (2014). Eye movement desensitization and reprocessing therapy in subsyndromal bipolar patients with a history of traumatic events: a randomized, controlled pilot-study. *Psychiatry Research, 219*(1), 122–128. https://doi.org/10.1016/j.psychres.2014.05.012

Pagani, M., Amann, B. L., Landin-Romero, R., & Carletto, S. (2017). Eye movement desensitization and reprocessing and slow wave sleep: A putative mechanism of action. *Frontiers in Psychology, 8*, 1935. https://doi.org/10.3389/fpsyg.2017.01935

Parker, A., Relph, S., &Dagnall, N. (2008). Effects of bilateral eye movements on the retrieval of item, associative, and contextual information. *Neuropsychology 22*, 136–145. https://doi.org/10.1037/0894-4105.22.1.136

Perez-Dandieu, B., & Tapia, G. (2014). Treating trauma in addiction with EMDR: A pilot study. *Journal of Psychoactive Drugs, 46*, 303–309. https://doi.org/10.1080/02791072.2014.921744

Raichle, M. E. (2015). The brain's default mode network. *Annual review of neuroscience, 38*(1), 433-447. https://doi.org/10.1146/annurev-neuro-071013-014030

Raine-Smith, H., & Rose, J. (2023). Psychedelic-assisted EMDR therapy (PsyA-EMDR): A memory consolidation approach to psychedelic healing. *ETQ, 4*, 1. https://doi.org/10.13140/RG.2.2.24683.35366

Rao, R. P., & Ballard, D. H. (1998). Predictive coding in the visual cortex: A functional interpretation of some extra-classical receptive field effects. *Nature Neuroscience, 2*, 79–87. https://doi.org/10.1038/4580

Rasch, B., & Born, J. (2013). About sleep's role in memory. *Physiological Reviews, 93*(2), 681–766. https://doi.org/10.1152/physrev.00032.2012

Rasolkhani-Kalhorn, T., & Harper, M. L. (2006). EMDR and low frequency stimulation of the brain. *Traumatology, 12*(1), 9–24. https://psycnet.apa.org/doi/10.1177/153476560601200102

Rubinov, M., & Sporns, O. (2010). Complex network measures of brain connectivity: Uses and interpretations. *Neuroimage, 52*,1059–1069. https://doi.org/10.1016/j.neuroimage.2009.10.003

Schore, A. N. (2015). *Affect regulation and the origin of the self: The neurobiology of emotional development.* New York: Routledge. https://doi.org/10.4324/9781315680019

Shapiro F., (Ed.) (2002). *EMDR as an integrative approach: Experts of diverse orientations explore the paradigm prism.* Washington, D.C: American Psychological Association. https://doi.org/10.1037/10512-000

Shapiro, F. (2007). EMDR, adaptive information processing, and case conceptualization. *Journal of EMDR practice and Research, 1*(2), 68–87. https://doi.org/10.1891/1933-3196.1.2.68

Shapiro, F. (2017). *Eye movement desensitization and reprocessing (EMDR) therapy: Basic principles, protocols, and procedures (3rd ed.).* New York: Guilford Publications.

Spiegel, D. (2012). Divided consciousness: Dissociation in DSM-5. *Depression and Anxiety, 29*(8), 667–670. https://doi.org/10.1002/da.21984

Steriade, M. (2016). Grouping of brain rhythms in corticothalamic systems. *Neuroscience. 137*(4), 1087–1106. https://doi.org/10.1016/j.neuroscience.2005.10.029

Stickgold, R. (2002). EMDR: A putative neurobiological mechanism of action. *Journal of Clinical Psychology, 58*, 61–75. https://doi.org/10.1002/jclp.1129

Stickgold, R. (2008). Sleep-dependent memory processing and EMDR action. *Journal of EMDR Practice and Research, 2*, 289–299. https://doi.org/10.1891/1933-3196.2.4.289

Takao, K., Nagatani, T., & Kitamura, Y. (1995). Chronic forced swim stress of rats increases frontal cortical 5-HT2 receptors and the wet-dog shakes they mediate, but not frontal cortical β-adrenoceptors. *European Journal of Pharmacology, 294*, 721–726. https://doi.org/10.1016/0014-2999(95)00620-6

Tesarz, J., Leisner, S., Gerhardt, A., Janke, S., Seidler, G. H., & Eich, W. (2014). Effects of eye movement desensitization and reprocessing (EMDR) treatment in chronic pain patients: a systematic review. *Pain Medications, 15*, 247–263. https://doi.org/10.1111/pme.12303

Van den Hout, M. A., Eidhof, M. B., Verboom, J., Littel, M., & Engelhard, I. M. (2014). Blurring of emotional and non-emotional memories by taxing working memory during recall. *Cognition and Emotion, 28*, 717–727. https://doi.org/10.1080/02699931.2013.848785

van den Hout, M. A., Engelhard, I. M., Rijkeboer, M. M., Koekebakker, J., Hornsveld, H., Leer, A., & Akse, N. (2011). EMDR: Eye movements superior to beeps in taxing working memory and reducing vividness of recollections. *Behaviour Research and Therapy Journal, 49*, 92–98. https://doi.org/10.1016/j.brat.2010.11.003

Van der Kolk, B. A., & Fisler, R. (1995). Dissociation and the fragmentary nature of traumatic memories: Overview and exploratory study. *Journal of Traumatic Stress, 8*, 505–525. https://doi.org/10.1002/jts.2490080402

Van der Kolk, B. A., & Van der Hart, O. (1989). Pierre Janet and the breakdown of adaptation in psychological trauma. *American Journal of Psychiatry, 146*(12), 1530–1540. https://doi.org/10.1176/ajp.146.12.1530

Vanderschoot, T., & Van Dessel, P. (2022). EMDR therapy and PTSD: A goal-directed predictive processing perspective. *Journal of EMDR Practice and Research, 16*(3), EMDR-2022-0009. https://doi.org/10.1891/EMDR-2022-0009

Varese, F., Sellwood, W., Pulford, D., Awenat, Y., Bird, L., Bhutani, G., Carter, L. A., Davies, L., Aseem, S., Davis, C., &Hefferman-Clarke, R., (2024). Trauma-focused therapy in early psychosis: results of a feasibility randomized controlled trial of EMDR for psychosis (EMDRp) in early intervention settings. *Psychological Medicine, 54*(5), 874–885, https://doi.org/10.1017/S0033291723002532

Vermetten, E., Doherty, M., & Spiegel, D. (2007). *Traumatic dissociation: Neurobiology and treatment*. Arlington, VA: American Psychiatric Publishing.

Vollenweider, F. X., & Preller, K. H. (2020). Psychedelic drugs: Neurobiology and potential for treatment of psychiatric disorders. *Nature Reviews Neuroscience, 21*(11), 611–624. https://doi.org/10.1038/s41583-020-0367-2

Von Helmholtz, H. (1866). *Concerning the perceptions in general. Treatise on physiological optics*. New York: Dover. https://doi.org/10.1038/s41583-020-0367-2

Whelan, A., & Johnson, M. I. (2018). Lysergic acid diethylamide (LSD) and psilo-cybin for the management of patients with persistent pain: A potential role? *Pain Management, 8*(3), 217–229. https://doi.org/10.2217/pmt-2017-0068

Zat Çiftçi, Z., Delibaş, D. H., Kaya, T., Kavakci, O., Savran, C., & Konuk, E. (2023). A randomized controlled trial of eye movement desensitization and reprocessing (EMDR) in the treatment of fibromyalgia. *Frontiers in Psychiatry, 15*, 1286118. https://doi.org/10.3389/fpsyt.2024.1286118

Zsoldos, E., & Ebmeier, K. P. (2016). Aging and psychological stress. In G. Fink (Ed.), *Stress: Concepts, Cognition, Emotion, and Behavior* (pp. 311–323). Washington, DC: Academic Press. https://doi.org/10.1016/B978-0-12-800951-2.00039-X

3 PsyA-EMDR protocol

Monoaminoxidase Inhibitor (MAOI)
Harmine ($C_{13}H_{12}N_2O$)

DOI: 10.4324/9781003431718-3

Ayahuasca is a traditional Amazonian plant medicine that has been used for centuries by indigenous communities in South America for spiritual and healing purposes (Frecska et al., 2016). Translated, ayahuasca means 'vine of the soul' or 'vine of the dead' (Halpern et al., 2008). Its therapeutic effects are best understood through the bio-psycho-social-spiritual model (Engel, 1977). The interplay of these factors contributes to the rich tapestry of experiences reported by those who participate in ayahuasca ceremonies, from intense introspection to a profound connection with nature and the spiritual realm.

Ayahuasca is renowned for the psychoactive effects rooted in its unique biochemistry. This psychoactive brew is prepared by simultaneously boiling an admixture of plants containing two key psychoactive agents. The *Banisteriopsis caapi* vine contains harmine, harmaline and tetrahydroharmine, which are potent monoamine oxidase inhibitors (MAOIs). This vine is brewed in conjunction with the leaves of the *Psychotria viridis* bush, which contains powerful tryptamine derivatives including N,N-dimethyltryptamine (DMT) (Hamill et al., 2019). DMT is a naturally occurring psychedelic compound that, when ingested, typically has little to no effect due to being rapidly metabolised by the enzyme monoamine oxidase in the digestive system. MAOI compounds play a crucial role in allowing the psychoactive effects of DMT to be orally active. The MAOIs in ayahuasca inhibit the effects of monoamine oxidase, allowing the prominent psychoactive chemical DMT to reach the bloodstream and exist for an extended period in the brain and central nervous system, inducing altered states of consciousness (Shen et al., 2010).

Another key element of this compound is the ceremonial contexts in which ayahuasca is traditionally consumed. Spiritual healing rituals are led by an experienced folk medicine practitioner (shaman), who guides participants through the experience, often with the support of traditional sacred songs called icaros. Religious organisations such as the Santo Daime and União do Vegetal syncretic Brazilian churches have been recognised for their cultural and religious significance, combining indigenous and Christian traditions. More recently, the therapeutic effects of ayahuasca have led to scientific interest about its psychological and pharmacological effects (Hamill et al. 2019). Studies have investigated the neurobiological effects of ayahuasca (dos Santos et al., 2016) and safety/adverse reactions (dos Santos, 2013), and it has been shown to be a promising treatment for depression (Palhano-Fontes et al., 2021). There has also been an explosion in Amazonian psychedelic tourism, and ayahuasca is now growing in popularity as a recreational drug (Winkelman, 2005).

This chapter outlines how to adapt the EMDR standard protocol to work in conjunction with psychedelics and enhance their therapeutic benefits. With the adaptive information processing (AIP) framework as a guide for clinical interventions, this cyclical model utilises the eight phases of EMDR across the preparation, medication and integration phases of psychedelic-assisted therapy. An evaluation of the most commonly used modalities in current PAP research reveals a deficit of trauma-informed care within existing practices. Harm reduction and stabilisation are central to the psychedelic-assisted EMDR therapy (PsyA-EMDR), and the transdiagnostic AIP model is equipped to support a wide range of psychological presentations. The development of the PsyA-EMDR protocol through clinical practice paves the way for formal research in this rapidly expanding field.

Humans have a long and rich history with medicinal plants, and it has been proposed that our multi-million-year relationship with psilocybin-containing fungi may have influenced our evolution (Sullivan et al., 2008). The profound neuropharmacological effects of entheogens on cognition, emotions and sociability have been associated with the development of pre-modern religion across the globe (Winkelman & Hoffman, 2015), and the once outlandish idea that the missing link between primate and modern man could be the humble magic mushroom is gaining weight within the field of consciousness research (Carhart-Harris et al., 2014). When compared with the traditional use of entheogens, the current incarnations of psychedelic therapies being developed through pharmaceutical research are unrecognisable. This is partly because protocols have been stripped right back to minimise variables in clinical research trials. This book does not have the scope to discuss the co-evolution of shamanism and ritual ingestion of entheogens in sufficient depth, but it is important to note that this may have played a central role in shaping our evolved psychology and therefore should not be overlooked (Winkelman, 2013).

EMDR uses repetitive rhythms comparable to traditional shamanic practices, to create an altered state of consciousness that facilitates healing, in what appears to be a modern adaption of an ancient healing mechanism. The flexibility of the AIP model means that it can readily be modified for use as an innovative transpersonal therapy (e.g. Parnell, 1996) and can be applied in contemporary clinical settings without the risk of cultural misappropriation. Through explorative clinical practice, adaptions have been made to the standard protocol so that it may be used alongside psychedelics. It is hoped that this will pave the way for formal research to validate PsyA-EMDR.

Current models of psychedelic-assisted psychotherapy

The format of PAP protocols implemented on the clinical trials can vary dramatically and is constantly evolving. This is due to insights gained throughout the ongoing research, which are then fed back to further develop research therapy protocols. Private treatment centres and underground settings add even more variability. Generally, the PAP format seen across the field consists of three main stages:

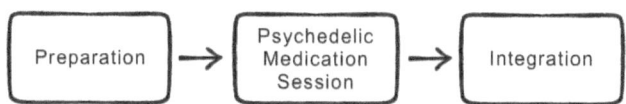

Figure 3.1 The three stages of psychedelic-assisted psychotherapy.

A brief outline of the PAP approach

Preparation phase: Varying from one to six hours of sessions, where goals for the therapy and intentions for change are defined. Psychoeducation is given regarding biographical memories that might emerge, and grounding techniques are taught.

Psychedelic medication phase: Generally, a client-led, non-directive, person-centred approach is used to support the individual with whatever emerges during their psychedelic treatment.

Integration phase: Across modalities, 'integration' of psychedelic material that has emerged during the treatment phase is achieved by non-directive exploration of content that is essentially person-centred in style (Rogers, 1942). This format is used irrespective of the therapeutic modality. For example, the cognitive behavioural PAP models engage in reflection of the psychedelic experience, and when this is complete, the therapist reverts to goal-oriented behavioural interventions.

In the context of clinical research, the number of integration sessions offered differs depending on the ethics committees' recommendations, the compound used and the number of doses offered. Phase 2a (first trials in a clinical cohort) will require more therapy than trials using healthy volunteers. For example, a phase 2 trial offering two doses could involve the following (in this order):

- One-hour recruitment telephone interview conducted by the recruitment team.
- One-hour psychiatric online pre-screen conducted by the therapy team.
- Two-hour in-person screening with the study psychiatrist.
- 3 × 1 ½ hour preparation sessions with the therapy team.
- A psychedelic treatment with the therapy team on day 0 and day 14.
- Integration therapy on day 0, +1 (in person), +7, +15, +23 (online), and a follow up call on day +90 (with the therapy team).

- Additional psychological support is often offered on request, should the need arise.

On UK trials, the therapy offered is dictated by a study therapy manual. Currently, the most practised protocol is a version of acceptance and commitment therapy (ACT; Hayes, 2004), a third-wave cognitive behavioural therapy (CBT) that was developed in response to the behavioural models of psychologist B.F. Skinner (Skinner, 1953). ACT has been adapted to be used in the psychedelic space, and is described as the 'accept, connect and embody' model (ACE; Watts & Luoma, 2020). In contrast to the future-focussed behavioural approach of ACT/ACE, the MAPS protocol for treating PTSD with 3,4-methylenedioxymethamphetamine (MDMA) employs a relational model designed for therapists from various training backgrounds. In this approach, the integration sessions also consist of non-directive exploration of the psychedelic session to facilitate emotional processing of the experience (Mithoefer et al., 2015). See Chapter 8, 'Integration.'

Preparation

Across the breadth of modalities in the field of PAP, there is inconsistency when it comes to preparing participants for the emergence of trauma during psychedelic therapy (Aday et al., 2021). One reason given for the lack of trauma-informed psychoeducation in the preparation and integration phases is that many of the treatments and trials are not classified as trauma-focussed interventions. Here we hit a common friction between the way that EMDR and the AIP model conceptualise pathogenesis and the way the medical model targets and treats different psychological presentations. Psychedelic studies often target specific DSM-5 presentations (e.g. treatment-resistant depression, Goodwin et al., 2023; anorexia, COMPASS, 2022) and do not explicitly target the individual's trauma history, despite mounting evidence suggesting that many psychiatric symptoms originate from the formation and consolidation of dysfunctionally stored implicit memory (Centonze et al., 2005). From an AIP perspective, it is illogical to treat depression without addressing the client's attachment and trauma history, and this approach is validated by a growing body of evidence that links depression to adverse life events (e.g. Kendler et al., 2003). Therefore, integration of an individual's adverse life experiences, combined with attachment-informed affect regulation interventions, should be considered the gold standard for achieving sustained positive psychological change. Some may argue that spontaneous healing can be achieved with psychedelics alone which, from an AIP perspective, may be due to the integration of pathogenic memories. However, overwhelming evidence suggests that accompanying psychotherapy is required to facilitate sustained change (Ko et al., 2022). This is likely linked to the potency of the psychotherapeutic relationship which is known to play a key role in psychotherapy outcomes across modalities (Flückiger et al., 2018).

The unifying stance across the majority of PAP studies is that a non-directive approach to preparation and integration during psychedelic-assisted therapy is sufficient. The person-centred emphasis on the core conditions of a strong therapeutic relationship and the development of rapport and trust are considered to be the critical psychotherapeutic components across different trials (Horton et al., 2021). Current PAP protocols do explore the possibility of historic trauma emerging during the psychedelic session with participants during preparation phases. There is often a lack of attachment/trauma-informed psychoeducation for participants and limited resourcing experiences, other than the use of deescalating breath, mantras, metaphors and the offer of physical support in the form of therapeutic touch.

As demonstrated in Chapter 6, 'Preparation,' some find that the interventions currently used to prepare clients for a psychedelic treatment are limited in depth and suitability. This is more of an issue for individuals with an impaired capacity to self-regulate. The potency of PAP means that a robust practical and theoretical framework is required to provide a container for the work and tools to enhance its effects.

(Mind)set and setting

Across substances and psychotherapeutic modalities, the preparation session generally refers back to the "nondrug parameters of psychopharmacology" (Feldman et al., 1963). The concepts of 'set' and 'setting' originated in the field of psychology and were later adopted and expanded upon by the psychedelic community. They are often associated with the use of psychedelic substances, but their applicability extends beyond this context.

The term 'set' refers to an individual's mindset, attitudes, expectations and psychological state. Indigenous use of entheogens involves preparatory mindset practices such as sexual abstinence, fasting, dream incubation and cleansing their system. The concept was first introduced into modern psychology by William James, who wrote about how our mental and emotional states – or what he referred to as "the set of mind" – can profoundly influence our perceptions, thoughts, and behaviours (James, 1863). The term 'setting' refers to the physical and social environment in which an individual's experiences occur. It has roots in various psychological theories, including Kurt Lewin's field theory (Lewin, 1936).

In the 1960s, Harvard psychiatrist Dr. Timothy Leary and his colleagues adopted these concepts to emphasise their importance in facilitating positive psychedelic experiences and minimising risk (Leary et al., 1964). The set and setting framework gained wider recognition and became an integral part of psychedelic research and harm-reduction practices. Researchers such as Stanislav Grof continued to explore the significance of set and setting in the context of psychedelic-assisted therapy, and these principles have expanded beyond psychedelic use and are now recognised as important considerations in various psychological, therapeutic and recreational contexts. Furthermore, they are employed in mindfulness practices, meditation retreats, psychotherapy and other transformative experiences (Fadiman & Kornfield, 2013). See Chapter 6, 'Preparation,' for more on set and setting.

Psychedelic treatment

In PAP research, it is common that the psychedelic dose phase is supported in a person-centred, non-directive manner (Horton et al., 2021). There are generally two trained therapists/sitters – one male and one female is considered best practice due to the transferential relationship of primary caregivers but sometimes this is deemed inappropriate depending on the participants' psychological profile. Economic and practical drivers are pushing towards using a one-therapist model, although the safety and efficacy of this are still being assessed. Whether it be a single therapist or co-therapists, the role involves supporting the participant with whatever emerges whilst under the influence of psychedelics and helping to ground them if they become dysregulated. The therapy protocols, and therefore all other aspects of the therapeutic approach, will depend upon the substance, the dose and the level of expertise of the therapists holding the space. For example, the aforementioned MAPS PTSD protocol with MDMA is one of the few trauma-focussed protocols where the therapist is more actively involved during the dosing phase, because the aim is to integrate pre-defined traumatic memories (Mithoefer et al., 2015). It centres around a non-directive approach and draws on 'internal family systems,' a version of ego state therapy, as a way of addressing dissociative elements should they arise (Schwartz, 1994). It is a strict protocol with clear adherence ratings, particularly during the dosing phase, and was primarily designed for therapists working on the MAPS-sponsored and investigator-initiated trials hence the levels of standardisation. There is more flexibility during preparation and integration phases, both of which may include the use of EMDR.

During the dosing, a range of psychotherapeutic interventions are offered such as interpersonal grounding, bodywork, psychotherapy and touch. However, many protocols don't mandate specialist training in these interventions, other than to instruct participants that it is a tool available upon request. The ethics, efficacy and logistical complexity of using touch in the psychedelic space is further explored in Chapter 4, 'Ethics.'

The combination of EMDR with MDMA (eMDMAdr) is a promising area of resource development that requires further research and is explored in more detail in Chapter 7, 'Psycholytic EMDR.'

Integration

In psychedelic research, integration is loosely defined as reflecting on the unusual thoughts and feelings that emerge from a psychedelic experience and exploring the implications of the experience for targeted areas of change (Johnson et al., 2008). There is a propensity within psychedelic research design to favour third-wave CBTs and the reason cited for this is the volume of empirical evidence of their efficacy gleaned from widespread use in the public health sector. CBTs have not yet been validated for use with psychedelics. However, CBT is deemed cost-effective because it is designed as short-term intervention (average 6–12 sessions) and because the protocols are easily manualised. There is also a focus on behavioural change and symptom management that is future oriented. There is a general trend to attempt to utilise the neuroplastogenic effects of substances by setting homework to elicit behavioural change. The metaphor of the drug acting like a fresh layer of snow over well-used tracks, enabling new pathways to be carved easily, is used to describe the neuroplastogenic effects that facilitate behavioural change (although some question whether using a skiing analogy is helpful for fostering a sense of inclusivity).

From an AIP perspective, attempting to change maladaptive behaviour in the present without fully addressing prior experiences that have caused the adaptions is often a futile exercise. This is because the information in the memory networks that is reactivated in the present and causing the symptoms is not integrated during the therapy. Behavioural interventions such as prolonged exposure only desensitise the client to the trigger (similar to EMD without the reprocessing) and do not address the root of the issue (maladaptively encoded information). Targeted reprocessing combined with attachment-informed interventions is a belt-and-braces approach to resolving maladaptive behaviour in the present, the merits of which are further explored in Chapter 8, 'Integration.'

Application of EMDR therapy in the psychedelic space

The integrative nature of EMDR therapy allows it to be combined with other models to support a breadth of client complexity rarely seen in other modalities. For example, the preparation phase can be enhanced with attachment-informed interventions to address attachment deficits and stabilise the client's nervous system. This is done through the cultivation of adaptive information in the memory networks by utilising the imaginal space to expand their repertoire of positive psychological and somatic experience (e.g. Knipe, 2018). This is then utilised during the reprocessing phase to facilitate regulation and the emergence of adaptive information in the memory networks (Korn & Leeds, 2002). These interventions are used specifically to treat cPTSD clients where there may not be an obvious single trauma, but instead there is cumulative trauma from emotional and/or physical needs not being met by primary caregivers in developmental years (Cloitre et al., 2009).

Other trauma-informed models can be integrated with EMDR to stabilise and support more complex clients. For example, ego state work can facilitate the integration of fragmented parts of the psyche (Gonzalez et al., 2012). Depending upon the practitioner's training, PsyA-EMDR therapy can be used as an integrative psychotherapy in conjunction with interventions from other therapeutic modalities, including but not limited to:

- Psychodynamic approaches.
- Ego state therapy/parts work.
- Somatic experiencing and exposure therapies.
- Cognitive behavioural therapies.
- Relational therapies and person-centred approaches.
- Creative, play and imaginal therapies.
- Mindfulness-based therapies.
- Group work and couples therapy.
- Breathwork.
- Shamanic and transpersonal therapies.
- Harm-reduction initiatives – the significance of which merits further exploration.

Harm reduction

Broadly speaking, harm reduction involves adopting a compassion-based, psychoeducational stance, and there are synergistic benefits to deploying harm-reduction techniques into all psychedelic treatments. Having a conceptual framework with strong theoretical foundations can help practitioners navigate high-risk situations in a coherent, standardised manner and minimise harm to both participants and practitioners. The AIP model is a transtheoretical case conceptualisation tool that has the potential to be utilised across all psychedelic settings to help prepare and guide the work. The focus of EMDR on stabilisation and preparation, through the development of adaptive information networks in the brain, indicates that it has the potential to be an accessible harm-reduction tool. There are examples of AIP-informed care, with a focus on resourcing and stabilisation being taught to paraprofessionals in developing countries and natural disaster zones with encouraging results (Eichfeld et al., 2019). Festival harm-reduction charities such as

PsyCare in the UK and the Zendo Project in the US may benefit from training their volunteers in the AIP model to facilitate a better understanding of service users' experiences. If volunteers are trained in this framework, the danger of re-enactments of past trauma can be identified and guarded against.

PsyA-EMDR protocol

Here we outline an adapted version of the standard protocol that is designed to augment psychedelic-assisted therapy. It is a cyclical model where the eight phases can be worked through in each of the preparation, medication and integration stages. This serves as an overview and each section is explored in more depth in later chapters. The table at the end of this section shows how all the eight phases are utilised before and after the psychedelic session. The PsyA-EMDR protocol has been developed through clinical practice and justifications for the interventions are based on existing EMDR and trauma research; however, further empirical validation is required to examine its efficacy.

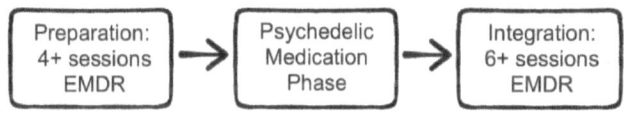

Figure 3.2 Three stages of psychedelic-assisted EMDR.

Preparation for psychedelics (4+ sessions)

Phase 1: History taking – The AIP model is used to create a case conceptualisation and develop a treatment plan:

- The complexity of the individual's trauma history and levels of psychological resources determine the pace of work and the amount of time spent in the preparation/resourcing phases.
- Exploration of the client's **goals for therapy** and more specifically for their psychedelic treatment (also referred to as 'intentions' in psychedelic therapy). Their presenting issues can be used as a starting point for this. For example, if they have a harsh inner critic, their intention might be 'to develop self-compassion.'
- Once a thorough history is taken, the therapist shares their conceptualisation of the link between the client's history and their presenting symptoms. This establishes the working relationship and is also used as an AIP-based **psychoeducation** intervention. The client can reflect on this and adjust the conceptualisation as they see fit.

- The co-created case conceptualisation facilitates insight through developing metacognitive skills and prepares them for what might emerge during the EMDR reprocessing (phase 4) and psychedelic treatment phases.
- **IMPORTANT:** Taking a full history in the first session can have a strong impact on the client's nervous system. This method of diving straight in (much like a psychiatric assessment) is useful because it is a good test of affect regulation capacity. Constant tracking of client's dysregulation in the session, **as well as in between sessions,** is important to determine the pace of the work.

See Chapter 5, 'Stabilisation,' for screening and assessing for risk.

Phase 2: Resourcing – Resources are developed to explicitly prepare for psychedelic dosing. Traditional resourcing interventions from phase 2 of the standard protocol can be followed, along with the following adaptions:

- The peaceful place and resource team are set up, and physical objects are chosen to represent these so they have a tactile reminder to facilitate grounding while potentially disoriented under the influence of psychedelics. Recruiting additional senses (touch, texture, shape, colour, scent etc.) enhances the potency of that resource during psychedelic treatments.
- An object can also be chosen to represent their goal/intention.
- This collection of symbolic items is then displayed in the psychedelic session with the aim of serving as a useful reminder to help refocus their internal process. This is similar to the 'altar' that is commonly used in the psychedelic space (Metzner, 1998).
- Preparing the client through psychoeducation about the psychedelic treatment and development of coping strategies. For example, the use of BLS, imaginal grounding techniques, parasympathetic breathing techniques, the use of mantras, weighted blankets and handheld beanbags.
- If the client is particularly anxious about the psychedelic treatment phase, it can be beneficial to 'tap in' memories of negotiating challenging situations to strengthen a sense of courage using slow, short sets of BLS.
- At this stage, the client's intentions for the psychedelic experience are solidified in response to the client's goals for therapy and case conceptualisation.

See Chapter 6, 'Preparation,' and Chapter 7, 'Psycholytic EMDR,' for more information.

Tip! The wisdom figure from their inner resource team can be utilised to explore their intention if they're struggling to define it.

Phases 3–7: Reprocessing as psychedelic preparation – Depending on the complexity of the client's psychological history, 1+ sessions of reprocessing with BLS are used as a tool to:

• Assess affect tolerance.
• Develop somatic awareness/mindfulness training.
• Practice embodiment through encouragement and coaching.
• Develop dual-attention skills.
• Develop emotional literacy.

This reprocessing test phase is used to assess the client's ability to tolerate moderately strong affect in preparation for the potential dysregulation to the nervous system caused by psychedelics. For this reason, it is suggested that **a target memory** is chosen with a **minimum SUD of 5** (out of 10) to sufficiently assess their ability to self-regulate during (and after) a reprocessing session. Although this potentially causes milder dysregulation than the psychedelic phase, it is deemed a good assessment of the individual's readiness to proceed to this phase. See Chapter 6, 'Preparation,' for more information on choosing a target for reprocessing as preparation.

This stage is particularly important for cPTSD clients who may require additional EMDR sessions to stabilise their nervous system sufficiently to warrant proceeding to the psychedelic treatment phase. Working in an attachment-informed manner is essential to facilitate reparative work, by reprocessing early biographical material and utilising the imaginal space to patch over attachment wounds, with the aim of strengthening their sense of self and increasing their ability to self-regulate (Parnell, 2013). This developmental work will develop their inner resources to navigate the potential dysregulation caused by psychedelic treatments.

Connecting with a figure from their resource team and/or their adult self in the imaginal space builds upon adaptive experiences in the memory networks that can be utilised in later phases. Beginning to acknowledge that emotional needs may have been missed in childhood can become part of the exploration to inform their choice of intention for the psychedelic phase. For example, if it becomes clear during the preparation phase that they were emotionally neglected in childhood, and as adults they have a harsh inner critic, an intention such as 'self-compassion' might be appropriate. Alternatively, the therapist and client can co-create an intention in response to the negative cognition (NC) of the memory network that is being targeted by the therapy. For example, if the NC that links to their trigger and corresponding trauma network is 'I should have done something,' their intention could be 'Self-forgiveness/I want to forgive myself.' See Chapter 7, 'Preparation,' for a more comprehensive list of intentions in response to memory networks/schemas.

Psychedelic therapy treatment phase

This phase will vary depending on the legal status and treatment pathway options based on geographical location. The rapidly expanding PAP market has created a 'Wild West' of emerging treatments that have become increasingly available to the general public, albeit often accessed at great personal expense. The quality of care offered across treatment centres varies dramatically because there is a distinct lack of a cohesive ethical framework, evidence-based practice and overseeing regulatory bodies. Ideally, a client would be accompanied by their EMDR therapist throughout all the stages of the treatment, but for many, this is neither logistically nor legally possible. See Chapter 7, 'Psycholytic EMDR,' for more on this treatment phase.

Possible treatment pathways:

- External treatment centre with wraparound EMDR therapy. For example, attending a legal (but currently off-label) ketamine treatment centre or taking part in a clinical trial.
- Legal self-administration, e.g. Ketamine and cannabis treatments that can be self-administered.
- Illegal underground group or 1:1 treatment.
- Illegal self-administration.

The above options have varying levels of risk and there are inevitable ethical considerations. From a harm-reduction perspective, therapists should be able to provide preparation and integration for a client. In many places, even a harm reduction is deemed unethical by accrediting bodies. As people travel long distances to treatment centres, there is often a lack of cohesion between the treatments being offered and the adjunctive therapy. This means that there can be a mismatch between modalities, and problems may arise from seeing more than one therapist at the same time.

Key points to consider as a practitioner are whether you are (a) working within your competency and (b) whether your insurance company will cover you. Underwriters will often update terms upon request so it is worth approaching insurance providers to adjust cover.

Warning: It is common for facilitators at legitimate treatment centres, in underground groups and even in research settings to have minimal psychotherapeutic training. Often this is attenuated by having a psychiatrist and psychologist on site. Many facilitators do not have a formal therapeutic training and may not be aware of trauma-informed care.

Post-psychedelic treatment integration (6 sessions) – Post-psychedelic therapy is where EMDR has the potential to enhance psychedelic therapy in a unique manner. The sensory material that emerges during treatment can be explored using techniques such as the somatic bridge to identify and integrate the corresponding subconscious material.

Phase 1: Debrief psychedelic treatment – Update AIP conceptualisation.

- The client debriefs the narrative of the psychedelic treatment with continuous BLS in the background, in a similar way to the recent traumatic events protocol (RTEP; Shapiro & Laub, 2015). Auditory BLS works well for this, particularly if working online, but visual or tactile BLS is also effective.
- Note down key moments of the experience that hold emotional charge/points of disturbance (PODs). Get the client to define the corresponding thought and feeling sensations and rate the SUDs for each item.
- The AIP case conceptualisation can be updated with any key themes that emerge during the treatment.
- Material from this initial processing can be used during phases 4, 5 and 6 integration.

Phase 2: Preparation – Any positive material from the journey can strengthened with slow BLS and used as a resource. If it was a difficult journey, grounding and resourcing can be used here to stabilise before reprocessing.

Phase 3: Assessment of target – Identifying psychedelic target for integration.

- Help the client to choose an appropriate target from the psychedelic therapy phase based on their intentions/goals for therapy and their case conceptualisation.
- **Note:** If they have had an underwhelming or disappointing psychedelic experience, this material can also be utilised. The response to a 'lack of material' can also be bridged from somatically to autobiographical material.
- **The somatic bridge** (Watkins, 1971) can be utilised to bridge into the memory network and identify the corresponding biographical material which is then reprocessed using the standard protocol. See Chapter 8, 'Bridging the Matrix.'
- Alternatively, the psychedelic material can be reprocessed and re-scripted directly without bridging. Treating the abstract material as if it is pre-verbal/perinatal or transpersonal maladaptively encoded information. See Chapter 11, 'Transpersonal healing.'
- For overwhelming psychedelic experiences that have caused PTSD-type symptoms, interventions such as the Flash technique (Manfield et al., 2017), EMDR 2.0 (Matthijssen et al., 2021), pendulation or similar to reduce the SUD to a low enough level to then bridge/reprocess with the standard protocol.

Phases 4, 5, 6: Desensitisation, installation, body scan – Utilising the standard protocol to integrate subconscious material that emerged during the psychedelic treatment.

- Use BLS (visual, auditory or tactile) to reprocess the identified target.
- Where appropriate, attachment-informed interventions such as re-scripting or inner child work can be used to find an adaptive resolution.
- Install the PC (which may just involve revisiting their initial intention for the therapy).

Phase 7: Closure – Debrief the session.

- If reprocessing is incomplete, use grounding visualisations such as the light stream or container to stabilise the client before ending the session.
- Encourage contemplative exercises such as journaling, being in nature and general self-care, as well as bodywork such as yoga or massage. Breathwork can also aid further integration, but beware that this can also overwhelm some clients.

Phase 8: Re-evaluation – Ensuring a thorough integration of psychedelic material in the past, present and future.

- In the following session, re-evaluate the target from the previous session. If SUDs are two or more, carry on reprocessing and bridge if necessary to earlier nodes in the network (touchstone memories) to facilitate the resolution of the network that has been activated.
- Then return to the psychedelic material and re-evaluate using SUDs. If there is still an emotional/somatic charge, the somatic bridge can be used to find additional biographical material that has been activated and reprocessed using the standard protocol as above.
- The psychedelic material is revisited in proceeding sessions until it no longer holds negative emotional charge and at this stage is deemed fully integrated.

Summary of PsyA-EMDR protocol

Phase	Description	Clinical justification
1 History taking	• AIP model used to create a case conceptualisation using information from history taking. • Psychoeducation linking symptoms to history using the AIP model. • Start exploring goals/intention setting – keep it specific, simple and tied in with the work. • Individualised treatment plan is created in reference to client's developing intentions (goals) for therapy.	• Establishing therapeutic alliance. • Developing metacognitive abilities and empowering client to understand their issues through an AIP lens. • Beginning to consider intentions for therapy and more specifically for the psychedelic journey.
2 Preparation	• Psychoeducation about the psychedelic space. • Explicitly prepare for use of resources in psychedelic space. • Peaceful place. • Resource team. • Goals/intention setting. • Choose physical objects/ images to represent resource team and intention(s). • Identify any blocks to the work that could be targeted in next phase.	• Preparing (mind)set. • Grounding training. • Developing adaptive networks of positive affect that can be accessed during medication phase to stabilise CNS. • Embodiment training (positive affect). • Physical objects act as a tactile reminder of their resources and intention that is easy to connect with during the dysregulation of the acute phase. This resembles the concept of the altar that is commonly used in psychedelic healing ceremonies.
3–8 Desensitisation, installation, body scan	• 2+ sessions of reprocessing with BLS. • A target is chosen by client based on: • Case conceptualisation • Goals/intention • Resource development • Blocks/anxiety about the work	• Embodiment training (negative affect). • Dual-attention training. • Testing affect regulation capacity in preparation for psychedelics. • Somatic awareness/ mindfulness training. • Development of emotional language.

PSYCHEDELIC MEDICATION PHASE

(Continued)

Phase	Description	Clinical justification
1 Debrief	• Initially talk through a narrative of the whole journey with BLS. • Explore how this links (or not) with intention/goals. • Explore any themes that emerge that link to core NCs, history and case conceptualisation.	• BLS while talking to begin to integrate the experience. • The therapist can add information to case conceptualisation and adjust focus to where the subconscious indicates there is a priority.
2 Preparation	• Strengthen any resources that were experienced during the journey by tapping in with BLS. • Grounding and resourcing are used to stabilise if it was a difficult journey.	• Strengthens adaptive information and ability to self-regulate.
3 Assessment of target	• Together, select appropriate target from the psychedelic journey based on intention/goals. • Define image, thought, emotion, sensation, NC and SUDs. • Use somatic bridge or reprocess and re-script the material directly as if a memory.	• Exploration of subconscious maladaptive material that emerges during psychedelic treatment.
4, 5, 6 Desensitisation, installation, body scan	• Standard protocol on target with attachment-informed re-scripting and ego state work.	• Utilising neuroplastic effects of the psychedelic treatment to facilitate the integration of emotionally salient material.
7 Closure	• Ensure stability before closing session. • Utilise grounding or container visualisations if necessary. • Debrief session.	• Minimising risk between integration sessions by activating the parasympathetic nervous system and sense of safety in the present.
8 Re-evaluation	• Re-evaluate target memory. • Re-evaluate psychedelic material. • Repeat previous stages until all targets in past, present and future have an SUD of 0/1.	• To ascertain whether all the maladaptively stored subconscious material has been reprocessed and integrated.

Additional training considerations for EMDR practitioners

The use of psychedelics in psychotherapy is a novel treatment; therefore, reflective practice and continuing professional development are highly advisable. Moreover, PsyA-EMDR employs advanced EMDR interventions and so the basic training alone may not be sufficient to hold the nuances required to do this work. As with practising standard EMDR, it is vital that practitioners have a solid understanding of the AIP model and how to create a case conceptualisation. EMDR accreditation, with experience of working with a range of psychological presentations, not just PTSD, can be useful preparation for practitioners learning about the intricacies and complexities of working with PsyA-EMDR protocols. A theoretical understanding of dissociation and practical training in working with this phenomenon is useful because of the potential for psychedelics to reactivate trauma. This is particularly important when working with HPPD and other dissociative presentations. Knowledge of how to work with structural dissociation using ego state interventions is also necessary as well as an understanding of the systemic and intergenerational impact of trauma may also be beneficial.

Mystical experiences are a common occurrence during psychedelic treatments and so practitioners should be open to working with transpersonal material as it emerges. Research has shown that exploration of transpersonal material can facilitate psychological healing (Ko et al., 2022). Consequently, there is an ongoing debate about whether practitioners who work in PAP should have personal experience of psychedelics, although for many this may not be possible due to legality, health, medication, religious views etc. Experiential training in altered state of consciousness also gives therapists an opportunity to do some of their own inner work. Breathwork can offer an alternative to psychedelics as it can elicit a similar subjective experience but is more controllable as the process can be stopped at any time.

The AIP model can also be utilised by those working in harm-reduction initiatives and community integration circles. AIP-informed supervision supports the effective application of such AIP harm-reduction initiatives.

Supervision

PsyA-EMDR supervision and opportunities for specialist reflective practice are recommended. Ongoing supervision with an accredited EMDR consultant who has experience of working with transpersonal content or psychedelic-assisted therapies can help with a multitude of issues, including developing effective case conceptualisations and harm-reduction support.

For more information on CPD and supervision, contact the authors directly via email.

References

Aday, J. S., Davis, A. K., Mitzkovitz, C. M., Bloesch, E. K., & Davoli, C. C. (2021). Predicting reactions to psychedelic drugs: A systematic review of states and traits related to acute drug effects. *ACS Pharmacology Translational Science, 4*, 424–435. https://doi.org/10.1021/acsptsci.1c00014

Carhart-Harris, R. L., Leech, R., Hellyer, P.J., Shanahan, M., Feilding, A., Tagliazucchi, E., Chialvo, D. R., & Nutt, D. 2014. The entropic brain: A theory of conscious states informed by neuroimaging research with psychedelic drugs. *Frontiers in Human Neuroscience, 8*, 20. https://doi.org/10.3389/fnhum.2014.00020

Centonze, D., Siracusane, A., Calabresi, P., & Bernardi, G. (2005). Removing pathogenic memories. *Molecular Neurobiology, 32*(2), 123–132. https://doi.org/10.1385/mn:32:2:123

Cloitre, M., Stolbach, B. C., Herman, J. L., Kolk, B. V. D., Pynoos, R., Wang, J., & Petkova, E. (2009). A developmental approach to complex PTSD: Childhood and adult cumulative trauma as predictors of symptom complexity. *Journal of Traumatic Stress, 22*(5), 399–408. https://doi.org/10.1002/jts.20444

COMPASS Pathways. (2022). Efficacy and safety of COMP360 psilocybin therapy in anorexia nervosa: A proof-of-concept study. Found at: https://www.clinicaltrials.gov/ct2/show/NCT05481736?term=comp360&draw=2.

Dos Santos, R. G. (2013). A critical evaluation of reports associating ayahuasca with life-threatening adverse reactions. *Journal of Psychoactive Drugs, 45*(2), 179–188. https://doi.org/10.1080/02791072.2013.785846

Dos Santos, R. G., Osório, F. L., Crippa, J. A. S., & Hallak, J. E. C. (2016). Classical hallucinogens and neuroimaging: A systematic review of human studies: Hallucinogens and neuroimaging. *Neuroscience & Biobehavioural Reviews, 71*, 715–728. https://doi.org/10.1016/j.neubiorev.2016.10.026

Eichfeld, C., Farrell, D., Mattheß, M., Bumke, P., Sodemann, U., Ean, N., & Mattheß, H. (2019). Trauma stabilisation as a sole treatment intervention for post-traumatic stress disorder in Southeast Asia. *Psychiatric quarterly, 90*, 63-88. https://doi.org/ 0.1007/s11126-018-9598-z

Engel, G. L. (1977). The need for a new medical model: A challenge for biomedicine. *Science, 196*(4286), 129–136. https://doi.org/10.1126/science.847460

Fadiman, J., & Kornfield, J. (2013). *The psychedelic explorer's guide: Safe, therapeutic, and sacred journeys.* Rochester, VT: Park Street Press.

Feldman, P. E. (1963). Non-drug parameters of psychopharmacology: The role of the physician. In M. Rinkel (Ed.), *Specific and non-specific factors in psychopharmacology* (pp. 149–158). New York: Philosophical Library.

Flückiger, C., Del Re, A. C., Wampold, B. E., & Horvath, A. O. (2018). The alliance in adult psychotherapy: A meta-analytic synthesis. *Psychotherapy, 55*(4), 316. https://doi.org/10.1037/pst0000172

Frecska, E., Bokor, P., & Winkelman, M. (2016). The therapeutic potentials of ayahuasca: Possible effects against various diseases of civilisation. *Frontiers in Pharmacology, 7*, 35. https://doi.org/10.3389/fphar.2016.00035

Gonzalez, A., Mosquera, D., & Morrison, M. R. (2012). *EMDR and dissociation: The progressive approach.* El-Bireh: A.I.

Goodwin, G. M., Aaronson, S. T., Alvarez, O., Atli, M., Bennett, J. C., Croal, M., & Malievskaia, E. (2023). Single-dose psilocybin for a treatment-resistant episode of major depression: Impact on patient-reported depression severity, anxiety, function, and quality of life. *Journal of Affective Disorders, 327*, 120–127. https://doi.org/10.1016/j.jad.2023.01.108

Halpern, J. H., Sherwood, A. R., Passie, T., Blackwell, K. C., & Ruttenber, A. J. (2008). Evidence of health and safety in American members of a religion who use a hallucinogenic sacrament. *Medical Science Monitor, 14*(8), SR15–SR22.

Hamill, J., Hallak, J., Dursun, S., M., & Baker, G. (2019). Ayahuasca: Psychological and physiologic effects, pharmacology and potential uses in addiction and mental illness. *Current Neuropharmacology, 17*(2), 108–128. https://doi.org/10.2174/1570159X16666180125095902

Hayes, S. (2004). Acceptance and commitment therapy, relational frame theory, and the third wave of behavior therapy. *Behavior Therapy, 35*, 639–665. https://doi.org/10.1016/S0005-7894(04)80013-3

Horton, D. M., Morrison, B., & Schmidt, J. (2021). Systematized review of psychotherapeutic components of psilocybin-assisted psychotherapy. *American Journal of Psychotherapy, 74*(4), 140–149. https://doi.org/10.1176/appi.psychotherapy.20200055

James's, W. (1863). *Principles of psychology*. New York: Henry Holt and Company.

Johnson, M., Richards, W., & Griffiths, R. (2008). Human hallucinogen research: Guidelines for safety. *Journal of Psychopharmacology, 22*(6), 603– 620. https://doi.org/10.1177/0269881108093587

Kapur, S., & Remington, G. (1996). Serotonin-dopamine interaction and its relevance to schizophrenia. *American Journal of Psychiatry, 153*, 466–476. https://doi.org/10.1176/ajp.153.4.466

Kendler, K., Hettema, J., Butera, F., Gardner, C., & Prescott, C. (2003). Life event dimensions of loss, humiliation, entrapment, and danger in the prediction of onsets of major depression and generalized anxiety. *Archives of General Psychiatry, 60*(8), 789–796. https://doi.org/10.1001/archpsyc.60.8.789

Knipe, J. (2018). *EMDR toolbox: Theory and treatment of complex PTSD and dissociation*. New York: Springer Publishing Company. https://doi.org/10.1891/9780826172563

Ko, K., Knight, G., Rucker, J. J., & Cleare, A. J. (2022). Psychedelics, mystical experience, and therapeutic efficacy: A systematic review. *Frontiers in Psychiatry, 13*, 917199. https://doi.org/10.3389/fpsyt.2022.917199

Ko, K., Kopra, E. I., Cleare, A. J., & Rucker, J. J. (2022). Psychedelic therapy for depressive symptoms: A systematic review and meta-analysis. *Journal of Affective Disorders, 322*, 194–204 https://doi.org/10.1016/j.jad.2022.09.168

Korn, D. L., & Leeds, A. M. (2002). Preliminary evidence of efficacy for EMDR resource development and installation in the stabilization phase of treatment of complex posttraumatic stress disorder. *Journal of Clinical Psychology, 58*(12), 1465–1487. https://doi.org/10.1002/jclp.10099

Leary, T., Metzner, R., & Alpert, R. (1964). *The psychedelic experience: A manual based on the Tibetan Book of the Dead*. New York: Citadel Press.

Lewin, K. (1936). *Principles of topological psychology*. New York: McGraw-Hill. https://doi.org/10.1037/10019-000

Manfield, P., Lovett, J., Engel, L., & Manfield, D. (2017). Use of the flash technique in EMDR therapy: Four case examples. *Journal of EMDR Practice and Research, 11*(4), 195–205. https://doi.org/10.1891/1933-3196.11.4.195

Matthijssen, S. J., Brouwers, T., van Roozendaal, C., Vuister, T., & de Jongh, A. (2021). The effect of EMDR versus EMDR 2.0 on emotionality and vividness of aversive memories in a non-clinical sample. *European Journal of Psychotrauma-tology, 12*(1), 1956793. https://doi.org/10.1080/20008198.2021.1956793

Metzner, R. (1998). Hallucinogenic drugs and plants in psychotherapy and sha-manism. *Journal of Psychoactive Drugs, 30*(4), 333–341. https://doi.org/10.1080/02791072.1998.10399709

Mithoefer, A., Jerome, L., Ruse, J., Doblin, R., Gibson, E., & Marcela Ot'alora, G. (2015). A manual for MDMA-assisted psychotherapy in the treatment of post-traumatic stress disorder, 7th version. Found at https://maps.org/research-archive/mdma/MDMA-Assisted-Psychotherapy-Treatment-Manual-Version7-19Aug15-FINAL.pdf.

Palhano-Fontes, F., Soares, B. L., Galvão-Coelho, N. L., Arcoverde, E., & Araujo, D. B. (2021). Ayahuasca for the treatment of depression. *Disruptive Psychophar-macology Current Topics in Behavioral Neurosciences, 56*, 113–124. https://doi.org/10.1007/7854_2021_277

Parnell, L. (1996). Eye movement desensitization and reprocessing (EMDR) and spiritual unfolding. *Journal of Transpersonal Psychology, 28*, 129-154.

Rogers, C. R. (1942). *Counseling and psychotherapy: Newer concepts in practice.* Boston: Houghton Mifflin.

Schwartz, R. C. (1994). *The internal family systems model.* New York: Guilford.

Shapiro, E., & Laub, B. (2015). Early EMDR intervention following a commu-nity critical incident: A randomized clinical trial. *Journal of EMDR Practice and Research, 9*(1), 17. 10.1891/1933-3196.9.1.17

Shen, H. W., Jiang, X. L., Winter, J. C., & Yu, A. M. (2010). Psychedelic 5-methoxy-N, N-dimethyltryptamine: Metabolism, pharmacokinetics, drug interactions, and pharmacological actions. *Current Drug Metabolism, 11*(8), 659–666. https://doi.org/10.2174/138920010794233495

Skinner, B. F. (1953). Some contributions of an experimental analysis of behav-ior to psychology as a whole. *American Psychologist, 8*(2), 69. https://doi.org/10.1037/h0054118

Sullivan, R. J., Hagen, E. H., & Hammerstein, P. (2008). Revealing the para-dox of drug reward in human evolution. *Proceedings: Biological Science, 275*, 1231–1241. https://doi.org/10.1098/ rspb.2007.1673

Watkins, J. (1971). The affect bridge: A hypnoanalytic technique. *International Journal of Clinical and Experimental Hypnosis, 19*(1), 21–27. https://doi.org/10.1080/00207147108407148

Watts, R., & Luoma, J. B. (2020). The use of the psychological flexibility model to support psychedelic assisted therapy. *Journal of Contextual Behavioral Science, 15*, 92–102. https://doi.org/10.1016/j.jcbs.2019.12.004

Winkelman, M. (2010). *Shamanism: A biopsychosocial paradigm of con-sciousness and healing.* Santa Barbara, CA: ABC-CLIO. https://doi.org/10.5040/9798216014133

Winkelman, M. (2013). Shamanism and psychedelics: A biogenetic structuralist paradigm of ecopsychology. *European Journal of Ecopsychology, 4*(1), 90–115.

Winkelman, M., & Hoffman, M. (2015). Hallucinogens and entheogens. In R. Segal and K. von Stuckrad (Eds.), *Vocabulary for the Study of Religion*, (Vol 2, pp. 126–132). Leiden, Boston, MA: Koninklijke Brill.

4   Ethics

Ketamine
2-(2-Chlorophenyl)-2-(methylamino) cyclohexanone ($C_{13}H_{16}ClNO$)

DOI: 10.4324/9781003431718-4

In pursuit of a safer anaesthetic than its predecessor phencyclidine (PCP), ketamine was first discovered as a novel compound in 1962 (Peltoniemi et al., 2016). It is a licenced dissociative drug, used for its anaesthetic and analgesic effects. Mechanistically, ketamine acts as an NMDA receptor antagonist. At anaesthetic doses, ketamine induces a trance-like state providing pain relief, sedation and amnesia. At lower, sub-anaesthetic doses, ketamine is a promising agent in the treatment of pain and mental disorders.

Ketamine appears to increase synaptogenesis and neuroplasticity (Joneborg et al., 2022) by promoting the growth of dendritic spines. 10–20% of adults (1–2% of children) experience psychiatric reactions to ketamine anaesthesia including vivid hallucinations, agitation, confusion, dysphoria, near death-like experiences and emergence delirium (Marland et al., 2013). It is thought that at varied doses, there may be therapeutic value to these psychological experiences which merits further investigation.

Ketamine is not currently licensed by the Medicines and Healthcare Products Regulatory Agency for the treatment of mental illness. However, in the UK and in parts of the US, ketamine is already being used 'off label' in private clinics and some self-pay/NHS services. The efficacy of ketamine as a treatment for mental health conditions such as PTSD (Philipp-Muller et al., 2023), treatment-resistant depression (Guo et al., 2023) and obsessive-compulsive disorder (Bandeira et al., 2022) is still being assessed. When used as an adjunct to psychotherapy, ketamine's neuroplasticity-promoting effects appear to strengthen cognitive restructuring, leading to long-lasting behavioural change (Greenway, 2020; Krystal, 2007). In America, some clinics are already using EMDR alongside ketamine therapy and describe synergistic benefits when combining these treatments.

Ketamine has powerful short-term antidepressant effects; however, its long-term therapeutic benefits have not yet been verified. It is physically and psychologically addictive and therefore has a major abuse potential (Davies, 2021). The long-term effects of repeated use are still unknown; however, evidence suggests that protracted use can cause damage to the bladder, kidney, liver, heart and respiratory system, as well as induce some psychological complications.

Ethics – The wider context

According to the US Drug Enforcement Agency (DEA), Schedule 1 drugs can be defined as "drugs with no currently accepted medical use and a high potential for abuse" (DEA, 2023). In many countries, including the US and the UK, Schedule 1/Class A drugs are regarded as the most harmful substances, making it illegal to take, carry, make, cultivate, sell or share these compounds. There is a growing body of evidence that suggests psychedelics may be powerful agents of psychological change (Nutt et al., 2019), calling into question the ethical and moral status of psychedelics as Schedule 1/Class A restricted drugs.

Ethical frameworks provide useful perspectives when evaluating which course of action may result in the most moral outcome. The current legislative restrictions have resulted in a largely utilitarian approach to ethical decision-making in the field of psychedelics. To do the least harm to all stakeholders involved, professional and governing bodies have not developed any ethical standards for working with psychedelic substances and continue to outlaw such practices. Whilst this reduces institutional risks, harm is done to those who are not adequately supported by robust ethical decision-making processes. As restrictions on the therapeutic use of psychedelics loosen, professional and regulatory bodies need to respond by setting out in policy the deliverables required to support this work.

Implementation of applied ethics needs to be a formulaic procedure executed through policy or law. Read and Papasypyrou (2021) suggest that "we may not need an entirely new set of ethical codes for working with expanded states, the intensity and complexities of this work call for an even finer attunement to the ethical pitfalls along the way." As psychedelic therapies begin to be delivered at scale in healthcare settings, clearly defined ethical standards will need to be expanded to mitigate potential risks. Ignoring such ethical pitfalls could be perilous. To illustrate, in the 1960s, amidst the era's cultural upheavals and burgeoning interest in consciousness expansion, ethical lapses emerged. These included inadequate informed consent procedures, questionable research practices and the indiscriminate use of psychedelics outside of controlled clinical settings. These ethical pitfalls underscored the need for responsible practices in contemporary PAP settings and highlighted the importance of ethical considerations in the development and delivery of psychedelic therapy at scale. This chapter unpacks some of these key themes.

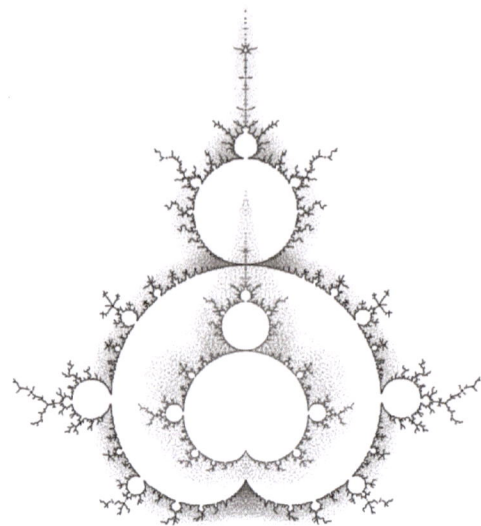

Figure 4.1 Much like the Mandelbrot Set, the concept of fractal epistemology in psychology (Marks-Tarlow, 2020) suggests that complex ethical and relational dilemmas repeat at every level within psychotherapy, manifesting in repeating patterns that shape the field's dynamics.

Identifying key ethical issues in PsyA-EMDR therapy

EMDR therapy is an integrative transdiagnostic approach that relies on other professional bodies to assert regulatory processes. Herein, a focused and comprehensive summary of the key ethical implications associated with PsyA-EMDR therapy delivery will be systematically explored.

The ethics of working inclusively

Exposure to childhood adversity has an impact on adult mental health, the outcomes of which are well documented throughout the literature (e.g. Felitti et al., 1998; Schofield et al., 2013). Adverse childhood experiences (ACEs) have been shown to increase the risk of a psychotic reaction in those using substances, and this risk effect is cumulative with a proportional increase in the odds of presenting a psychotic experience for each lifetime ACE exposure (Bórquez-Infante et al., 2022). Many downplay the severity of their mental health to access psychedelic treatments, and difficult psychedelic experiences are routinely underreported (Breeksema et al., 2022). Psychedelic treatment options need to better support those with trauma and undiagnosed psychopathologies.

Contemporary research trials are duty bound to comply with ethical committee guidance. Strict exclusion criteria prohibit participation of those with complex mental health diagnoses, comorbidity or (in some PTSD research) those whose trauma profile relates to adversity during childhood. Those who have a first-degree relative with a diagnostic label that has been named as an exclusion criterion are also screened out. Many of the legal retreat settings abroad also exclude those deemed most at risk. This results in the most vulnerable people seeking underground treatment alternatives. Some clinical research does operate inclusive treatment pathways for those who would not be deemed as suitable participants in other clinical trials (Mitchell et al., 2021). Therapist training, boundary transgression and working safely with the erotic transference have led to inconsistencies in treatment outcomes for these populations (Nickles & Kay-Ross, 2021). Making treatment options more inclusive will only improve psychological outcomes and reduce associated risks if those interventions are consistently robust and provide sufficient preparation, containment and integration.

Reducing the risk of adverse drug effects, widening participation, increasing efficacy and supporting inclusion in PAP need to be prioritised. Environmental, social and economic factors play into mental health outcomes later in life, yet pharmaceutical interests through the DSM have led us to believe that the problem is with our brain chemistry. Individuals who have had adverse reactions to psychedelic treatments should be supported using non-pathologising, trauma-informed treatment modalities to facilitate inclusion, widen participation and reduce risk.

The ethics of diversity

Psychological mindset is often referred to as the 'set,' and the importance of 'set and setting' is long-established essentials in PAP delivery (Pollan, 2018). Psychosocial factors, such as gender, sexuality, ability, class, the social stigmas of diagnostic labelling and racial differences, constitute meaningful variations to the 'set' for those in receipt of psychedelic treatments. The identity of that individual and the identity of the therapist are both components of the set and setting. During psychedelic preparation and integration therapy, such identifications may also contribute to practitioner variation in framing and interpreting psychedelic experiences (Neitzke-Spruill, 2019). Healthcare delivery is cumbersome, as the process of acculturation impacts both social and psychological wellbeing. Developing protocols that work within diversity, incorporating whole, inclusive and embedded practice *(WIEP) whilst also educating practitioners on how to best meet the needs of diverse patient populations is essential (The Anti-discrimination Focus, n.d.). Professional frameworks and protocols need to incorporate anti-discriminatory competency wherever possible, and the professional and relational structures need to be robust enough to mitigate the inevitable shortfalls.

Cultural trauma harms individuals. If we are to mend hearts and bodies, cultural components must be healed too (Menakem, 2021). Anti-oppressive therapeutic pathways that challenge power differentials, and do not alienate or exclude, are integral in the development of any new psychedelic treatment. Privilege blinding makes challenging the existing institutional frameworks difficult. There is a need for greater diversity and improved cultural competency within PAP development. The lack of diversity in mental health professionals (Gopalkrishnan, 2018), lack of diversity in research participants (Michaels, 2018) and lack of cultural representation within the transpersonal, collective and spiritual movements (Turner, 2014) need to be challenged. Destigmatising psychedelics as medicines will also improve engagement and inclusion where religious or cultural factors might otherwise be preclusive. Trauma-focused PAP frameworks are designed to widen participation and improve accessibility. Working within diversity using anti-oppressive practice also requires culturally competent language, and this language will continue to evolve. PsyA-EMDR supports diversity by fostering a climate of cultural appreciation, without the need for cultural appropriation or cultural extractivism, but in order to remain anti-oppressive, its frameworks will need to match the pace and direction of cultural change. EMDR exists in the public domain, challenging power differentials by making PAP a widely accessible treatment option. The PsyA-EMDR protocol should be adjusted/extended to support and accommodate any significant issues that present in the 'set and setting.'

*WIEP – An umbrella term for difference, diversity, race, cultural and structural competence, equality diversity & inclusion, relational (re)inclusion, anti-discrimination & anti-oppressive practice, social chance and action. All of which are designed to contribute to a better society for all.

The ethics of bodywork and touch

Joyce Martin was amongst the first to describe the use of bodywork and touch in psychedelic therapy (Martin, 1957; Martin, 1964). Therapeutic touch has now become a common aspect of psychedelic work (McLane et al., 2021). Behind every instance of therapeutic touch, there is an intention, either conscious or unconscious. When considering the use of touch, body psychotherapist Shoshi Asheri asks a useful question for *client* and *therapist* to hold in awareness *"who is touching, and who is being touched?"* (Asheri, 2009). Deciphering which part of the therapist is motivated to offer touch (and possibly seeking gratification in so doing) and which ego states of the client are being served in that offer (and which parts might be wounded or retraumatised) requires training, trustworthiness, sensitivity and a dedication to reflective practice.

Bodywork and touch require specialist training and may not be suitable in every situation, for all practitioners, with every patient or in many scalable healthcare settings.

According to Asheri's aforementioned question, touch also demands that the client is able to hold in awareness both a sense of self and the capacity for decision-making processes. Research has shown that psychedelics impair cognitive executive function and memory (Barret et al., 2018) and undermine a client's capacity to make informed decisions (Healy, 2021). Therefore, for touch to be used in psychedelic therapy, there is a heavy reliance on pre-agreed consent, the practitioner's intuition, the depth of the practitioner's training and how well the client's needs are known by the practitioner. Uncertainty remains as to how well we are ever able to really know a client and whether providing/receiving touch is remedial, compensative or even therapeutic. Some question the potential for trauma by omission caused by denied touch, although there is little evidence to support this claim (Devenot et al., 2022; O'Mathuna et al., 2002). Any benefits of touch need to be weighed against the potential harm caused by trauma enactments (Van Der Kolk, 1989) and therapeutic abuse (Hall, 2021).

Even with well-meaning practitioners, Read and Paparspyrou (2021) describe how "ethical pitfalls and vulnerabilities tend to present themselves when practitioners have not tended to their own material sufficiently, [have] unresolved personal issues or inadequate self-care so that [they] are [un]able to provide a solid enough container for all material that emerges". How do we assess whether practitioners have attended to their own material sufficiently? And how do we reduce the risk of practitioner malpractice during a psychedelic treatment, which enhances suggestibility (Carhart-Harris et al., 2015) and impairs memory (Healy, 2021), increasing the patient's susceptibility to manipulation? Psychedelic therapy abuse has a history that reaches back to the early days of LSD research (Hall, 2021), a continuum of abuse that stretches from therapist idolisation and therapeutic inappropriateness to boundary transgressions and sexual activity (Goldhill, 2020; Hausfeld, 2019; Nickles & Kay-Ross, 2021). Numerous reports of therapist transgressions indicate that proactive approaches to prevention are required and that an emphasis should be made on greater boundary definition and boundary maintenance, not less (Hausfield, 2019).

The precautionary principle in psychedelic therapy advocates that in the absence of evidence to support the benefits of touch or harm of denied touch, alongside acknowledging any potential risks, ideally, a risk-adverse approach should be adopted (Devenot et al., 2022). Potential harm from a refusal to provide touch in trauma therapy can be successfully mitigated by skilful therapist responses (Daleberg, 2000). Until the impact of consensual touch and interpersonal grounding in psychedelic therapy is scientifically verified, the precautionary principle advocates that the therapeutic frame should be held with rigidity. Organisations and those delivering psychedelic therapy need clear guidelines when working with people in altered states. For now, some are calling for urgent ethical guidance, or even an ethical freeze, on the use of touch in psychedelic therapy (Devenot et al., 2022).

EMDR is a body-orientated psychotherapy which incorporates somatic experience without the need for touch. Following EMDR protocols ensures that a balance of rightness is consistently maintained. Ecologist Aldo Leopold defined right relationship as "A thing is right when it tends to preserve the integrity, stability, and beauty of the biotic community. It is wrong when it tends otherwise" (Leopold, 1949). Right relationship extends to our interactions with ourselves, others and the world (Taylor, 1995). In respect of the importance of right relationship to self, EMDR keeps processing internal, reducing therapist influence and supporting the emergence of adaptive information. With rigorous resourcing and BLS, clients are encouraged to provide their own containment needs whilst reprocessing any caregiving deficiencies as they emerge. Grieving the shortcomings of primary caregivers is integral to healing and supports the real work that needs to be done. Any attempts at remediation would ultimately be futile and ineffectual and could get in the way of therapeutic process. In respect of right relationship to others, reprocessing with EMDR does not compromise client or practitioner safety. Weighted blankets and handheld bean bags can be offered to those requiring greater levels of physical containment. In respect of right relationship to the world, EMDR therapy ensures therapeutic consistency, minimising the impact of practitioner variability and therapeutic abuse. If used at all, any offer of safe touch to maintain physical safety (such as supporting toilet breaks) during PsyA-EMDR should be discussed and contracted for in advance and if needed, physical support should be kept to a minimum.

The ethics of harm reduction

Outside of clinical research settings, most psychedelic therapy is an illegal practice. There have been some remarkable efforts by those working in the field to develop an ethical stance (Brennan & Belser, 2022; Taylor, 1995). Many of the professional bodies that govern ethical frameworks have not been able to be developed for practices that remain illegal and harm-reduction initiatives have been left to pick up this ethical shortfall. Harm reduction highlights the importance of adequate preparation and integration and safe settings for dosing, minimising harm primarily through psychoeducation.

In healthcare settings, psychedelic therapy already occupies some grey areas that remain ethically contentious. As outlined at the start of this chapter, ketamine is a licenced anaesthetic and analgetic drug which also has powerful antidepressant secondary effects. Whilst the evidence base for ketamine therapy is not yet complete, private clinics (and in the UK, self-pay NHS ketamine treatment services) are already offering treatments. Ketamine has been approved for specific indications such as treatment-resistant depression, but it is also being used off label for several other psychiatric conditions. Using drugs off label is legal and is common practice, although off-label prescribing can expose patients to risky and ineffective treatments. Reducing the number of doses by optimising the therapeutic value of each dose delivered reduces potential risks and therefore reduces exposure to harm. However, many clinics are offering repeated ketamine therapy without any psychological support. Whilst ketamine therapy appears to be pharmacokinetically and pharmacodynamically safe, it is costly and remains inaccessible for many, with its full therapeutic potential often remaining untapped.

Psychedelic advocacy and psychedelic justice initiatives propagate awareness and support those who have been adversely affected by ethical issues associated with psychedelic use. For example, PsyPan is a UK-based non-profit organisation advocating for improvements to participant safety and wellbeing globally (https://www.psypanglobal.org). In the US, Chacruna Chronicles offers supportive frameworks for publications relating to whistle blowing, education, academic research, protection and reciprocity (https://chacruna.net/chronicles/).

Proactive approaches to harm reduction are needed. Leaving harm reduction to whistle-blowers, culturally relativistic applications and the fallout from malpractice leaves those who are most vulnerable at risk. Ethical frameworks and codes of conduct are essential. In the UK, EMDR therapists are registered with EMDR-UK (EMDRIA, EMDR-institute, EMDR-Europe, EMDRAA and EMDRASIA are some of the global equivalents). To train in EMDR, individuals must be an accredited mental health practitioner with a minimum of two years' experience of providing one-to-one psychotherapy, in addition to their professional training. The professional bodies that provide accreditation for therapists are registered with a legislating 'arm's length body' (ALB), who's clear focus is on overseeing the delivery of specific outputs, with a framework of accountability to the relevant government minister. This chain of accountability supports both patient and practitioner safety. More specific and sophisticated frameworks for safe and effective PAP need to be developed and legislated for in order that the public bodies can then disseminate out the requirements of what constitutes ethically sound practice.

Picking up the fallout from those adversely impacted by the shadow aspects of psychedelics will require delicacy, curiosity and a dedication to reflective practice. Harnessing the authority of pre-existing professional bodies, training programmes and accreditation processes will be essential. Professional bodies are already well versed in providing safe, objective, commissionable, trauma-informed treatment options that offer a good (enough) framework to be applied to PAP. PsyA-EMDR is a treatment that adheres to the frameworks of its regulatory bodies wherever possible, despite the current lack of clear guidance.

Case material

An underutilised stroke of insight

At 43-years-old, Lawrence suffered a near-fatal stroke. Some months later, he presented at therapy, hoping to work through what he described as a "monumental shift in identity" following his recent experiences. During history taking and preparation, Lawrence described how he had experienced acute "paranoia and vivid hallucinations" whilst on the stroke treatment unit and that he "had not felt the same since." The therapist encouraged Lawrence to access his medical notes for the time that he spent in critical care. The medical notes uncovered the use of ketamine as a neuroprotective agent. The medical staff had not specifically told Lawrence about the ketamine treatment or its potential effects. During EMDR therapy, the somatic bridge technique was applied to the paranoid hallucinatory symptoms that Lawrence experienced whilst on the ward. These symptoms linked back to memories of not feeling safe during his infancy. Tactile BLS was used to reprocess his experiences according to the EMDR therapy's three-pronged approach. Despite his new physical and cognitive disabilities, Lawrence has now been able to make meaning of his experiences. He described a newfound sense of peace, acceptance and appreciation for his new life. Whilst Lawrence continues to receive support with the physical and cognitive symptoms associated with his stroke recovery, he has found meaning and gratitude for his new identity and values the additional time that he now gets to spend with his children, prioritising the relationships that are important to him. Whilst he says that he "wouldn't wish it to happen to anyone else," he is grateful for the opportunity that he has had to redesign his life according to his "new set of values."

Lawrence's experiences are not uncommon. Ketamine is administered to many, without people being educated about the potential psychological effects. These medically induced psychedelic experiences can be life changing, yet their therapeutic value remains largely untapped due to this lack of awareness, the lack of holistic care within standard medical practice and the lack of effective integration therapy. Lawrence's case illustrates a necessity for comprehensive psychoeducation and informed consent in medical treatments involving psychoactive substances. It highlights the potential benefits of utilising these experiences therapeutically and a potential for turning medical events into opportunities for personal discovery.

The ethics of standardisation

In the UK, the National Institute of Clinical Excellence (NICE) quality standards "set out priority areas for quality improvement (QI)" and "highlight areas with identified variation in current practice." NICE indicators then "measure outcomes that reflect the quality of care, or processes linked by evidence to improve outcomes" (NICE, n.d.). In terms of QI and standardisation, ethical frameworks constitute the bare minimum, and yet because of the legal status of psychedelic drugs, professional ethical frameworks do not yet exist. Building an evidence base for drug development has attracted support from investors, but building an evidence base to demonstrate optimal therapeutic delivery of PAP is unlikely to attract sufficient funding. QI in therapeutic provision is already a contentious area, as therapeutic outcomes are highly individualised and notoriously difficult to measure. Some question the value of inserting PAPs into a broken healthcare system, a psychiatric model in paradigmatic crisis or using ineffectual scientific methods to research and assess therapeutic efficacy. Yet providing psychedelic treatment options in healthcare settings will help to eradicate psychedelic elitism and widen accessibility of PAPs to those most in need. Clearly, some standardisation and adherence to QI will be required for commissioners to deploy psychedelic therapies at scale.

Historically, psychedelic therapy has largely been delivered using non-manualised interventions. Some therapists have been resistant to adopt what they see as restrictive standardised treatments, which reduce professional autonomy and prevent individuals from receiving individualised treatments. Delivering psychedelic therapy at scale presents us with a clinical and ethical dilemma. Higher authority figures such as governments, healthcare organisations and commissioners and the scientific method used in medical research act on evidence to determine the larger goals, which then filter down improving the consistency of those delivering and developing clinical interventions. In the West, we are restricted by strict governance, scientific and clinical reasoning, as well as access to funding which demands a top-down approach to psychedelic therapy applications. Non-clinical and non-westernised settings may be able to provide opportunities for less rigidity, where clinicians and those with expertise in the field communicate their qualitative assessment of what works, and this then features in the design and decision-making processes of PAPs. The systems of power make such bottom-up approaches difficult to implement. Ideally, developing treatment options which fit the expectations of top-down models, but are informed and shaped by bottom-up influences, stand the best chance of being both a viable and a 'good enough' accessible treatment option for most. At least initially, it is important that PAPs are conducted in hospitals and other controlled settings to enable appropriate monitoring and ensure ease of access to acute care services in the event of adverse effects (APA, 2022) which will demand some form of standardisation.

Understandably, some are concerned that manualisation of PAP will lead to a focus on corporate priorities over therapeutic outcomes. Indeed, in the rapidly expanding field of psychedelic capitalism, some companies have already applied for patents of intellectual ownership for basic components of the psychedelic experience, for example, the use of soft furniture or muted decorations (Love, 2021). Some pharmaceutical companies are seeking to manualise the therapy so that drug licences are only awarded alongside their own patented therapeutic treatment options (Marks & Cohen, 2022). Clinical trials do require some stand-ardisation to reduce compounding variables and expectancy effects, but uncertainty remains around how far to take this. McDonaldization is the process by which the principles of the fast-food restaurant – efficiency, calculability, predictability and control come to dominate health-care provision (Miller, 2021). Questions have been asked as to whether an appetite for fast fixes is a consumerist approach and constitutes a method of applying a corporate method to psychedelic healing. What is certain is that as psychedelic therapies are scaled up, marketing and branding will lead to profiteering. Developing a psychedelic brand without substance or solid enough foundations does not lead to good therapeutic or investment outcomes (Evans, 2023). Some psychedelic therapies are in the public domain, but these manuals remain vague, or client led, labelling the mechanics of the non-specific therapeutic intervention as "integrative psychotherapy" (MAPS, 2015). Such protocols fall short of full standardisation.

Proponents of non-manualised therapies suggest that healing needs to be highly individualised and that reducing practitioner autonomy leads to suboptimal healing outcomes. Bespoke treatment options remain a therapeutic ideal but are expensive, unsustainable, inconsistent and perhaps overly idealistic. Reducing the risks associated with non-standardised practices, such as practitioner variability and therapeutic abuse, needs to be weighted alongside the positive outcomes that can be achieved using more precautionary manualised alternatives. Questions remain around how to do the greatest good whilst doing no harm (Miles, 2004). A risk-adverse approach to PAP recognises that participation can be widened and 'good enough' outcomes can be achieved using manualised interventions. In trauma-informed practice, the therapeutic frame needs to be held with rigidity to facilitate deliverable outcomes, without causing unnecessary risk. Whilst it is important to recognise that some people desire or would benefit from a non-manualised bespoke approach to PAP provision, balancing people's needs and preferences without doing harm to anyone, and minimising the impact on the planet, might just be an impossible balance to strike. Standardisation through manualisation of PAPs supports the precautionary application of psychedelic treatments and provides healthcare systems with an opportunity to justify scaling PAP provision.

The procedures used in PsyA-EMDR therapy are a manualised approach to healing through memory reconsolidation (Raine-Smith & Rose, 2023). For those not familiar with EMDR, it is important to highlight that, whilst the protocol is a systematic approach to PAP delivery, once a client is inducted into the procedure (phases 1–3) and begins reprocessing with bilateral stimulation of the brain (phase 4), the sessions transition from a therapist-led to a client-led intervention, becoming less structured and highly individualised. During reprocessing, the therapist is encouraged to 'stay out of the way' allowing the space for client's own inner healing processes to emerge. If reprocessing becomes blocked, the use of cognitive interweaves provides the therapist with an opportunity to deliver highly personalised interventions that promote the emergence of adaptive information in the memory networks. If a client has attachment deficits that impair their ability to self-regulate, resourcing techniques during the preparation phase (phase 2) can be used to bolster their affect tolerance during reprocessing. The use of the AIP case conceptualisation to guide the work makes it more individualised. Alongside the PsyA-EMDR protocol, the strength of the therapeutic relationship is a key component in holding space and supporting the client with whatever arises.

The ethics of sustainability

Responding to climate change requires coordinated actions guided by strategic planning. In healthcare, embedding sustainability into QI indicators will be the most impactful strategy, and this requires a sustainable quality improvement (SusQI) agenda. SusQI encourages practitioners to respond to the ethical challenges faced such as climate change and social inequalities. As outlined in Chapter 1, sustainable healthcare happens when we meet the interdependent financial, social and environmental agendas, which are often referred to as the 'triple bottom line' (Centre for Sustainable Healthcare, n.d.). Herein, we unpack how the sustainable value of PsyA-EMDR can be established by identifying and measuring the outcomes for patient populations, then dividing this value by the costs of these interventions to the factors implicated in the triple bottom line.

$$\text{Sustainable value of PsyA - EMDR} = \frac{\text{Outcomes for patients and population}}{\text{Environmental, social and financial impacts}}$$

(Triple bottom line)
(Centre for Sustainable Healthcare, n.d.)

To improve the sustainable value of any intervention, we need to address the issues implicated in the triple bottom line. For this to happen, social determinants need to sit at the heart of our understanding of mental distress, with supportive social and welfare interventions re-politicising our views of what constitutes a treatment for an individual in the context of the wider societal discourse (Davies, 2021). This challenges western conceptions of mental health. Interventions need to focus on social foundations and lifelong societal measurables rather than the short-term effect of an intervention or drug. Short-term funding cycles support short-term interventions but cannot support an evidence base for long-term mental health outcomes. As we move towards net zero carbon initiatives, the commissioning of healthcare services needs to shift from annual or political funding cycles to generational funding cycles which are supportive of health, social and welfare provision. Until this happens, trauma will continue to be experienced disproportionately by society's most disadvantaged, and mental health provision will continue to pick up the fallout of this imbalance, with an ever-increasing environmental impact. A safe and just place for humanity means balancing the conflicting needs of the social global foundations, whilst minimising the environmental ceilings reached by implementing these interventions (Raworth, 2017). See Chapter 12, The Future of PsyA-EMDR. Put simply, social inequality harms individuals and damages the environment. In the short term, this underpins the need for inclusive trauma-focused interventions, whilst highlighting the need to continue to address the power differentials and inequality in society that would eventually lead to large scale reform. PsyA-EMDR is a trauma-focused intervention which is a cost-effective short-term treatment. We anticipate that evidence will show that it is a largely tolerable intervention and leading to improved accessibility and widened participation in psychedelic treatments for those who are most disadvantaged by the current milieu.

Unpacking how PsyA-EMDR therapy supports the proposed SusQI agenda and how this leads to more sustainable healthcare practice can be established by knitting PsyA-EMDR therapy into the four principles for achieving sustainable healthcare. In order of importance, the four principles for achieving sustainable healthcare are prevention, patient empowerment/supported self-care, lean service pathways and low-carbon treatment alternatives (Mortimer, 2010).

The table overleaf illustrates the four principles for achieving sustainable healthcare in PsyA-EMDR.

Low-Carbon Alternatives	Lean Service Pathways	Patient Empowerment	Prevention
– Travelling abroad to treatment centres is not sustainable and has wider social, cultural and economic implications. PsyA-EMDR could be a local service, minimising the need for travel. – PsyA-EMDR works psychologically with destabilised individuals, keeping people out of inpatient services. – PsyA-EMDR works well with both pharmaceutically developed and naturally occurring psychedelic compounds. Naturally occurring psychedelics reduce the costs and environmental impacts associated with drug research and development and patented PAP protocols. – PsyA-EMDR can occur in both NHS inpatient treatment centres and in naturalistic, non-medical settings, which are significantly less carbon intensive.	– PsyA-EMDR optimises the therapeutic value of every dose, minimising the number of doses required. This is in line with the NHS-UK's 'getting it right first time' and 'making every contact count' initiatives. – Outcomes from G-TEP and G-REP protocols demonstrate that EMDR provides good treatment outcomes when provided in group interventions. Further research is needed to assess the value of group PsyA-EMDR therapy. – Psychedelic treatments need to be financially sustainable. PsyA-EMDR uses a one-therapist model during dosing (with floating support staff). This reduces costs and makes these treatments more accessible to more people. – PsyA-EMDR uses tolerance testing, psycho-educative and harm minimization approaches to reduce the risk of needing to access further services.	– PsyA-EMDR is a trauma-focused PAP. Trauma-focused PAPs widen participation and make psychedelic treatments available to those with complexity; this empowers those who are most at risk of poor mental health outcomes and those with high levels of ACEs. In so doing, PsyA-EMDR challenges the power differentials in psychedelic therapy provision. – If necessary, PsyA-EMDR therapy can use the PC associated with a memory network to support the client to identify and set their intention(s) for their dosing session. – PsyA-EMDR is a manualised PAP that adopts an ideographic approach during phase 4 reprocessing, putting the individual's inner healing intelligence at the heart of the healing intervention, and reducing the potential of therapeutic subjugation.	– PsyA-EMDR produces long-term positive treatment outcomes by addressing the root cause of a condition, rather than providing a sedation/maintenance programme. – PsyA-EMDR assesses patients' tolerability for the intensity of the psychedelic experience. This identifies and prevents those at risk of adverse reactions from unnecessary exposure. – When experiencing adverse reactions, PsyA-EMDR therapy is the only trauma-focused PAP, working to stabilise clients psychologically rather than using medications. This prevents the need for ongoing carbon-intensive treatments.

(*Continued*)

Low-Carbon Alternatives	Lean Service Pathways	Patient Empowerment	Prevention
– PsyA-EMDR can occur in both NHS inpatient treatment centres and in naturalistic, non-medical settings, which are significantly less carbon intensive. – Working online using PsyA-EMDR preparation and integration interventions are safe, effective and reduce the need for travel. – Group protocols can be used to efficiently deliver group integration and minimise the carbon footprint per intervention. – PsyA-EMDR uses tolerance testing, psycho-educative and harm minimalization approaches to reduce the risk of needing to access further services.	– PsyA-EMDR is a manualised treatment improving practitioner consistency leading to leaner service pathways. – PsyA-EMDR can be used as a short-term intervention. This is more efficient than ongoing, open-ended therapeutic alternatives. – PsyA-EMDR therapy delivers measurable outcomes so that efficacy can be more easily assessed. – Finding ways of optimising PAP delivery would prevent the need for additional dosing, lengthy therapy and reduce the risk of adverse reactions. More needs to be done to assess the synergistic effects of PsyA-EDMR therapy, but early indicators from clinical practice look promising.	– PsyA-EMDR improves the therapeutic impact of each preparation and integration session, reducing the number of sessions required. – PsyA-EMDR is universally applicable providing psychedelic treatments without the need for appropriation or cultural extractivism. PsyA-EMDR is a culturally competent approach to delivering psychedelic therapy at scale, empowering individuals by being inclusive and appreciating difference and diversity. – PsyA-EMDR is a body-orientated trauma-focused PAP which supports a client's unfolding process without the need for physical touch. – PsyA-EMDR is suitable for those with trauma profiles, which may otherwise prohibit access to PAP.	– PsyA-EMDR therapy objectively measures psychedelic integration using cognitive, emotional, behavioural, somatic and psychometric indicators, reducing the need for unnecessary onward treatments. – PsyA-EMDR integration therapy is impactful on historic, treatment-resistant psychedelic content and can be used to integrate material from adverse reactions from many years ago, preventing the need for ongoing treatment. – Healthcare settings need to ensure that service provision does not lead to practitioner burnout or vicarious traumatisation, which is more easily acheived when using manualised therapies. – Theoretically, interventions could be shared across several practitioners if deemed necessary.

Conclusion

Any exploration of ethics in field of psychedelics illuminates a complex landscape fraught with historical abuses and contemporary challenges. From the shadowy history of unethical experimentation during the 1950s and 1960s, as exemplified by the disturbing MKUltra project (United States Senate, 1977), to modern-day dilemmas such as patient vulnerability, or profiteering from patented medications, ethical breaches remain a significant concern. As we navigate these murky waters, it becomes increasingly evident that uncovering such ethical considerations is paramount in ensuring the safety, integrity and efficacy of psychedelic-assisted therapies. While this chapter provides an overview of a few of the core issues, it also acknowledges the myriad of ethical complexities that will continue to shape the evolving landscape of psychedelic-assisted EMDR therapy.

References

American Psychological Association (APA). (2022). Psychologists and psychedelic-assisted therapy. Found at: https://psychology.org.au/getmedia/1549bc9d-69da-4085-91b6-68e489ba696d/050922aps-ps-psychedelics-p2.pdf

Asheri, A. (2009). To touch or not to touch: A relational body psychotherapy perspective. In L. Hartley (Ed.), *Contemporary body psychotherapy, the Chiron approach* (pp. 106–120). London: Routledge. https://doi.org/10.4324/9780203892640

Banderira, I. D., Lins-Silva, D. H., Cavenahi, V. B., Dorea-Banderira, I., Faria-Guimaraes, D., Barouh, J. L., Jesus-Nunes, A. P., Beanes, G., Aouza, L., Leal, G. C., Sanacora, G., Miguel, E., Sampaio, A.S., & Quarantini, L. (2022). Ketamine in the treatment of obsessive-compulsive disorder: A systematic review. *Harvard Review of Psychiatry, 30*(2), 135–145. https://doi.org/10.1097/hrp.0000000000000330

Barrett, F., Carbonagro, T., Hurwitz, E., Johnson, M., & Griffiths, R. (2018). Double-blind comparison of the two hallucinogens psilocybin and dextromethorphan: Effects on Cognition. *Psychopharmacology (Berl), 235*(10), 2915–2927. https://doi.org/10.1007/s00213-018-4981-x

Bórquez-Infante, I., Vasquez, J., Dupre, S., Undurraga, E. A., Crossley, N. A., & Undurraga, J. (2022). Childhood adversity increases risk of psychotic experiences in patients with substance use disorder. *Psychiatry Research, 316*, 114733. https://doi.org/10.1016/j.psychres.2022.114733.

Breeksema, J., Bouwe, W. K., Kamphuis, J., van den Brink, W., Vermettern, E., & Schoevers, Ro. (2022). Adverse events in clinical treatments with serotonergic psychedelics and MDMA: A mixed-methods systemic review. *Journal of Psychopharmacology, 36*(10), 1100–1177. https://doi.org/10.1177/02698811221116926

Brennan, W., & Belser, A. (2022). Models of psychedelic-assisted psychotherapy: A contemporary assessment and an introduction to EMBARK, a transdiagnostic trans-drug model. *Frontiers in Psychology: Sec. Psychology for Clinical Settings, 13*, 866018. https://doi.org/10.3389/fpsyg.2022.866018

Carhart-Harris, R., Kaelen, M., Whalley, M. G., Bolstridge, M., Fielding, A., & Nutt, D. (2015). LSD enhances suggestibility in healthy volunteers. *Psychopharmacology*, 232(4), 785–794. https://doi.org/10.1007/s00213-014-3714-z

Centre for Sustainable Healthcare (n.d.). Sustainable Quality Improvement (SusQI). Found at https://sustainablehealthcare.org.uk/susqi

Daleberg, C. J. (2000). Therapy as a unique human interaction: Management of boundaries and sexual countertransference. In C. J. Dalenberg (Ed.), *Countertransference and the treatment of trauma* (pp. 199–239). Washington, NE: American Psychological Association. https://doi.org/10.1037/10380-000

Davies, J. (2021). *Sedated. How modern capitalism created our mental Health Crisis*. London: Atlantic Books.

Devenot, N., Tumilty, E., Buisson, M., McNamee, S., Nickles, D., & Ross, L. K. (2022). Bill of health. Examining the intersection of health, law, biotechnology and bioethics. *Law Harvard Education*. Found at https://blog.petrieflom.law.harvard.edu/2022/03/09/precautionary-approach-touch-in-psychedelic-assisted-therapy/

Evans, J. (2023). Synthesis and the shadow of psychedelic capitalism. Found at https://www.ecstaticintegration.org/p/synthesis-and-the-shadow-of-psychedelic?utm_source=substack&publication_id=1072242&post_id=107808599&utm_medium=email&triggerSave=true

Felitti, V. J., Anda, R. F. & Nordenberg, D. (1998). Relationship of childhood abuse and household dysfunction to many of the leading causes of death in adults: The Adverse Childhood Experiences (ACE) Study. *American Journal of Preventive Medicine*, 14(4), 245–258. https://doi.org/10.1016/s0749-3797(98)00017-8

Goldhill, O. (2020). Psychedelic therapy has a sexual abuse problem. Found at https://qz.com/1809184/psychedelic-therapy-has-a-sexual-abuse-problem-3

Gopalkrishnan, N. (2018). Cultural diversity and mental health: considerations for policy and practice. *Frontiers in Publish Health*, 6, 179. https://doi.org/10.3389/fpubh.2018.00179

Greenway, K. T., Garel, N., Jerome, L., & Feduccia, A. A. (2020). Integrating psychotherapy and psychopharmacology: Psychedelic-assisted psychotherapy and other combined treatments. *Expert Review of Clinical Pharmacology*, 13(6), 655–670. https://doi.org/10.1080/17512433.2020.1772054

Guo, J., Gu, H. W., Wang, X. M., Hashimoto, K., Zhang, G. F., & Yang, J. J. (2023). Efficacy and safety of perioperative application of ketamine on postoperative depression: A meta-analysis of randomised controlled studies. *Nature Molecular Psychiatry*, 28(6), 2266–2276 https://doi.org/10.1038/s41380-023-01945-z

Hall, W. (2021). Ending the silence around psychedelic therapy abuse. Found at https://www.madinamerica.com/2021/09/ending-silence-psychedelic-therapy-abuse/

Hausfield, R. (2019). As legal psychedelic therapy emerges, ethicists urge for more comprehensive frameworks to address sexual abuse. *Psymposia*. Found at https://www.psymposia.com/magazine/psychedelic-therapy-ethics-sexual-abuse/

Healy, C. J. (2021). The acute effects of classic psychedelics on memory in humans. *Psychopharmacology*, 238, 639–653. https://doi.org/10.1007/s00213-020-05756-w

Hoeffer, C.A., & Klann, E. (2010). mTOR signalling: At the crossroads of plasticity, memory and disease. *Trends Neuroscience*, 33, 67–75. https://doi.org/10.1016/j.tins.2009.11.003

Joneborg, I., Lee, Y., Di Vincenzo, J. D., Ceban, F., Shakila, M., Lui, L. M. W., Fancy, F., Rosenblat, J. D., & McIntyre, R. S. (2022). Active mechanisms of ketamine assisted psychotherapy: A systematic review. *Journal of Affective Disorders, 315*, 105–112. https://doi.org/10.1016/j.jad.2022.07.030

Krystal, J. H. (2007). Neuroplasticity as a target for the pharmacotherapy of psychiatric disorders: new opportunities for synergy with psychotherapy. *Biological Psychiatry, 62*(8), 833–834. https://doi.org/10.1016/j.biopsych.2007.08.017

Leopold, A. (1949). *A Sand County Almanac.* New York: Oxford University Press.

Love, S. (2021). Can a company patent the basic components of psychedelic therapy. Found at https://www.vice.com/en/article/93wmxv/can-a-company-patent-the-basic-components-of-psychedelic-therapy

Multidisciplinary Association for Psychedelic Studies (MAPS). (2015). A manual for MDMA-assisted psychotherapy in the treatment of posttraumatic stress disorder. Found at https://maps.org/research-archive/mdma/MDMA-Assisted-Psychotherapy-Treatment-Manual-Version7-19Aug15-FINAL.pdf

Marks, M., & Cohen, I. G. (2022). Patents on psychedelics: The next legal battlefront of drug development. *Harvard Law Review.* Found at https://harvardlawreview.org/forum/no-volume/patents-on-psychedelics-the-next-legal-battlefront-of-drug-development/

Marks-Tarlow, T. (2020). *Mythic Imagination and Modern Psychotherapy: The Psyche in Transformative and Healing Relationships.* Routledge.

Marland, S., Ellerton, J., Andilfatto, G., Strapazzon, O., Thomassen, O., Brandner, b., Weatherall, A., & Paal, P. (2013). Ketamine: Use in anaesthesia. *CNS Neurosci Therapy, 19*(6), 381–389. https://doi.org/10.1111/cns.12072

Martin, J. (1954). L. S. D. lysergic acid diethylamide_ treatment of chronic psychoneurotic patients under day-hospital conditions. *Journal of Social Psychology, 3*(3), 188–195. https://doi.org/10.1177/002076405700300304

Martin, J. (1964). L. S. D. analysis. *Journal of Social Psychiatry, 10*(3), 165–169. https://doi.org/10.1177/0020764064010000301

McLane, H., Hutchinson, C., Wikler, D., Howell, T., & Knighton, E. (2021). Respecting autonomy in altered states: Navigating ethical quandaries in Psychedelic therapy. *Blog Journal of Medical Ethics.* Found at https://blogs.bmj.com/medical-ethics/2021/12/22/respecting-autonomy-in-altered-states-navigating-ethical-quandaries-in-psychedelic-therapy/

Menakem, R. (2021). *My grandmother's hands. Racialized trauma and the pathway to mending our hearts and bodies.* London: Penguin.

Michaels, T., Purdon, J., Collins, A., & Williams, M. (2018). Inclusion of people of color in psychedelic-assisted psychotherapy: A review of the literature. *BMC Psychiatry, 18*, 245. https://doi.org/10.1186/s12888-018-1824-6

Miles, S. H. (2004). *The Hippocratic Oath and the ethics of medicine.* New York: Oxford University Press.

Mitchell, J., Bogenschutz, M., Lilienstein, A., Harrison, C., Kleinman, S., Parler-Guilbert, M., Garas, W., Paleos, C., Gorman, I., Nicholas, C., Mithoefer, M., Carlin, S., Poluter, B., Mithoefer, A., Quevedo, S., Wells, G., Klaire, S., Van der Kolk, B., Tzarfaty, K., Amiaz, R., Worthy, R., Shannon, S., Woolley, J.D., Marta, C., Gelfand, Y., Hapke, E., Amar, S., Wallach, Y., Brown, R., Hamilton, S., Wang, J., Coker, A., Matthews, R., Boer, A., Yazar-Klosinski, Y., Emerson, A., &

Doblin, R. (2021). MDMA-assisted therapy for severe PTSD: a randomized, double-blind, placebo-controlled phase 3 study. *Nature Medicine, 27*(6), 1025–1033. https://doi.org/10.1038/s41591-021-01336-3

Miller, R. (2021). From mao to mcdonaldization? Assessing the rationalisation of healthcare in China. *Sociology of Health & Illness, 43*(7), 1643–1659. https://doi.org/10.1111/1467-9566.13351

Mortimer, F. (2010). The sustainable physician. *Clinical Medicine, 10*(2), 110–111. https://doi.org/10.7861/clinmedicine.10-2-110

National Institute for Health and Care Excellence (NICE), (n.d.). Improving access to psychological therapies, national institute for health and care excellence. Found at https://www.nice.org.uk/about/what-we-do/our-programmes/nice-advice/iapt

National Institute for Health and Care Excellence (NICE). (n.d.). Standards and Indicators. Found at https://www.nice.org.uk/standards-and-indicators. Accessed 15.5.24

Neitzke-Spruill, L. (2019). Race as a component of set and setting: How experiences of race can influence psychedelic experiences. *Journal of Psychedelic Studies, 4*(1), 51–60. https://doi.org/10.1556/2054.2019.022

Nickles, D., & Kay-Ross, L. K. (2021). Bad Hug. Cover Story. Power Trip. Found at https://podcasts.apple.com/us/podcast/bad-hug/id1594675355?i=1000545625279

Nutt, D. (2019). Psychedelic drugs – A new era in psychiatry? *Dialogues in Clinical Neuroscience, 21*(2), 139–147. https://doi.org/10.31887/DCNS.2019.21.2/dnutt

O'Mathuna, D. P., Pryimachuk, S., Spencer, W., Stanwick, M., & Matthiesen, S. (2002). A critical evaluation of theory and practice of therapeutic touch. *Nursing Philosophy, 3*(2): 163–176. https://doi.org/10.1046/j.1466-769X.200200089.x

Peltoniemi, M. A., Hagelberg, N. M., Olkkola, K. T., & Saari, T. I. (2016). Ketamine: A review of clinical pharmacokinetics and pharmacodynamics in anaesthesia and pain therapy. *Clinical Pharmacokinetics, 55*(9), 1059–77. https://doi.org/10.1007/s40262-016-0383-6

Philipp-Muller, A. E., Stephenson, C. J., Moghimi, E., Shirazi, A. H., Milev, R., Vazquez, G., Reshetukha, T., & Alavi, N. (2023). Combining ketamine and psychotherapy for the treatment of posttraumatic stress disorder: A systematic review and meta-analysis. *The Journal of Clinical Psychiatry, 84*(2), 22br14564. https://doi.org/10.4088/JCP.22br14564

Pollan, M. (2018). *How to change your mind. The new science of psychedelics.* Bristol: Allen Lane.

Raine-Smith, H., & Rose, J. (2023). Psychedelic-assisted EMDR therapy (PsyA-EMDR): A memory consolidation approach to psychedelic healing. *ETQ, 4*, 1. https://doi.org/10.13140/RG.2.2.24683.35366

Raworth, K. (2017). *Donut economics – seven ways to think like a 21st century economist.* New York: Random House.

Read, T., & Papaspyrou, M. (2021). *Psychedelics and Psychotherapy – The healing potential of expanded states.* Paris, ME: Park Street Press.

Schofield, T. J., Lee, R. D., & Merrick, M. T. (2013). Safe, stable, nurturing relationships as a moderator on intergenerational continuity of child abuse and neglect: A meta-analysis. *Journal of Adolescent Health, 52*(5), S32–S38. https://doi.org/10.1016/j.jadohealth.2013.05.004

Taylor, K. (1995). *The ethics of caring. honouring the web of life in our healing professional relationships.* Santa Cruz, CA: Hanford Mead Publishers.

The Anti-discrimination Focus (n.d.). Found at: https://tadf.co.uk/

Turner, D. (2014). Searching for Afrocentric spirituality within the transpersonal. Found at https://nectar.northampton.ac.uk/7074/3/Turner20147074.pdf

United States Drug Enforcement Administration (DEA). (2023). Drug Scheduling. Found at https://www.dea.gov/drug-information/drug-scheduling#:~:text=Schedule%20I%20drugs%2C%20substances%2C%20or,)%2C%20methaqualone%2C%20and%20peyote

United States Senate. (1977, Aug 3). Project MKULTRA, the CIA's program of research in behavioral modification: Joint hearing before the select committee on intelligence and the subcommittee on health and scientific research of the committee on human resources, United States Senate, Ninety-Fifth Congress, First Session. Found at https://www.intelligence.senate.gov/sites/default/files/hearings/95mkultra.pdf

Van Der Kolk, B. (1989). The compulsion to repeat the trauma. Re-enactment, revictimization, and masochism. *Psychiatric Clinics of North America,12*(2), 389–411. https://doi.org/10.1016/S0193-953X%2818%2930439-8

5 Stabilisation and risk reduction

5-MeO-DMT
5 Methoxy-N, N-dimethyltryptamine ($C_{13}H_{18}N_2O$)

DOI: 10.4324/9781003431718-5

5-MeO-DMT is a naturally occurring tryptamine which differs structurally from DMT by a single methoxy group, and yet its acute drug effects are markedly different. There are some parallels in that they are both short acting and very intense; however, the subjective intensity of the psychedelic experience is stronger in 5-MeO-DMT compared to that induced by DMT. The phenomenological effects of 5-MeO-DMT are also very different to DMT and other nonselective serotonin (5-HT) agonists. The phenomenological uniqueness of 5-MeO-MET might be caused by its pharmacokinetics, that indicate a 1000-fold greater binding affinity for the $5-HT_{1A}$ receptor over the 5-HT2A (Ray, 2010). It causes a potent suppression of firing in the dorsal raphe, an area in the brainstem densely populated with serotonergic neurons that modulate a wide range of processes including mood and motor functions (Rogawski et al., 1981). Additional mechanisms of action are also likely to be involved, including the inhibition of monoamine reuptake (Nagai et al., 2007). A single dose of 5-MeO-DMT has also been demonstrated to induce neurogenesis in mice (Lima da Cruz et al., 2018).

The acute effects of 5-MeO-DMT vary but range from a radical shift in perspective, perception of new insights, euphoria, sensual/erotic enhancement, dissociation or non-responsiveness, dysphoria, fear, terror and panic. Some have likened the 5-MeO-DMT experience to a white light, non-dual or to near-death experiences.

5-MeO-DMT occurs naturally in a variety of plants, seeds and animals (most notably the Sonoran Desert toad, *Bufo Alvarius*) and has even been found in the cerebrospinal fluid, blood and urine of humans (Christian et al., 1975). It was first synthesised in Japan in 1936, and its use has since been made illegal in the US, in 2011, and shortly followed by the UK government in 2015.

A European study with 42 volunteers in 2019 showed that single inhalation of 5-MeO-DMT produced sustained enhancement of satisfaction with life and easing of anxiety, depression and post-traumatic stress disorder (PTSD) (Uthaug et al., 2019). 5-MeO-DMT is currently being developed and evaluated in a multi-site, multinational phase 2b RCT for its potential therapeutic effects in patients with treatment-resistant depression (TRD).

An important question remains unanswered

Can psychedelic-assisted psychotherapy (PAP) become a fully accessible and well-tolerated treatment option for all?

This question is likely to persist, until,

- Psychological interventions are designed to address the challenges that arise from implementing large-scale psychedelic treatments.
- There is a comprehensive evidence base to support working inclusively in diverse clinical populations.

The field of psychedelics is gradually becoming more inclusive, opening to ever wider and more diverse populations (Mitchell, 2023). As discussed in Chapter 4, widening participation and addressing the power differentials in healing outcomes are important goals for individuals, family systems, organisations, society, humanity and ecology at large.

Giving psychedelic treatments to individuals with high levels of agitation, or those who do not have sufficient insight into their condition, would likely be countertherapeutic and may cause significant harm (Breeksema et al., 2022). However, even for the most unwell and treatment-resistant presentations, much can be learned from trauma-focused practice to support safety and stabilisation, thus widening access to trauma-focused psychedelic treatments.

In the aftermath of the first world war, Pierre Janet was the first psychologist to formulate a systematic approach to explain and treat post-traumatic pathology (Janet, 1919). His three-stage methodology included:

1 Stabilisation with symptom-orientated treatments and preparation for trauma memory resolution.
2 Trauma confrontation, involving identification, exploration and modification of traumatic memories.
3 Post-traumatic growth and resilience, addressing relapse prevention, residual symptom relief, personality integration and rehabilitation.

These early foundations paved the way for studies and methodologies in trauma-oriented psychological therapies. In her formative paper 'The work of stabilisation in trauma treatment,' Janine Fisher highlights that psychoeducation about trauma symptoms, grounding techniques, coping strategy development, shifting from self-blame to narrative construction, viewing symptoms as potential bodily memories, distinguishing past trauma from a secure present and establishing safety contracts are important tools in trauma recovery (Fisher, 1999). In an interview in 2002, Babette Rothschild described how "Trauma is a feeling of not having any resources," indicating that resourcing and relational security enhance the sense of safety and improve patient stability for safe trauma recovery.

In EMDR therapy, history taking (phase 1) and preparation (phase 2) are synonymous with stabilisation and act as gateways to accessing safe treatment. It is possible that once stabilised using non-psychedelic trauma-focussed interventions such as EMDR, those with more complex diagnoses could be accommodated in carefully designed psychedelic treatment pathways. Regardless of necessity, ample resourcing is universally beneficial; a spectrum of benefits that ranges from enhanced patient empowerment to reduced risk for those accessing inclusive treatment pathways. A Dutch version of EMDR called 'EMDR 2.0' shows promise with unstable cohorts, because working memory is taxed to the extent that even the most overwhelming traumatic memories can be accessed and reprocessed quickly and effectively (Alting Van Geusau et al., 2023). Paul Mansfield's flash technique is a similar EMD (without the reprocessing) intervention designed to rapidly desensitise overwhelming material (Manfield et al., 2024). Flash also shows promise as a scalable, group intervention (Manfield et al., 2021) and has the additional accessibility of being simple enough for non-EMDR mental health workers to execute successfully if adequately trained.

Humanitarian research projects have highlighted the efficacy of EMDR's stabilisation and resourcing phases as the sole psychological intervention in the aftermath of natural disasters. It has been demonstrated that such strategies can even be utilised by non-clinicians treating PTSD in the immediate aftermath of a traumatic event. For example, paraprofessionals in disaster zones have been trained in resourcing techniques, grounded in the AIP model, yielding favourable outcomes (Eichfield et al., 2019; Mattheß et al., 2019). The translation of this into psychedelic therapy could prove valuable as a harm-reduction strategy when used by facilitators at festivals, in acute mental health care settings, by police and security officials who are dealing with people who are under the influence of psychedelics, as well as in underground PAP settings.

Defining stabilisation

Medical ethics uphold the principle of non-maleficence. Establishing psychological stability serves as the primary basis for prioritising non-maleficence in psychedelic treatments. Achieving adequate states of stability is pivotal when working with those with enhanced risk and psychological complexity. To avoid conflation, the concept of stabilisation would merit clear distinction:

Safety and stabilisation – Before treatment, helping individuals to develop skills to self-soothe and self-rescue. Establishing and increasing their 'window of tolerance.' Establishing an environment that is suitable for trauma work. **EMDR equivalent** – procedures and techniques used in EMDR standard protocol phase 2 "preparation and resourcing."

Grounding and (re)stabilisation – After treatment, helping individuals to self-soothe and self-rescue. Re-establishing nervous system stability using grounding techniques such as awareness of the immediate environment and awareness of self. **EMDR equivalent** – procedures and techniques used in EMDR standard protocol phase 7 "closure."

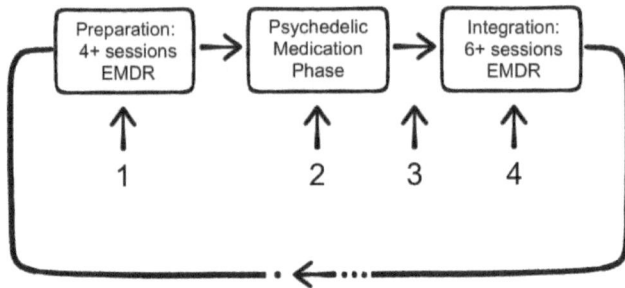

Figure 5.1 Diagram of the four critical cornerstones that underpin the foundations of stabilisation.

Four critical cornerstones underpin the foundations of stabilisation in PsyA-EMDR:

1 **Preparation**

Increasing the patient's capacity to tolerate stress is a core harm-reduction intervention in preparation for a psychedelic medication. Several strategies can be deployed to enhance psychological stability and therefore widen access. Positive therapeutic outcomes are best achieved by reducing risk through rigorous screening and emphasising pre-dose stabilisation. This is more comprehensively explored in Chapter 6, 'Preparation.'

2 **Medication phase**

Several strategies can be deployed to enhance psychological stability during dosing to reduce the risk of extended adverse drug effects. This is explored in more detail in Chapter 3 on the PsyA-EMDR protocol and in Chapter 7 on psycholytic EMDR.

3 **Post-dose grounding and (re)stabilisation**

There are numerous strategies in EMDR therapy that can be used to support post-dose psychological stability to reduce the need for additional pharmacological interventions. In addition to this, treatment-specific interventions tailored for PsyA-EMDR are explored later in this chapter, and also in Chapter 9 on integration, and in Chapter 12 on the future of PsyA-EMDR.

4   Integration

Integration is a nuanced, lifelong process. From a memory consolidation perspective, integration occurs when material from psychedelic therapy is reprocessed according to the three-pronged approach (past, present, future) across the somatic, emotional and cognitive domains, as measured by the SUDS, VOC and body scan. Thorough integration can also enhance safety outcomes when preparing for subsequent psychedelic treatments. A comprehensive overview of integration is explored in Chapter 8.

NB – PsyA-EMDR therapy can be used as an integrative psychedelic therapy whereby PsyA-EMDR stabilisation techniques can assist individuals to stabilise at cornerstones 3 and 4, regardless of their preparation and medication experiences.

Developing inclusive psychedelic treatments

With the right psychological and relational support, appropriate substance and dose, adequate preparation and tolerance testing, support in developing the right mindset and creating an adequately containing setting, it is believed that many more people, if not most, could be adequately supported to access psychedelic medications. Widening the treatment domain to promote access to psychedelic interventions requires client engagement, therapeutic skill, relational rapport, and the availability (if required) of a supportive interdisciplinary clinical team and/or inpatient treatment setting. The following two sections outline the practical application of PsyA-EMDR for stabilisation and risk reduction.

Assessment of risk

Risk mitigation in PsyA-EMDR therapy demands thorough evaluation of the risk factors involved. This is achieved by utilising screening tools and cultivating an awareness of key contraindications.

The screening toolkit

The following psychometric and psychological assessments can help to ascertain readiness versus risk in preparation for psychedelic administration:

- Psychedelic Preparedness Scale (PPS) that measures modifiable pre-treatment preparatory behaviours and attitudes (McAlpine et al., 2023).

- Dissociation screening tools such as the dissociative experiences scale (DES II; Carlson & Putman, 1993).
- Clinical Administered PTSD Scale Checklist (CAPS) is a 30-item structured interview that corresponds to the DSM V criteria for PTSD (Weathers et al., 2015).
- Adverse Childhood Experiences Questionnaire (ACE-Q) is a 10-item measure used to assess childhood trauma (Felitti et al., 1998).
- Psychedelic therapy practitioners' own screening/assessment tools/intuition to assess for client's ability to self-regulate, particularly within the psychotherapeutic dyad.

- Psychiatric screening to include (but not limited to):

  - Personal history to provide a more nuanced view of past traumas, attachment history and relational issues. Exploration of any risk factors described.
  - GP summary.
  - The Mini-International Neuropsychiatric Interview (M.I.N.I.) to screen for major psychiatric symptoms and evaluate suicidality (Sheehan et al., 1998).
  - Assessment to ensure capacity to give the informed consent required for administering psychedelic medication (and the possibility also for the use of rescue medication), including an ability to understand, appreciate, reason and express their own choices.

For individuals considered unsuitable, traditional trauma-focussed work deserves further consideration. The following psychometrics can be employed to evaluate areas where trauma-focussed interventions (such as standard protocol EMDR) can be specifically targeted to enhance tolerability for subsequent psychedelic treatments.

- Post-Traumatic Stress Disorder Check List (PCL-5) PTSD Checklist for DSM-V (Weathers et al., 2013).
- International Trauma Questionnaire (ITQ) is an 18-question self-report measure focusing on the core features of PTSD and complex PTSD (cPTSD) (Cloitre et al., 2018).
- Psychological Mindedness Scale (PMS) is a 45-item self-report instrument intended to assess capacity to engage in psychological therapies (Conte et al., 1996).
- Self-Reflection and Insight Scale (SRIS) is a 20-item self-report scale to ascertain the metacognitive capacity to inspect and evaluate one's own thoughts, feelings and behaviour (Grant et al., 2002).
- Psychological Flexibility Scale (Psy-Flex) as a measure to assess the impact of the intervention and where to target future interventions (Gloster et al., 2021).

Scores outside of pre-determined thresholds on any of these psychometric measures may indicate a need for additional preparation in that area. Once the psychometric scores reach parameters indicating sufficient resourcing, patients may then be rescreened and signposted to the appropriate treatment pathway.

Note: MDMA could also be considered as a tool for stabilisation at this stage as discussed in Chapter 6, 'Preparation.'

Wider context

It is important to pay careful consideration to the need for highly bespoke, individualised treatment plans, where the most appropriate psychedelic substance is selected, along with an appropriate dose. If multiple doses or multiple drug options are needed, it is important that these occur in the appropriate sequence. The pace and timing of the work need to be dictated by the individual's needs and external factors, as well as the resources available. Preparatory discussions play a crucial role in empowering individuals to make informed decisions about their treatment options, and the therapist's AIP case conceptualisation is used to guide this process and ensure that the client chooses the most beneficial treatment option available. If required, the risks and benefits of travelling abroad to access psychedelic treatments can also be considered.

Contraindications

Highlighting the contraindications for PsyA-EMDR therapy is paramount for providing responsible, safety-informed therapeutic practice. The following items can be used to guide the pacing of the work and determine how much time is spent in the preparatory EMDR sessions before progressing to a psychedelic treatment. In some cases, the psychedelic phase would be omitted completely due to several risk factors listed below.

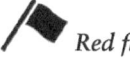 *Red flags*

- *Do not proceed* where there is an imminent risk of suicide or harm to self or others. Prioritise stabilisation through resource enhancement and psychiatric support.
- *Do not proceed* if the individual is unable to tolerate the dysregulation caused by EMDR reprocessing (phases 3–7). Severe abreaction during reprocessing could indicate an inability to tolerate the intensity of a psychedelic treatment. If this is the case, consider slowing down the work and staying at the PsyA-EMDR preparation phase until the capacity to tolerate intense emotions has been established.

- *Do not proceed* without a strong therapeutic container. A greater emphasis on interpersonal dynamics is required when working with psychedelics/expanded states. There is a need for a solid relational container for the work to happen. Discuss how any emergent infantile content (such as paranoia) might be worked through with the client ahead of dosing.
- *Do not proceed* where the practitioner's training is not suited to the client's content. It is important for participant and practitioner safety to work within the clinician's skill set.
- *Do not proceed* where there are dual relationships between the patient and the therapist or medical staff involved in their care.
- *Do not proceed* where the enhanced erotic transferences may interrupt the holding of the therapeutic frame. Close adherence to ethical frameworks is necessary both during the psychedelic session as well as when holding clear professional boundaries when responding to emails, correspondence, timings, contracting etc.
- *Do not proceed* where there are signs of vicarious trauma in the practitioner. It is important to foster a culture where there is a greater awareness of the potential impact of trauma work on practitioners. Self-care and self-reflective practices should be central to the work.
- *Do not proceed* where a practitioner's unresolved trauma may interrupt the client's process. Practitioners need to have sufficient insight into their own material, being aware of potential blind spots, hotspots and soft spots that could get magnified by the strong counter-transferential material emerging.
- *Do not proceed* where supervision processes are not in place.
- *Do not proceed* when the care team has ongoing relational or situational ruptures that might get in the way of the formation of a solid therapeutic container.
- *Do not proceed* where there are high levels of instability and low levels of self-awareness/psychological insight. When necessary, the patient can be supported by a multidisciplinary team, with access to medication and inpatient care if required.
- *Do not proceed* where the individual displays physical symptoms in a pre-dose resting state that might interfere with patient or practitioner safety. For example, movement disorders with violent tics or convulsions, physical collapse, non-epileptic seizures, severe migraines etc.
- *Do not proceed* where hyper/hypo-arousal may interrupt a patient's capacity to engage with the process. Use stabilisation/resourcing techniques to increase capacity for dysregulation.
- *Do not proceed* where patients lack capacity to make informed decisions about their own care needs. Patients need to be active in decision-making processes related to their care.
- *Do not proceed* where a previous difficult psychedelic experience is still agitating or concerning *and* where there has been an inability or unwillingness to work through the emergent material using psychological methods.

- *Do not proceed* where a patient discloses ongoing abuse. Challenging abuse through therapeutic change can lead to relational instability and increased risk. If appropriate, signpost those who are vulnerable to abuse on to other service options until their situation has stabilised.
- *Do not proceed* where age restrictions apply. Further research is needed to assess the risks when working with children, young people, the elderly and some individuals with cognitive impairments.

Please note that this list of contraindications is illustrative but not exhaustive and that a practitioner's professional judgement and policy/legal procedures should always be followed as a priority.

Warning

A history or family history of mania and psychosis (including drug-induced psychosis) can heighten the risks associated with psychedelic medications. EMDR therapy as a stand-alone could offer safer and more suitable therapeutic alternative. Ongoing suitability needs to be assessed on a case-by-case basis and may depend upon several external factors. See 'Widening the treatment domain decision-making matrix' in Chapter 12, 'The Future of PsyA-EMDR.'

Stabilisation

Previously, we explored the four critical cornerstones that underpin the foundations of stabilisation. The first, second and fourth cornerstones are unpacked in later Chapters 6–8 on preparation, psycholytic EMDR and integration. This section explores the third cornerstone and outlines strategies that can be implemented to bolster stability directly after the acute effects of the psychedelic medications have subsided.

Post-dose grounding and (re)stabilisation toolkit

Standard tools for stabilisation:

- Practitioners to support a slow and nourishing re-entry, with ample time for reorientation before higher levels of functionality are required.
- Client-led language should be adopted.
- Work with sensitivity in the wider contextual setting, as undefended ego states can be easily traumatised.

- Minimise exposure to emotionally charged situations, social interactions or media content.
- Use of a weighted blanket can be helpful if greater physical containment is required.
- Fresh fruit might be offered to help get people back into their bodies, whilst providing some light sustenance to restore energy levels.
- A gentle (accompanied) walk in nature or EMDR walking therapy (walking as BLS) may also be helpful (Nondu, 2024).
- Art, journaling, music and gentle movement can be grounding.
- Psychoeducation to normalise post-dose vulnerability. Oversharing during the medication session can heighten vulnerability and lead to overwhelm/paranoia.
- Relationships appear to be crucial in retethering those destabilised by psychedelic experiences. Strategies that promote relationship building (such as humour, movement, music and art) can be deployed to support stabilisation. These can also include enhancing relationality to their body, their identity, to work, to nature, to loved ones and the clinicians present. Enhancing these relationships can reduce the symptoms of derealisation.
- There are various methods that can be used to reinstate balance in the nervous system, such as the use of internal and external resources, deactivating breathwork, calming mantras and focusing on their inner resources.
- Interpersonal grounding through bodywork or touch might be considered, but only after the acute drug effects have subsided, and only introduced by practitioners suitably trained and qualified in bodywork-orientated therapies where prior consent has previously been obtained.

Another noteworthy contemporary approach that serves as an adjunct to EMDR is resource-oriented trauma therapy (ROTATE, Wöller et al., 2016). This method activates positive personal resources within a secure therapeutic relationship, drawing from affective neuroscience, resilience research and attachment theory. The manual outlines a compilation of diverse stabilisation techniques to achieve this with a focus on enhancing resilience and coping capacities.

ROTATE-informed stabilisation tools (Adapted from the ROTATE manual) (Wöller et al., 2016)

- Relationship orientation – psychodynamic attachment-informed, trauma-focussed formulations using AIP model.
- Neurobiological reorientation (see ROTATE manual) to modulate hyper/hypo-arousal of the nervous system.

- Strengthen resilience and coping capabilities by activating positive personal resources including activating:

  Internal resources which include:

  - Capabilities and competencies.
  - Pleasant activities.
  - Positive memories of the past.
  - Positive visions of the future.
  - Positive visions from previous psychedelic journeys.
  - Positive inner images created by guided imagery.

  External resources include:

  - Family members.
  - Partner.
  - Friends.
  - Organisations etc.

- Absorption technique – modification of resource development and installation (RDI; Hofmann, 2009).
- Not solely language based – also focus on somatic aspects and bodily reactions.
- Rebuilding impaired ego-functions by challenging maladaptive introjected parts.
- Monitoring therapist's own counter-transferential content can provide further insight.

Advanced tools for stabilisation

- The 'Google search' intervention from the recent-traumatic events protocol (R-TEP, Shapiro & Laub, 2015) can be used to identify significant points of distress (PODs).
- The standard protocol can then be used to reduce the PODs identified.
- Alternatively, the PODs can be processed using rapid memory reconsolidation/EMD techniques such as:

  - The Flash Technique. Note: this can be taught to non-clinicians as a harm-reduction tool.
  - EMDR 2.0
  - Four blinks, a version of the flash technique is available free of charge at www.fourblinks.com (Zimmerman, n.d.).

- Disconfirming experiences using the two-handed interweave (Shapiro, 2006).

- It is hypothesised that the 'empathogen' MDMA could be helpful in supporting stabilisation through a pharmacologically enhanced relational safety, although further research is required.

Systemic adaptations for enhanced stabilisation

- Information can be shared about community-run integration circles that provide peer support through horizontal models of care.
- Prioritising early access to acute care is crucial for individuals destabilised by psychedelic treatments. Fast-tracked, trauma-informed pathways into acute care services need to be made available. There is a risk of traumatisation if attempts to access services are impeded by lengthy waiting lists.
- Specialist training in psychedelic stabilisation made available to clinicians working across mental health settings, third-sector organisations, festival staff, police and security officials and suicide helpline operatives.
- Efforts need to be made (through psychoeducation and the media) to destigmatise those who experience acute adverse drug effects. This improves safety outcomes for all and supports the work of stabilisation for those most in need of emergency care.

There may be times when psychological stabilisation is not achievable, and there are significant risks to self/others, at which point rescue medication might be deemed necessary. In cases of persistent anxiety and distressing depersonalisation/derealisation, where psychological grounding interventions have been tried and nothing has helped, the prescribing psychiatrist may prescribe an antidepressant (such as an SSRI) with consideration of using this in combination with an anti-dissociative medication. If anxiety is high with predominantly somatic symptoms, then beta-blockers could also be of help. If closer to the event, where the distress is more acute and the risk of harm to self and/or others is more pronounced, benzodiazepines and antipsychotics show the potential to provide symptom relief. Sedative medications such as benzodiazepines and beta-blockers have the potential to induce avoidance behaviours. The impact of these strong medications on the nervous system can adversely impact the efficacy of the BLS. Benzodiazapines are contraindicated for EMDR because they have been shown block the degrading effects of the eye movements during memory reconsolidation (Littel, 2017). Recent unpublished research in the Netherlands had a similar outcome for beta blockers (Propranolol), indicating that this might be because of the impact these medications have on accessing (and reprocessing) the somatic component of trauma. Assessment and therapeutic attunement remain the best indicators for positive patient outcomes, and reprocessing versus medication should be evaluated on a case-by-case basis, depending on service availability.

Therapist self-care is an essential element that underpins PsyA-EMDR, and there is a need for greater awareness to reduce the risk of vicarious traumatisation and practitioner burnout. For further guidance, see Chapter 12, 'The Future of EMDR.'

Case material

Psychedelic preparation and integration EMDR therapy

Stabilisation – Cornerstone 1
  "I am <u>not</u> Spiderman"

Ray was a self-confessed adrenaline junkie who was widely known for his willingness to do anything for anyone. The eldest of five children, he was raised in a deprived area of London, in a family of mixed Romani Gypsy descent. Ray was active in his community, offering martial arts classes and using his love of adventure to raise funds for charity. On one occasion, Ray abseiled off a high-rise building dressed as Spiderman and was "mobbed and chased by a pack of kids at the bottom," having to demask to emphatically reveal to them that "I am not Spiderman!"

During his working life, Ray had served in the army in the Queens Parachute Regiment. His tours of duty included Cypress, the Falkland Islands, and Northern Ireland. Upon discharge from the army, he worked for 14 years in the London Ambulance Service. In 1998, Ray was diagnosed with cPTSD and since then described how he had "not stopped seeking professional help so that I may reclaim my lost mental balance and peace of mind damaged by the emotional trauma of my life experiences." In 2001, Ray was the paramedic in attendance at a road traffic accident that changed everything. Deeply traumatised by his experiences, he left the scene and never returned to his post. It transpired that even superheroes are not infallible.

Ray described his time between the ages of 36 and 60 as "years of swinging from darkness and light." His PTSD symptoms cost him his relationships with his family, his friends and his community and got him in trouble with the law. His blind rage and suicidality had a deep and lasting impact on his family, where both of his children would later be diagnosed with trauma-related disorders. Proactive in his 22-year healing journey, now aged 61, Ray described how he had "gone to the end of every trauma pathway offered." Ray had received five counselling sessions offered by his GP; he had completed the British Legion Combat Stress and Warrior programmes. He was later supported by Hillingdon mental health unit and then by London Veterans Trauma Clinic at St Pancras Hospital, where he took part in their PTSD research programme. Ray also accessed a range of alternative therapies including Emotional Freedom Technique, Reiki and

Hypnosis. Ray described that his PTSD symptoms were so bad that they had "made me resentful of my wife's love for keeping me alive."

In 2003, Ray read an article in a magazine in his GP surgery by the UK TV host Trisha. In the article, Trisha spoke about her own experiences of using MDMA to support her mental health. Inspired by what he had read, Ray described how over the next 20 years "MDMA saved my life." Whilst MDMA had helped to moderate the worst of his symptoms, he was still unable to work because his mood was unstable and "the monster" rage was still unpredictable. Ray would have been unable to access the PTSD clinical research trials as his trauma was linked to childhood adversity as well as his adult experiences in public uniformed services. He described that accessing PsyA-EMDR therapy was his "last throw of the dice."

Due to the complexity and severity of Ray's psychological presentation, an extended PsyA-EMDR protocol was required. In total, 32 sessions of PsyA-EMDR therapy were applied. Initially, three preparation sessions (phase 1–3) were used along with harm minimisation, psychoeducation and psychological resourcing. One reprocessing session (phase 4) was then used to prepare for the dosing mindset and assess his affect tolerance capacity. After which, Ray attended the first of two underground retreats, with ayahuasca offered on the first night and San Pedro (mescalin) offered on the second night. On ayahuasca, Ray experienced his sitter as a benevolent version of his "sociopathic-narcissistic mother." The following night on mescalin, Ray experienced a unification with the cosmos, a non-dual experience where he saw the ultimate perfection and interconnectivity of all things, which appeared to repair his attachment deficits. In the following nine sessions, attachment-informed EMDR was used to reprocess each of the key targets identified from his childhood.

After session 12, with his key childhood targets reprocessed, Ray attended his second underground retreat, this time accompanied by his wife. On the first night on ayahuasca, Ray struggled to let go, feeling very protective of other members of the group. On the second night on mescaline, in what he described as "a blood splatter," Ray re-experienced all his trauma in an instant. This distanced perspective gave him the insight needed to get a handle on the totality of his experiences. Upon his return, during PsyA-EMDR session 13, we used BLS whilst applying the Google search from R-TEPs to identify the key PODs from his most recent psychedelic retreat and unpacked how this related to his trauma history timeline. Standard protocol was then used against this list to address all the targets identified during history taking. The SUDs scored at a 0 and the VOC at a 7 for each of the targets before moving on to the next. At session 31, all significant adult traumas were addressed, and one final relational session was used to close.

Ray describes this intervention as "marking the end of his healing journey." At 61 years, he can now emotionally retire from his term in service. He intends to use the time and money that he has been using on getting psychological support to take his wife to Africa on safari.

For the medication phase

Stabilisation – Cornerstone 2
  "Tapping through spiders"

Jane, age 27, had been accessing EMDR therapy with a practitioner in private practice. Jane supplemented her therapy with therapeutic psychedelic experiences which she either did on her own or assisted by an untrained sitter. She also intermittently attended a local psychedelic community integration circle. Community integration circles are a group space that promotes the integration of psychedelic experiences into everyday life in a way that is meaningful to the individual. During Jane's 20-minute share with the integration group, she disclosed that she had been using psychedelics for over a decade. She described how she had found them helpful in healing trauma from childhood. Jane described herself as being disturbed from a young age. After spending time in foster care as an infant, Jane was later expelled from various schools, intermittently attending a pupil behavioural unit which she described as a "brutal environment." Healing from these experiences had come from exploring the inner depths of her psyche. A self-declared psychonaut, Jane had found LSD helpful in her early explorations but had changed to working with multi-dose smoked DMT sessions. She explained to the group that this had helped to "expose the latent unconscious content." During a recent experience, she had set the intention to experience unconditional love. To qualify love, the experience showed her everything that love was not. She described to the group how she was dragged through hellish realms, devoured by giant spiders and consumed by darkness only to be reborn and then devoured over and over again. Jane outlined how she had used the skills from her EMDR therapy to "tap her way through" the challenges that had emerged during her psychedelic sessions. She described how she had found this technique especially helpful as it stopped her avoidance of the difficult experiences. She also described how her resourcing figures and parts work had been especially helpful and that these resourcing experiences frequently appeared in her psychedelic dosing sessions. Jane continues to use EMDR therapy and the psychedelic integration community to integrate the content that emerges during the psychedelic sessions and to heal her deep relational wounds.

For psychedelic post-dose grounding and (re)stabilisation

Stabilisation – Cornerstone 3
"There is no such thing as a healthy Norm"

Norm was a healthy normal volunteer in his early 60s who had taken part in a safety testing phase 1 psychedelic clinical research trial. During screening, his mental health history had flagged up a diagnosis of autism, but this was not an excluding criterion for his participation. Physiologically, all had gone as expected for assessing the drug safety, with Norm's heart rate rising to 163 and blood pressure of 171 at the peak of the experience in what the physician described as a "reasonable stress response." These measures were within the study protocol safety parameters and matched Norm's phenomenological experience, albeit he described this as "difficult." For the first 15 minutes during drug administration, Norm exhibited extreme physical movement, tremors in his arms and hands and vigorous kicking to the extent that both of his legs left the bed. He was very aware of the physicality of his experience and described the somatic reaction as "distracting." Ten minutes in, Norm removed his blindfold and communicated with the clinical team present that he was experiencing a sense of fear/terror. Despite the high dose, Norm maintained full ego integrity throughout, although he experienced sense of a dread, which he later interpreted as a fear of his own death and described as a "deeply uncomfortable position." He also described how in that moment, his acute paranoia had led him to question "…This is so horrific… is this part of a cult? am I being sacrificed…?". "Blind terror" was how he referred to his emotional state.

Before the experience, Norm had described himself as a 'proud man.' Now, he grappled with a shift in his identity which he attributed to changes to his state of mind. He was experiencing somatic reactivations connected to the terror that he had experienced during the psychedelic dosing session. These somatic reactivations were especially pronounced when Norm fell asleep or when he transitioned between sleep states throughout the night. The terror state was frequently waking him up, and the resulting sleep deprivation was impacting his daily functioning and mental health. Reactivations causing sleep interruption were reported as a potential side effect of this psychedelic compound. Norm agreed that he needed extra support but was struggling to engage therapeutically with the framing of the experience in terms of either his current or historic problems. The clinical team were questioning how best to work with the energetic/somatic integration of the difficult experiences, which appeared to relate to transpersonal or somatically stored content.

Challenging psychological experiences/reactions are often unreported in psychedelic drug research. This participant was medically stabilised using pharmacological methods and signposted on to work with other healthcare agencies. The study psychiatrist expressed their frustration at not being able to offer EMDR to this participant as he sat outside of the clinical trials therapy manual. EMDR therapists would be well versed to work with such somatic reactivations. The traumatic psychedelic experience could be the target for reprocessing with the aim of resolving the flashbacks. Alternatively, a more comprehensive approach could utilise the somatic bridge to identify the pathogenic memories that correspond with the persistent death anxiety that he was experiencing. The standard protocol could then be used to reprocess and integrate this material and extinguish the fear response. This is similar to the way HPPD can be treated with EMDR.

Whilst many trials do offer good aftercare, the continuing unfolding nature of integration means that there may be times when participant follow-up is insufficient. Public healthcare services and community-led psychedelic integration circles continue to provide support to former participants, the exact cost of which remains to be determined. Psychometric assessments and study protocols don't assess for archetypal, intergenerational and cultural trauma that resides in the hearts and bodies of individuals. Underinvestigated epigenetic stressors will likely continue to put research participants and patients at risk as such issues will not be flagged up during history taking and case conceptualisation. This interpersonal trauma can be worked with using cognitive interweaves during EMDR reprocessing, giving positive outcomes to those adversely affected by their psychedelic experience. Greater awareness is needed within clinical teams and on the boards of ethics committees to build in more robust screening processes and to offer psychological alternatives for treating adverse reactions induced by psychedelic drugs.

For psychedelic integration

Stabilisation – Cornerstone 4
  "A model student, hungry for more"

Ofelia reached out for therapy following a difficult relationship break-up. At assessment, she described herself as a "perfectionist" with a "fear of failure," who needs to be "told what to do" and went on to describe how at times, she felt "completely overwhelmed." At 25, she was living at home with her mother, whom she described as "controlling." As a teenager, Ofelia had been hospitalised with anorexia nervosa. Although she described her eating disorder as "historic," Ofelia worked as a model and continued to struggle with body image and food restriction.

Ofelia was resistant to engage in conventional treatments relating to her eating disorder and exhibited symptoms of medical trauma that stemmed from her previous hospitalisations. After engaging with private talk therapy for several weeks, Ofelia recognised the potential benefits of reengaging with eating disorder services. She was told that she faced a long waiting list for accessing NHS support. In the interim, her privately funded therapy continued, and some standard protocol EMDR was introduced (intermittently) to facilitate trauma reprocessing (where tolerable). During which time, Ofelia was signposted to some novel clinical research investigating the potential of psychedelics in the treatment of anorexia. Six months into therapy, Ofelia was accepted as a research participant in the psilocybin for anorexia (Panorexia) clinical trial at Imperial College London (Spriggs, 2021). Ofelia was able to continue with her therapist alongside the trial, but EMDR reprocessing was paused to avoid introducing confounding variables into the data set.

The psychedelic research involved 3 closed-label doses of psilocybin, along with preparation and integration therapy and follow-ups. During these sessions, Ofelia experienced profound shifts in perspective, gaining insights into the underlying emotional and systemic triggers of her anorexia. Symbolic representations of her eating disorder emerged, manifesting as the Pale Man, a grotesque child-eating monster from Guillermo del Toro's film Pan's Labyrinth. From start to finish, the trial took place over a nine-month period, where the final follow-up took place six months after Ofelia's final dose of psilocybin. Ofelia found this research hospital setting to be a really triggering environment. The blue trays on which food was served illustrate one example of how her medical trauma manifested within the setting of the psychedelic experience. At the end of her participation in the trial, Ofelia was instructed to get some further CBT in relation to her disordered eating. As a model student, she buried herself in the self-help CBT for anorexia literature, until the NHS provision became available. Ofelia found the materials interesting but described how they didn't really address the somatic/strong emotional responses linked to her condition. Subsequently, the NHS provision became available; however, this CBT intervention was terminated after only a few sessions due to her medical trauma being retriggered by the hospital setting, rendering her unable to engage. She explained that CBT failed to address the underlying feelings of powerlessness or lack of control that she believes sit behind her eating disorder.

After disengaging from NHS services, Ofelia felt better able to fully embrace EMDR as a psychedelic integration tool. PsyA-EMDR was applied using the AIP-informed psychedelic integration procedure. Ofelia was clear from the outset that "she didn't want to do it" and this defence was the first target to be reprocessed using standard protocol EMDR. After which, the most distressing part of her psychedelic experience, the hallucination reminiscent of Pan's Labyrinth's Pale Man, was identified as a target for reprocessing. Using the somatic bridge technique, we traced this hallucination back to an early touchstone memory from childhood. In this memory, she had been overwhelmed by feelings of powerlessness when shopping for a pair of school shoes with her mother. This target took some time to reprocess and took her on a journey through her memory networks, exploring the complex attachment relationship with her mother and the intergenerational trauma of having had a parent who had been an adoptee. Once reprocessed, key elements of the trauma clusters relating to her intense academic schooling experiences and her later hospitalisations were also addressed. Upon revisiting the psilocybin experience, the previous processing had had a generalising effect. Psychedelic integration is an ongoing process, and the work has now shifted to address other pathological NCs present in her personality construct. A movement from "I am powerless" and "I am not in control" to "I am a failure" and "I did something wrong." The work systematically continues, following the 3-pronged approach, and EMDR is now well tolerated.

Integrating her psychedelic experiences has been a slow and unfolding process, demanding a significant degree of painful behavioural change. These behavioural shifts created blocks to recovery, uncovering systemic and secondary gains which retriggered disordered eating patterns. It has been a journey of two steps forwards and one step back. EMDR has been used to process each of these blocks as they emerge. To illustrate, the realisation that behavioural change would inevitably lead to a change in body shape emerged and was reprocessed. Behavioural change also led her to disentangle herself from co-dependent relationships. This was especially difficult. The gaslighting by professionals working in the modelling industry and a suicide attempt by her mother were especially triggering and could have derailed her recovery. EMDR has helped to reduce the triggers that would have previously caused sustained dysregulation. These layers of integration and recovery have been complex and multifaceted.

PsyA-EMDR integration therapy has facilitated a journey of integration through behavioural change that has taken her on a path through family breakdown, changes to financial security, temporary housing, relationship renegotiations, reconciliation with estranged family members, career changes, physical and menstrual changes and an identity metamorphosis. She recognises that at the time, her ED behaviours had become a resource, which she was able to turn to if she didn't feel that she was able to cope and that new resources needed to be found, as well as tools for widening her window of tolerance for stress. Indeed, it seems that the Pale Man has now become rich fertiliser for other resources that better support her. Ofelia no longer works as a low-BMI model. She has returned to education, went travelling in India and has trained as a yoga teacher. She is rebuilding her relationship with her body and routinely challenges her need for perfectionism and is moving towards financial independence. She has developed new friendships and has recently enrolled at university. None of these changes were captured in the Panorexia data set at the nine-month follow up (Spriggs, et al., 2021). This questions a need for longitudinal data sets when measuring the therapeutic impact of these treatments when coupled with long-term psychedelic integration therapy. Ofelia continues to make sense of her experiences; she volunteers for a UK-based psychedelic harm-reduction charity and is on a path to become a clinical psychologist.

References

Alting van Geusau, V. V. P., de Jongh.z, A., Nuijs, M. D., Brouwers, T. C., Moerbeek, M., & Matthijssen, S. J. M. A. (2023, Nov 9). The effectiveness, efficiency, and acceptability of EMDR vs. EMDR 2.0 vs. the Flash technique in the treatment of patients with PTSD: Study protocol for the ENHANCE randomized controlled trial. *Frontiers in Psychiatry, 14,* 1278052. https://doi.org/10.3389/fpsyt.2023.1278052.

Bernstein, E. M., & Putnam, F. W. (1986). Development, reliability and validity of a dissociation scale. *Journal of Nervous & Mental Disease, 174*(12), 727–735. https://doi.org/10.1097/00005053-198612000-00004

Breeksema, J., Kuin, B., Kamphuis, J., Van de Brink, W., Vermetten, E., & Schoevers, R. (2022). Adverse events in clinical treatments with serotonergic psychedelics and MDMA: A mixed-methods systematic review. *Journal of Psychopharmacology, 36*(10), 1100–1117. https://doi.org/10.1177/02698811221116926.

Carlson, E. B., & Putnam, F. W. (1993). An update on the Dissociative Experience Scale. *Dissociation, 6*(1), 16–27.

Christian, S. T. Benington, F., Morin, R. D., Corbett, M., & Corbett, L. (1975). Gas–liquid chromatographic separation and identification of biologically important indole alkylamines from human cerebrospinal fluid. *Biochemical Medicine, 14,* 191–200. https://doi.org/10.1016/0006-2944(75)90036-8

Cloitre, M., Shevlin, M., Brewin, C., Bisson, J., Roberts, N., Maercker, A., Karatzias, T., & Hyland, P. (2018). The international trauma questionnaire: development of a self-report measure of ICD-11 PTSD and complex PTSD. *Acta Psychiatrica Scandinavica, 138*(6), 536–546. https://doi.org/10.1111/acps.12956

Conte, H., Ratto, R., & Karasu, B. (1996). The psychological mindedness scale: Factor structure and relationship to outcome of psychotherapy. *Journal of Psychotherapy Practice and Research, 5*(3), 250–259.

DMT-Nexus Wiki Contributors. (2015). 5-MeO-DMT. *DMT-Nexus Wiki.* Found at https://wiki.dmt-nexus.me/w/index.php?title=5-MeO-DMT&oldid=14270. Accessed 20.12. 2023

Eichfeld, C., Farrell, D., & Mattheß, M. (2019). Trauma stabilisation as a sole treatment intervention for post-traumatic stress disorder in southeast Asia. *Psychiatry, 90,* 63–88. https://doi.org/10.1007/s11126-018-9598-z

Felitti, V. J., Anda, R. F., Nordenberg, D., Williamson, D. F., Spitz, A. M., Edwards, V., Koss, M. P., & Marks, J. S. (1998). Relationship of childhood abuse and household dysfunction to many of the leading causes of death in adults. The adverse childhood experiences (ACE) study. *American Journal of Preventive Medicine, 14*(4), 245–258. https://doi.org/10.1016/s0749-3797(98)00017-8

Fisher, J. (1999). The work of stabilisation in trauma treatment. The trauma centre at HRI, Boston, MA paper presented at the trauma centre lecture series 1999. Found at https://www.complextrauma.uk/uploads/2/3/9/4/23949705/the_work_on_stabilization_in_trauma_work.pdf. Accessed 29. 01. 2024

Gloster, A., Block, V., Klotsche, J., Villanueva, J., Rinner, M., Benoy, C., Walter, M., Karekla, M., & Bader, K. (2021). Psy-Flex: A contextually sensitive measure of psychological flexibility. *Journal of Contextual Behavioural Science, 22*, 13–23. htts://doi.org/10.1016/j.jcbs.2021.09.001

Grant, A. M., Franklin, J., & Langford, P. (2002). The self-refection and insight scale: a new measure of private self-consciousness. *Social Behaviour and Personality: Society for Personality Research, NSW, Australia, 30*(8), 821–836. https://dx.doi.org/10.2224/sbp.2002.30.8.821

Hofmann, A. (2009). The absorption technique. In M. Luber (Ed.), *Eye Movement Desensitization (EMDR) Scripted Protocols: Special Populations* (pp. 275–279). New York: Spinger Publishing Corporation. htts://doi.org/10.1891/9780826122452.0023

Janet, P. (1919). *Les médications psychologiques* (Vol. 3). Paris: Félix Alcan. (Reprint: Société Pierre Janet, Paris, 1984). English edition: Principles of Psychotherapy (Vol. 2)

Lima de Cruz, R. V., Moukin, T. C., Petiz, L. L., & Leão R. N. (2018). A single dose of 5-MeO-DMT stimulates cell proliferation, neuronal survivability, morphological and functional changes in adult mice ventral dentate gyrus. *Frontiers in Molecular Neuroscience, 11*, 312. https://doi.org/10.3389/fnmol.2018.00312

Littel, M., Kenemans, J. L., Baas, J. M., Logemann, H. A., Rijken, N., Remijn, M., & Van den Hout, M. A. (2017). The effects of β-adrenergic blockade on the degrading effects of eye movements on negative autobiographical memories. Biological *Psychiatry, 82*(8), 587–593. https://doi.org/10.1016/j.biopsych.2017.03.012

Manfield, P. E., Engel, L., Greenwald, R., & Bullard, D. G. (2021). Flash technique in a scalable low-intensity group intervention for COVID-19-related stress in healthcare providers. *Journal of EMDR Practice and Research, 15*(2), 127–139. https://doi.org/10.1891/EMDR-D-20-00053

Manfield, P. E., Taylor, G., Dornbush, E., Engel, L., & Greenwald, R. (2024). Preliminary evidence for the acceptability, safety, and efficacy of the flash technique. *Frontiers in Psychiatry, 14*, 1273704. https://doi.org/10.3389/fpsyt.2023.1273704

Mattheß, C., Farrell, D., Mattheß, M., Bumke, P., Sodemann, U., & Mattheß, H. (2019). The therapeutic value of trauma stabilisation in the treatment of post-traumatic stress disorder: A Southeast Asian study. *Asian Journal of Psychiatry, 41*, 45–49. https://doi.org/10.1016/j.ajp.2018.09.010

McAlpine, R., Blackburne, G., & Kamboj, S. K. (2023). Development and psychometric validation of a novel scale for measuring 'psychedelic preparedness'. Clinical Pharmacology Unit, University College London. Found at https://psyarxiv.com/gw9jp/ Accessed 29.01.2024

Medford, N., Sierra, M., Baker, D., & David, A. S. (2005). Understanding and treating depersonalisation disorder. *Advances in Psychiatric Treatment, 11*(2), 92–100. https://doi.org/10.1192/apt.11.2.92

Mitchell, A. (2023). *Ten Trips. The new reality of psychedelics.* London: Bodley Head.

Nagai, F., Nonaka, R., & Satoh Hisashi Kamimura, K. (2007). The effects of non-medically used psychoactive drugs on monoamine neurotransmission in rat brain. *European Journal of Pharmacology, 559*(2–3), 132–137. https://doi.org/10.1016/j.ejphar.2006.11.075

Nondu, L. (2024). Walking EMDR therapy (WET). Found at https://www.lorrainetindale.com/walking-emdr-therapy. Accessed 29.1.24

Ray, T. S. (2010). Psychedelics and the human recetorome. *PLOS One, 5*(2), e9019. https://doi.org/10.1371/journal.pone.009019

Rogawski, M. A., & Aghajanian, G. K. (1981). Serotonin autoreceptors on dorsal raphe neurons: structure-activity relationships of tryptamine analogs. *Journal of Neuroscience, 1* (10), 1148–1154. https://doi.org/10.1523/JNEUROSCI.01-10-01148.1981

Rothschild, B. (2002). The body remembers: An interview with Babette Rothschild. *Psychotherapy in Australia,* 8(2). Found at https://www.somatictraumatherapy.com/the-body-remembers-an-interview-with-babette-rothschild/. Accessed 29.1.24.

Shapiro, F. (2014). The role of Eye Movement Desensitization and Reprocessing (EMDR) therapy in medicine: Addressing the psychological and physical symptoms stemming from adverse life experiences. *The Permanente Journal, 18*(1), 71–77. https://doi.org/10.7812/TPP/13-098

Shapiro, R. (2005). The two-hand interweave. *EMDR solutions: Pathways to healing,* W.W. Norton & Company. 160–166. Shapiro, E., & Laub, B. (2015). Early EMDR intervention following a community critical incident: A randomized clinical trial. *Journal of EMDR Practice and Research, 9*(1), 17. https://doi.org/10.1891/1933-3196.9.1.17

Sheehan, D., Lecrubier, Y., & Sheehan, K. (1998). The mini-international neuropsychiatric interview (M.I.N.I.): The development and validation of a structured diagnostic psychiatric interview for DSM-IV and ICD-10. *Journal of Clinical Psychiatry, 59*(Suppl 20), 22–33.

Spriggs, M. J., Douglass, H. M., Park, R. J., Read, T., Danby, J. L., de Magalhães, F. J. C., Alderton, K. L., Williams, T. M., Blemings, A., Lafrance, A., Nicholls, D. E., Erritzoe, D., Nutt, D. J., & Carhart-Harris, R. L. (2021, Oct 20). Study protocol for psilocybin as a treatment for anorexia nervosa: A pilot study. *Frontiers in Psychiatry,12,* 735523. https://doi.org/10.3389/fpsyt.2021.735523.

Uthaug, M. V., Lancelotta, R., & van Oorsouw, K. (2019). A single inhalation of vapor from dried toad secretion containing 5-methoxy-*N*, *N*-dimethyltryptamine (5-MeO-DMT) in a naturalistic setting is related to sustained enhancement of satisfaction with life, mindfulness-related capacities, and a decrement of psychopathological symptoms. *Psychopharmacology, 236,* 2653–2666. https://doi.org/10.1007/s00213-019-05236-w

Varese, F., Sellwood, W., Aseem, S., Awenat, Y., Bird, L., Bhutani, G., Carter, L.A., Davies, C., Horne, G., Keane, D., Logie, R., Malkin, D., Potter, F., van den Berg, D., Zia, S., & Bentall, R. (2021, Oct.). Eye movement desensitization and reprocessing therapy for psychosis (EMDRp): Protocol of a feasibility randomized controlled trial with early intervention service users. *Early Intervention in Psychiatry, 15*(5), 1224–1233. https://doi.org/10.1111/eip.13071

Weathers, F. W., Blake, D. D., Schnurr, P. P., Kaloupek, D. G., Marx, B. P., & Keane, T. M. (2015). The clinician-administered PTSD scale for DSM-5 (CAPS-5) – Past Week [Measurement instrument]. Found at https://www.ptsd.va.gov/. Accessed 29.01.2024

Weathers, F. W., Litz, B. T., Keane, T. M., Palmieri, P. A., Marx, B. P., & Schnurr, P. P. (2013). The PTSD checklist for DSM-5 (PCL-5) – Standard [Measurement instrument]. Found at https://www.ptsd.va.gov/. Accessed 29.01.2024

Wöller, W., & Mattheß, H. (2016). ROTATE. Resource-orientated trauma therapy combined with EMDR resource installation. *Trauma Aid Germany*. Version 1.0, July 2016.

Zimmerman, C. (n.d.). Four blinks version of flash: An open approach to trauma reprocessing rapid memory reconsolidation resources. Found at https://fourblinks.com/. Accessed 23.01.2023

6   Preparation

MDMA
3,4-Methylenedioxymethamphetamine ($C_{11}H_{15}NO_2$)

DOI: 10.4324/9781003431718-6

3,4-Methylenedioxymethamphetamine, also known as MDMA or 'ecstasy,' was patented in 1914 by German pharmaceutical company Merck but was never marketed. The psychedelic chemist Alexander Shulgin introduced the compound to the psychedelic therapist Leo Zeff in 1976 in the wake of the government crackdown on the therapeutic use of LSD in the 1960s. Shulgin specialised in the phenethylamine family of drugs, a class of compounds with psychoactive and stimulant effects and said that MDMA was the closest he got to fulfilling his ambition of finding the perfect therapeutic drug (Shulgin & Shulgin, 1991). Meanwhile, its non-clinical use on the club scene expanded, and in response to this, the Drug Enforcement Administration (DEA) categorised it as a Schedule I drug in 1985, which restricted any further opportunities for research. The Multidisciplinary Association for Psychedelic Studies (MAPS) was set up in response to the embargo on clinical research and is now at the forefront of global research into the therapeutic uses of MDMA.

MDMA is not a 'classic' psychedelic but is an entactogen that predominantly impacts the serotonin system in the brain. It has a gentler, shorter acting effect than LSD and is easily tolerated. It acts by releasing serotonin, noradrenalin and dopamine, attenuating feelings of depression and anxiety and reducing the amygdala fear response. The relaxation effect of its effects at the alpha-2 receptors is thought to be beneficial for trauma-induced hypervigilance and the raised levels of awareness and empathy are thought to promote fear extinction (Sessa et al., 2019). MDMA has been shown to increase levels of the neuropeptide oxytocin, a hormone that plays a pivotal role in early mother-infant bonding, which is key to its potential use in attachment-informed EMDR therapy. This is thought to be linked to the action of MDMA on 5-HTP$_{1A}$ receptors in areas of the hypothalamus that are responsible for exerting control over the release of oxytocin (Thompson et al., 2007).

Its widespread use as an illicit drug is attributed to MDMA's acute effect on sociability. It has been suggested that modern rave culture is a continuation of group ritual seen across the globe in indigenous cultures, involving dancing to repetitive drum beats combined with psychoactive substances (Winkelman, 2021). Fatal overdoses are rare, but there are risks posed by increases in blood pressure, dehydration (when used in combination with vigorous exercise) and hypothermia. It is considered psychologically but not physically addictive, and chronic administration of MDMA has been linked to cardiac valvulopathy (Droogmans, 2007).

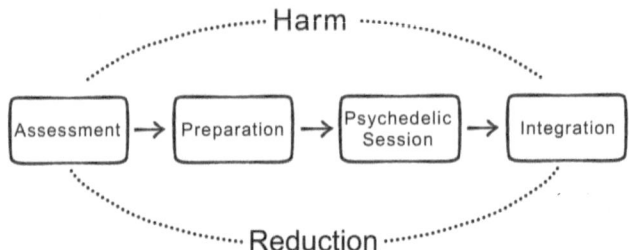

Figure 6.1 Harm reduction throughout the stages of psychedelic assisted therapy.

Preparation in psychedelic-assisted therapy is a term that broadly refers to the phase prior to a psychedelic medication session and aims to ready the individual for the upcoming psychedelic treatment. Psychedelic preparation has a rich history that intertwines historical contexts with cultural and spiritual practices. Contemporary psychedelic preparation is informed by threads that originate from religious ceremonies dating back to ancient civilisations, rituals from countless indigenous cultures, westernised social and cultural influences from the mid-20th century, techniques from psychedelic therapy research, as well as initiatives from contemporary drug harm-reduction strategies. Whilst preparation methods vary, and continue to evolve, the shared element that is interwoven throughout is that a thoughtful and intentional approach to embarking upon a psychedelic experience can enhance positive outcomes and minimise potential risks. The importance of this preliminary phase was highlighted during research in the mid-20th century, and current clinical research reveals that comprehensive preparation is associated with positive outcomes in PAP (Thal, et al., 2022). Despite a growing body of evidence, the length and depth of preparation for psychedelic therapy varies dramatically across the field, and some settings do not offer it at all.

In PAP trials, a full psychiatric assessment is used as a screening tool and is generally carried out prior to the preparation phase. Any additional information that is gleaned during preparation is also used to screen participants. Despite this, significant psychological factors such as adoption and dissociated childhood trauma have reportedly been missed on trials and are likely to have contributed to some of the adverse reactions reported. In private practice, underground settings and in other contexts where a full psychiatric assessment (conducted by a psychiatrist) is not available, the preparation phase is the only opportunity to screen people for suitability. Many underground PAP providers only include a basic screening process, which may include a short health questionnaire and a brief overview of mental health/trauma history. See Chapter 5, 'Stabilisation,' for an overview of screening and a list of contraindications.

Consistent preparation is crucial, because it aims to optimise the effects of any treatment, by creating optimal conditions (internal and external) for the experience. The core elements of the preparation phase include:

Establishing the therapeutic relationship – The need for relational containment is essential, irrespective of whether the therapist is able to accompany the individual during a psychedelic medication phase. The therapeutic relationship will contain any challenges that arise before, during and after a psychedelic experience.

Gathering information – This is a way to develop a deeper understanding of the participant's presenting issues and history whilst strengthening the therapeutic relationship. It also gives a sense of what may emerge during the dosing session.

Educating the participant – AIP-focused, trauma-informed psychoeducation is a baseline to any preparatory work. Clarifying expectations about the experience and exploring what might be expected, including the logistics of the session. Familiarisation with the setting, such as seeing the treatment room, can be helpful at this point.

Establishing harm-reduction measures – Mindfulness-based attentional training. Teaching grounding techniques and training embodiment through guided visualisations. Explaining practicalities of safety measures e.g., how the therapist/sitter will intervene if the participant becomes distressed. A contracted commitment to stay in the session throughout the duration of the acute drug effects is also essential at this stage.

Contracting – Establishing agreed boundaries of interaction between the participant and therapist during medication session. The use of safety touch will be rehearsed, along with discussions about how toilet breaks and physical needs will be navigated. This includes discussions around the use/absence of 'therapeutic touch.' See Chapter 4, 'Ethics,' for further discussion.

Obtaining informed consent – This is a legal requirement for all treatments in medical settings. In medical contexts, consent is described as an ongoing process and can be withdrawn at any time. The dynamic nature of PAP adds complexity to these dynamics which need to be explored during preparation.

(Mind)set and setting

The set and setting hypothesis asserts that a drug experience can be significantly influenced by crucial factors in the physical environment and in the psychological mindset. This is at odds with the basic principle of pharmacology that drugs exert relatively standardised effects on individuals to whom they are administered (Farinde, 2021). Research into the phenomena of the 'placebo effect' highlights the importance of mindset, and it is widely accepted within the field of pharmacology that this is responsible for a significant part of the therapeutic benefits of a wide variety of drug treatments (e.g. Brown, 2012).

In traditional healing rituals with entheogens, shamans influence the set and setting through the performance of traditional songs, smoke/burning rituals, chanting and drumming. The internal mindset is also shaped through preparation by fasting, sexual abstinence and engaging in customs and rituals in the lead up to a plant medicine ceremony (Winkelman & White, 1987). Some of these rituals have made their way into western PAP, for example, the use of smudging sticks, an indigenous tool for energy cleansing, but there is some debate about the cultural misappropriation of such methods.

The restriction of food prior to a treatment often forms part of PAP protocols and for good logistical reasons (such as reducing nausea, vomiting and other purgative reactions). The reintroduction of 'clean foods' after a psychedelic treatment is often overlooked in western PAP, albeit this is often ritualised in indigenous cultures (e.g. the 'dieta' in the ayahuasca traditions). This book does not have the scope to explore this area in sufficient depth; however, there is a wealth of literature available on this topic and it remains an untapped topic for future investigation.

The set (or mindset) refers to a participant's inner psychological processes but also extends to include the psychological processes of sitter/therapists, the personalities of those who are present, as well as any intentions for the treatment, and any preparation work that has been done prior to the psychedelic session. In research settings, there is a focus on the (mind) set whilst the impact of the setting is somewhat underinvestigated. In part this is due to constraints of RCTs which aim to minimise any variables in order that the compounds can be rigorously assessed. This is regrettable, because the evidence suggests that optimising the setting can improve psychotherapeutic effects and minimise the harm that is experienced during drug testing.

The use of eye masks, often combined with music, reduces the impact of variability in experimental settings. Stanislav Grof was credited as the first to use this combination as a means of encouraging participants to engage with their own internal process. This developed from his early work where the therapist engaged more with the client, which he later believed detracted from the deeper internal work that was deemed to be necessary for healing outcomes (Grof, 1980). Psychedelic administration rooms in clinical trials are often adorned with various new-age paraphernalia, such as mandala wall hangings, tie-dyed throws, cushions, salt lamps and faux-plants. However, soft lighting and comfortable furnishings in a relaxed atmosphere, with minimal interruption from external stimulus, is considered to be an adequate setting for PAP delivery, encouraging participants to go inwards into their own internal process. Safe access to an outdoor/natural environment might also be beneficial, should the need for nature-based stabilisation arise.

PsyA-EMDR preparation

History taking and preparation (phases 1 and 2) form a key tenant of standard EMDR protocol. These screening and preparatory processes have developed in complexity over the past 30 years to meet the needs of increasingly complex presentations. The stabilisation and resourcing interventions that have developed are based on developmental neuroscience, utilising the therapeutic relationship and the imaginal space to heal attachment wounds and increasing the client's capacity for self-regulation. The concept of preparing a client for potential dysregulation, caused by any trauma that re-emerges during reprocessing, is emphasised as a fundamental element during the basic EMDR training. Below illustrates how the core components of EMDR align with those of the preparation phase in PAP:

Assessing readiness

- o Screening
- o Building relational rapport
- o Psychoeducation to establish boundaries, contracting and informed consent
- o Co-creating an AIP informed case conceptualisation
- o Setting intention based on the goals for therapy
- o Resourcing
- o Embodiment training

PsyA-EMDR phase 1: history taking/assessment

The history-taking phase of PsyA-EMDR should resemble a psychiatric evaluation and form part of the psychotherapeutic process, whilst also acting as a screening tool. The main goals of history taking are:

- to evaluate the severity of symptoms;
- to establish the most prominent underlying negative beliefs about the self and negative emotions that manifest in response to the trauma/attachment history;

- to establish the most prominent underlying negative beliefs about the self that manifest in response to triggers in the present;
- to assess personality structure and use the AIP model to cocreate a case conceptualisation, highlighting emergent patterns of behaviour (self-awareness through psychoeducation enhances patient empowerment);
- to explore the healthy and resilient parts of the self (strengthening adaptive networks with bilateral stimulation of the brain [BLS]);
- to understand motives for change (goals for therapy/intentions) and motives for not changing (secondary gain);
- and to assess levels of dissociation/fragmentation of the psyche.

The interpersonal dynamic of 'client as the expert of their own experience' is a core psychotherapeutic intervention and fosters an environment of co-creation, trust and mutual respect which serves to fortify the therapeutic relationship. The therapist invites the client to share their experience with non-judgemental curiosity, deepening the core themes by asking questions about the felt experience. The therapist facilitates a psychodynamic exploration of the material through the lens of the AIP model, highlighting patterns and linking these back to their formative childhood experiences.

Revealing the fractals

Throughout phase 1 history taking, a skill that merits special mention is the ability to identify the patterns of experience that emerge in the information that is given. In other words, having the ability to zoom out from complex information and observe the broader themes of strong emotions and self-referencing beliefs that emerge from the networks, paving the way for the phenomenology of the psychedelic experience. In amongst the chaos there will be repeating, self-similar patterns that can often be traced back to early childhood (and beyond!).

"As above, so below"

Case conceptualisation

The process of individualised case conceptualisation, using the AIP model, is a fundamental component of EMDR that can be adapted for psychedelic-assisted therapy to optimise outcomes by keeping the work focused on the client's goals. In addition to the basic EMDR training, a solid understanding of the AIP model is required for this phase to effectively tailor the work to the client's goals for therapy/presenting issue(s).

The therapeutic alliance can be strengthened through the process of co-creating a treatment plan. The strength of the therapeutic relationship is particularly important if the therapist is accompanying them during the psychedelic session, but it is also vital for stabilisation, risk reduction and ongoing integration therapy. Relational safety is necessary for the participant to trust and relinquish control of the situation, allowing them to engage with the experience on a deep emotional level. The case conceptualisation process is broadly the same as in standard EMDR, whereby the client's presenting symptoms and goals for therapy are cross-referenced with their trauma and attachment history to clarify the associative memory networks that are to be targeted. As in standard EMDR, the memory network that is to be targeted is defined by the feeling and negative cognition (NC) that represents it. For example, a client states that their goal for treatment is to 'have better relationships.' The symptoms that they present within their interpersonal relationships is that they struggle to commit to partners for fear of getting hurt. The NC that they choose that represents this issue is 'I cannot trust anyone.' During the history-taking phase, there are a number of memories that have the same theme of trust, the earliest of which is their father leaving suddenly when they were six years old. The NC they ascribe to this memory is also 'I cannot trust anyone.'

As with standard EMDR, the history-taking phase is used to assess the levels of trauma and fragmentation of the psyche, either through use of dissociation scales (e.g. DES-II) or questioning around the topic whilst monitoring the client's presentation in the room (particularly their capacity to disclose difficult material). Dissociation is also assessed by asking the client to check in with their body, assessing the levels of embodiment experienced when talking about traumatic material. The amount of previous trauma-focussed therapy, including alternative therapies, will impact their levels of embodiment. Assessing their emotional vocabulary can also be helpful. Any indicators can then be cross-referenced with information about their early childhood and attachment history. Information gathered about the complexity of the individual's presentation will determine the initial pacing of the work. The suggested four preparation sessions with EMDR should be extended if necessary. The following case conceptualisation tool can support the harvesting of any such information.

See Chapter 5, 'Stabilisation and Risk Reduction,' for contraindications, screening tools and assessment scales. See Chapter 12, 'The Future of PsyA-EMDR,' for information about the PsyA-EMDR decision-making matrix.

Another core aim of this phase is to understand the client's relationship with psychedelics. Were any previous psychedelic experiences spontaneous or planned? Were they taken in a therapeutic setting with intention or recreationally? What was the experience like for them and what emerged? Is

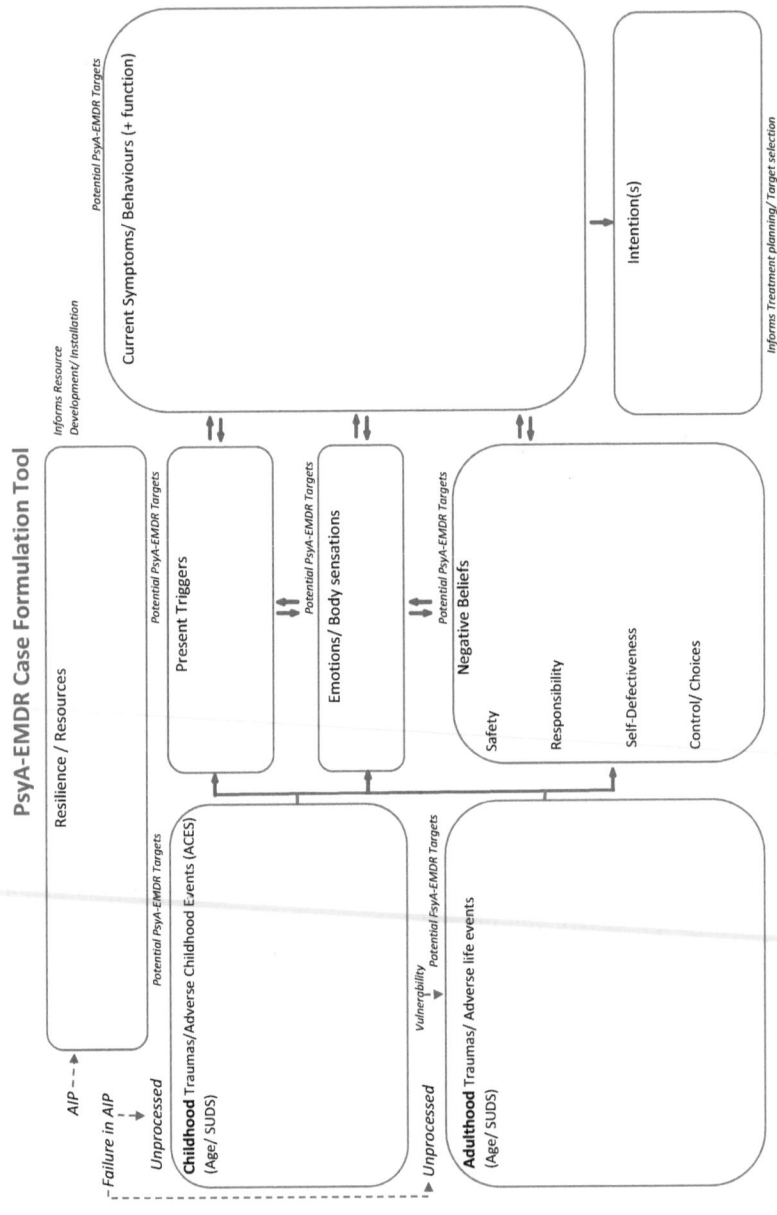

Figure 6.2 Case conceptualisation tool. Adapted from Santos (2019).

there any unresolved content that they are unable or unwilling to address? It is possible to work with any material from historic psychedelic experiences with EMDR? (as it is likely to inform subsequent work). If there are positive experiences, these can be installed using BLS. If there are any difficult experiences, an image, sound, thought or feeling can be bridged from to access the unconscious material. See Chapter 10, 'Working with Historic content.'

Intention setting

In the field of psychedelic therapy, participants are encouraged to formulate an 'intention' for the psychedelic experience with the aim of keeping the work focused on their goal for therapy. In PAP trials, the intention is rarely revisited during the treatment phase and can be overlooked during integration. Such intentions are phrased into statements, questions or requests, for example, 'what is holding me back in my career?' The AIP model can be used to dig deeper into this and identify the NC that corresponds with the block to progressing in their career, for example, 'I am a failure' or 'I'm not good enough.' In PsyA-EMDR, co-exploration of the client's goals, through the AIP lens, can elucidate their intention to keep the work focused, particularly in the psychedelic treatment phase. Dig down into the issue and encourage the client to clarify the NC that's been imprinted by their past traumas or the NC that is stopping them from overcoming their presenting issue(s). They can then create an intention (similar to the positive cognition [PC] used in standard EMDR) in response to this.

In standard protocol EMDR, defining the memory network that is being targeted, and the corresponding NC and PC, is key to the individualised case conceptualisation process. In PsyA-EMDR, defining the client's intention for the psychedelic treatment is an adapted version of this process that uses languages adopted from the field of PAP. The co-created case conceptualisation is used to formulate the intention in the same way that they are used traditionally (looking for themes in your life that you want to change). However, using the AIP model will hone into the theme and the root of the issue more precisely. For example, instead of vague, non-specific intentions such as 'to heal from my past traumas' or to 'overcome my depression,' ask the client "what is the negative belief that you have about yourself now, based upon these experiences?" or "what is the negative belief that you have about yourself that stops you from overcoming your depression?" It can be helpful to have a list of generic positive and negative beliefs (schemas) to show the client so they can see what might best fit.

Goal	To have better relationships
Presenting issue	Struggles to commit to partners for fear of getting hurt
Negative cognition for presenting issue	'I cannot trust anyone'
Touchstone memory (same network)	Father leaving suddenly at age six
Targeted PsyA-EMDR intention	'To learn to trust others'

During psycholytic PsyA-EMDR, the intention can be used to activate the memory network that corresponds with the client's treatment goal(s) at the beginning of the acute stage of a psychedelic session. See Chapter 7, 'Psycholytic EMDR.' The intention replaces the PC and acts as adaptive information in the network. It serves as a reminder of the purpose of the work and to keep things on track. It is common for participants' minds to wander under the influence of even low-medium dose psychedelics, so having a solid intention that can be reconnected with throughout the experience can refocus the work back to therapeutic purposes and help maintain the window of tolerance. The intention can be revisited throughout the work, but it is suggested that the VOC scale is only useful in the preparatory and integration sessions (as in child and adolescent protocols), because it can cause confusion when swapping between VOC and SUD scales during the psychedelic medication phase.

Examples of intentions

Targeted memory network	*Intention*
Responsibility – Guilt	
I should have done something	Self-compassion
I did something wrong	To love myself without fear of judgement
I should have known better	To connect with/forgive my inner child
Responsibility – Self-defectiveness	
I'm a bad person	Self-forgiveness
I am shameful	Learn to love myself
I do not deserve	Learn to make my needs known
Safety/venerability	
I'm in danger	To connect with the safety of the present
I cannot stand up for myself	To safely connect with my body/emotions
I cannot trust...	Learn to trust myself
Control/choice	
I'm not in control	Learn to trust myself/trust others
I am powerless	Improve my relationships
I do not trust myself/others	To trust the process and let go

PsyA-EMDR phase 2: resourcing and stabilisation

Traditional PAP prepares participants to navigate strong emotional content that may surface during a psychedelic treatment by encouraging radical acceptance of what emerges, with the belief that whatever is happening is supposed to happen (Cosimano, 2021). Participants are taught specific self-regulation techniques such as breath awareness, positive mantras such as the famous Bill Richards' quote: "trust, let go and be open" and interpersonal grounding such as hand holding. Other mindfulness-based interventions are utilised in an effort to encourage embodiment but inadequately prepare people for strong somatic and psychological responses to psychedelics. We propose that the resourcing phase of EMDR therapy supplements these interventions, offering a comprehensive range of interventions to regulate affect that can be targeted to meet individualised needs. In addition, information from the case conceptualisation can be used to target specific deficits of care in early attachment relationships which led to the formation of these maladaptive memory networks and increase affect regulation capacity.

Resourcing in PsyA-EMDR aims to develop adequate psychological resources to be able to navigate any dysregulation experienced during a psychedelic session. Establishing intersubjective safety in the present through the development of a stable therapeutic relationship, based on trust, is core to any trauma work but is particularly important if the therapist is accompanying the client during a psychedelic session. This highlights an area of risk, where the requirement for continuity of care cannot be fulfilled, particularly in situations where individuals attend retreats or treatment centres and their primary therapist is either absent, or there is a lack of adequate handover between care teams. This lack of cohesion erodes the therapeutic container, increasing the risk of harm.

Achieving psychological stability prior to a psychedelic treatment is essential to optimise the psychotherapeutic outcomes. During the stabilisation phase, EMDR clients are trained in various mindfulness-based grounding and relaxation exercises as well as distancing and stress-management practices. Imaginative distancing techniques aim to reduce dysregulation by increasing their sense of control and safety, for example, the well-established 'safe place' and 'container' exercises and interventions to refocus attention away from activating internal material in order to reduce distress. The client choses the strategies that work best for them, perhaps creating a self-care plan to make it part of their daily routine. This can also include activities like journaling, yoga and physical exercise. Therapists should encourage clients to practise their chosen techniques prior to a psychedelic treatment so they are familiar with the interventions. See Chapter 5, 'Stabilisation and Risk Reduction.'

Peaceful place: a personalised visualisation designed for grounding.

Resource team: nurturing, protective and wise figures.

Ideal parents: if the client struggles to create an adequate resource team, for example, some people with severe attachment trauma may only choose animals. Co-create a list of qualities that they would have liked their parents to have, then use this to construct parental figures.

Mastery experiences: if the client is anxious about their psychedelic treatment, adaptive information from mastery experiences can be strengthened.

Tip!

Research has shown that the vividness of sensory details of the mental imagery determines the number of brain subregions recruited (Schmidt & Blankenburg, 2019). Therefore, the more detail in the imagery resources the better (e.g. the peaceful place), so that all the senses are recruited when describing a resource, to elicit the strongest felt sense possible = more adaptive information encoded.

Use of the imaginal space

Neuroimaging studies have shown that imagining an experience fires up the parts of the brain that correspond with actually having that experience. The somatosensory motor regions have been repeatedly shown to be activated when imagining engaging in activities that would activate these regions (Schmidt & Blankenburg, 2019). This is why we utilise the imaginal space to stabilise the nervous system through neurobiologically informed, trauma-focused visualisations. The combination of ego state work and attachment-informed interventions empower the client to tend to their attachment wounds and stabilise their own nervous system in preparation for their psychedelic session. For clients with more complex trauma histories that impair their affect regulation capacity, EMDR interventions that target structural dissociation, such as 'The Progressive Approach' (Gonzalez & Mosquera, 2012), 'Ego State Interventions' (Shapiro, 2016) or complex PTSD interventions designed to work with dissociation from the 'EMDR Toolbox' (Knipe, 2018), can be used to work with structural dissociation. Other ego state modalities such as transactional analysis (Berne, 1961) or Internal Family Systems (Schwartz, 1997) can also be integrated with EMDR to stabilise individuals in preparation for a psychedelic treatment.

During this phase, psychological resources are enhanced by recalling positive memories, personal achievements and role models who embody nurturing, protective or wise qualities (Korn & Leeds, 2002). The addition of slow BLS is used during resource instillation to enhance memory representation, increase comfortable feelings about pleasant memories and facilitate relaxation. Slow BLS can also be used as a grounding tool, because it has been shown to downregulate the prefrontal cortex (Amano & Toichi, 2016). A comprehensive guide to attachment-informed EMDR resourcing can be found in a number of publications by Laurel Parnell (e.g. Parnell, 2013)

The Inner Healer (Grof, 1980)

The concept of the inner healer is described in the MAPS manual as an individual's "innate capacity to heal wounds of trauma" (Mithoefer, 2017). This concept is presented in both EMDR and psychedelic literature, because both establish the optimum conditions to evoke positive change and engage what Shapiro referred to as the 'inherent system' (Shapiro, 2002) that moves towards integration. This inner healing intelligence can be embodied in the 'wise' figure of the inner resource team through the minor adjustment of the name and their qualities.

Collection of objects

In the 1960s, Grof encouraged PAP participants to bring pictures of family members with them into sessions to activate unconscious memories underlying the symptoms. In neo-shamanic psychedelic ceremonies, the facilitators often construct an 'altar' that consists of items of personal significance, along with symbolic items from various indigenous and religious settings. Even in westernised settings, incense, sage smudging sticks, drums, statues of deities and spiritual iconography from across the globe are commonplace in psychedelic ceremonies. Some of these items are also found in clinical research settings. PsyA-EMDR participants are encouraged to bring a collection of physical objects that represent their resources and symbolise their intention(s) into the psychedelic session. For example, they might choose a heart-shaped rock to represent their intention to learn to trust others. Photos or images are also useful, but multi-sensory physical objects (that recruit multiple brain subregions) can be especially useful in the throes of a difficult psychedelic experience. For example, an item from childhood like a security blanket or teddy bear can be useful, or something that represents a significant event or person in their life. These resource items can be used for grounding whereby the physical sensation of an object can be particularly useful during the acute period when eyesight might be compromised in a dimly lit room or when vision might be compromised by acute drug effects. As well as being items for grounding, they can also be used to activate targeted memory networks and allow the corresponding maladaptive memories to emerge. The items can be arranged as a constellation and explored before dosing or with the therapist during psycholytic therapy if appropriate.

Establishing boundaries/expectations

This section is most relevant if the therapist is going to be supporting the client during the psychedelic session, but such psychoeducation is also useful for individuals attending treatments elsewhere.

Establishing clear boundaries and managing expectations is of paramount importance. All modalities necessitate a deliberate and comprehensive contractual agreement between the therapist, the participant and the psychedelic medication setting. This contractual framework serves as a foundational guide that delineates the scope and limits of the therapeutic encounter. Roles, responsibilities, rights, limitations and expectations all need to be explored to foster a secure and containing environment. Well-defined boundaries promote the safety and wellbeing of the individual, the therapist and the setting, so that all parties can navigate the emotionally intense experiences with grace. Psychedelics intensify emotional content, and so there is a need for a robust structure where vulnerabilities are clearly communicated and adaptions negotiated, all of which serve to further enhance the therapeutic alliance. Cultivating a culture where potential challenges can be worked with, and where all post dose experiences are all welcome, merits special attention. Mistake-friendly environments engender this outcome, through transformative reflective practice, maximising the potential of each experience as an opportunity to learn can further develop and refine the transformative effects of these treatments.

Touch

While the use of pre-contracted therapeutic touch is often utilised in PAP, trauma-informed practice necessitates a wider discussion around the implications of using bodywork during the psychedelic encounter. EMDR therapists work without the need for therapeutic touch so as to mitigate for any risk of therapeutic intrusion into the individual's process. Safer alternatives such as grounding objects, weighted blankets and handheld beanbags can be used to ensure adherence to consensual boundary management. The use of safety touch (such as physical support to access a toilet) needs to be agreed and rehearsed where possible. Where there is a personal preference for the use of therapeutic touch, body psychotherapists who are adequately trained to deliver such interventions can be accessed through alternative specialised treatment pathways. For a more comprehensive discussion on this subject, see Chapter 4, 'Ethics.'

PsyA-EMDR phases 3–8 (pre medication): reprocessing as a preparation and screening tool

PAP guidelines indicate that participants should be prepared for the range of somatic and emotional subjective experiences that may arise during a psychedelic treatment. This is achieved through the use of metaphor, guided visualisations, breathwork, sharing testimonials from prior participants or through psychoeducation.

We propose that PsyA-EMDR offers an alternative, comprehensive preparatory phase for psychedelic treatments, because reprocessing trauma using BLS can be used to assess readiness on a number of levels:

- It tests the client's tolerance for dysregulation of the nervous system. How they react during and after the session is an indicator of this.
- It flags any missed dissociation issues in a more controlled environment than a psychedelic session (EMDR can be stopped at any point).
- EMDR is a somatic therapy and therefore the client is not just practising embodiment through a guided visualisation, instead they are connecting with stored somatic stress responses and directly faced with negotiating embodiment whilst the nervous system is activated. This prepares the client for the potential dysregulation cause by a psychedelic treatment.
- If a client severely abreacts during well-managed reprocessing, this indicates that they may need further preparation sessions and may need to postpone the psychedelic treatment.
- An alternative to this is opting for a psychedelic medication that is more conducive to working with complex trauma, such as MDMA.
- Or they may consider microdosing/macrodosing alongside therapy as a safety precaution to ascertain their tolerability.

The key reason for using EMDR reprocessing as a precursor to psychedelic therapy is for risk reduction and harm minimalisation. The transient hyperplastic states caused by serotonergic psychedelics appear to remove psychological barriers to past trauma that were originally constructed to avoid overwhelm. The developmental differences between individuals means not everyone is able to withstand the impact of removing their defence mechanisms. This is particularly acute when there is a large volume of unintegrated/compartmentalised trauma, as is often seen in clients with extensive trauma histories, in whom there is a risk of overwhelm and flooding of the nervous system. A common saying heard in the field of PAP is that 'there is no such thing as a bad trip' and any adverse effects are just a 'spiritual emergence,' in which, if handled correctly, the individual can be guided through to a place of stability. But in practice this is not the case, and this belief can lead to secondary victimisation of those who already have an impaired ability to re-establish themselves into their window of tolerance.

Choice of target for preparation phase reprocessing

It can be helpful to choose a target for the preparation phase that is oriented towards the client's intention (goal for therapy), their connection with psychological resources or blocks preventing their connection to their resources. Alternatively, if they have anticipatory anxiety about the psychedelic treatment, the somatic bridge can be used to identify the biographical material that is being reactivated, or a flash forward can be used to process their anticipatory fear. For example:

- Identify the thought (NC), feeling and sensation and image that are triggered by the prospect of psychedelic treatment.
- Rate the strength of activation using the SUD scale.
- Use the somatic bridge to identify the biographical information that has been reactivated.
- The standard protocol, with attachment-informed re-scripting, can be used to desensitise and reprocess the maladaptively stored material.
- Ask the client to re-assess the trigger (the prospect of psychedelic therapy) using the SUD scale. If the target is sufficiently reprocessed, the SUDs will be lower. **This also serves as the perfect opportunity to demonstrate the AIP model experientially.**

If the SUDs are not completely reduced, you can:

- Bridge back again and reprocess another target
  and/or
- Use the flash forward protocol (Logie & De Jong, 2014)

Then a future template can be installed of them handling the psychedelic treatment in a way they would like following the three-pronged approach. Alternatively, if the client has already defined their goal/intention, define the NC linked to this and target this memory network using the somatic bridge with the standard protocol.

Troubleshooting – and Indications to slow down!

The indicators below can be used to determine the pacing of the work and whether to extend the beyond four sessions for preparation. If in doubt, err on the side of caution. See Chapter 5, 'Stabilisation and Risk Reduction,' for a list of contraindications.

Issue	*Action*
Significantly impaired affect regulation capacity	Delay psychedelic treatment until able to tolerate reprocessing.
Prone to dissociation	Delay psychedelic treatment until sufficient amount of attachment-informed EMDR to develop capacity for embodiment.
No previous integration of trauma	Closely monitor reaction to pre-psychedelic EMDR reprocessing to ascertain tolerance.
Significant amount of blank memory from childhood	Be very cautious. This can lead to flooding/overwhelm during psychedelic therapy. Spend more time doing EMDR before proceeding.
Abreaction to reprocessing in between sessions	Stabilise and slow down. Spend more time on resourcing phase before proceeding.
Lack of support network	Work on this in preparation phase. Introduce to group integration circles etc. if appropriate.
Unable to tap into felt sense of safety	Spend more time resourcing with attachment-informed interventions until enough adaptive information created in memory networks.
Difficulty creating resource team	Spend more time in preparation phases before proceeding.

Note Any of the above alone do not necessarily indicate that the individual is unsuitable for psychedelic therapy. It is suggested that these issues, combined with information the clinician has obtained from the assessment session, should be added to the AIP-informed case conceptualisation to determine the pacing of the work and help the client make an informed choice about their treatment. Certain issues, such as severe dissociation, may warrant pausing any plans for psychedelic therapy until enough attachment-informed EMDR has been done to stabilise the nervous system. Psychedelics are not necessarily completely ruled out; instead treatments such as the empathogen MDMA might be more appropriate to first develop a felt sense of safety.

eMDMAdr – MDMA-assisted EMDR as a preparation tool

MDMA creates a sense of safety and sociability (Bedi et al., 2009) and can be used in conjunction with attachment-informed EMDR interventions to target attachment deficits. Reports suggest that the feelings of safety and connectedness elicited by MDMA can be used to enhance the resourcing phases of EMDR therapy by creating adaptive memories in the networks with a strong embodied component. The mild psychedelic effects, combined with an increased sense of wellbeing, mean that it is gentler than typical psychedelics like psilocybin or LSD. This PAP is an ideal candidate for the treatment of clients with complex trauma histories because of its suppression of amygdala activation, resulting in a decreased fear response. In a psychotherapeutic setting, this can be used to target attachment deficits by creating emotionally salient experiences (Schmid & Liecht, 2018). For example, connecting with the nurturer from their resource team in the imaginal space (Parnell, 2013) can be used to create an embodied memory of a co-regulating attachment relationship. The felt sense of connectedness and relational safety can be enhanced through the addition of MDMA to create a memory of that feeling. A variety of attachment-informed interventions can be used in the stabilisation and resourcing phase of PsyA-EMDR to create adaptive information/felt experiences in the memory networks to facilitate stabilisation of the nervous system during reprocessing.

Subjective reports of 'eMDMAdr' state that the substance allowed a deeper connection with feelings of safety that had not been experienced due to unstable attachments in childhood. An anonymous individual, who shared their experience of eMDMAdr, stated:

> "I noticed how infrequently I allow myself to feel safe,
> and it felt really nice"

Support messages from the resource team

When the client connects with their resource team/ideal parents in the peaceful place, it can be useful to encourage them to ask their team for any messages of encouragement or wisdom to take with them on their psychedelic journey. The feelings of sociability and wellbeing elicited by MDMA, combined with the activation of a previously specified memory network, encourage messages of support that counteract the trauma. For example, in a case of pathological independence, the resource team said:
> "You've got this, and we've got you!"

Summary

EMDR therapy is well established in the field of trauma and the approach been honed over the past 40 years to treat a wide range of psychological presentations. Over this time, the three-pronged approach has been refined through experimental clinical practice to support individuals with varying levels of dysregulation, and progressive approaches have emerged to address structural dissociation and facilitate reprocessing with complex cases. The preparation phases of EMDR have been developed to support clients to withstand the dysregulation caused by reprocessing traumatic memories and can easily be adapted to support people embarking on psychedelic treatments. Creative use of the imaginal space can resource clients and prepare them for psychedelics. The combination of EMDR with specific compounds, such as MDMA, to enhance the effects of EMDR resourcing holds great promise, although further research is required to empirically validate this intervention.

References

Amano, T., & Toichi, M. (2016). The role of alternating bilateral stimulation in establishing positive cognition in EMDR therapy: A multi-channel near-infrared spectroscopy study. *PloS one, 11*(10), e0162735. https://doi.org/10.1371/journal.pone.0162735

Bedi, G., Phan, K. L., Angstadt, M., & De Wit, H. (2009). Effects of MDMA on sociability and neural response to social threat and social reward. *Psychopharmacology, 207*, 73–83. https://doi.org/10.1007/s00213-009-1635-z

Berne, E. (1961). *Transactional Analysis in Psychotherapy*. New York: Grove Press.

Brown, W. A. (2012). *The Placebo Effect in Clinical Practice* (1st ed.). Oxford: Oxford University Press. https://doi.org/10.1093/med/9780199933853.001.0001

Cosimano, M. (2021). The role of the guide in psychedelic-assisted therapy. In C. Grob and J. Grigsby (Eds.), *Handbook of medical hallucinogens* (pp. 377–394). New York: The Guilford Press.

Droogmans, S., Cosyns, B., D'haenen, H., Creeten, E., Weytjens, C., Franken, P. R., Scott, B., Schoors, D., Kemdem, A., Close, L., & Vandenbossche, J. L. (2007). Possible association between 3, 4-methylenedioxymethamphetamine abuse and valvular heart disease. *The American Journal of Cardiology, 100*(9), 1442–1445. https://doi.org/10.1016/j.amjcard.2007.06.045

Farinde, A. (2021). Dose-response relationships. Found at: https://www.msdmanuals.com/en-gb/professional/clinical-pharmacology/pharmacodynamics/drug%E2%80%93receptor-interactions. Accessed 23.10.23

Gonzalez, A., & Mosquera, D. (2012). *EMDR and dissociation: The progressive approach*. El-Bireh: AI.

Grof, S. (1980). *LSD psychotherapy*. Alameda, CA: Hunter House.

Knipe, J. (2018). *EMDR toolbox: Theory and treatment of complex PTSD and dissociation*. New York: Springer Publishing Company. https://doi.org/10.1891/9780826172563

Korn, D. L., & Leeds, A. M. (2002). Preliminary evidence of efficacy for EMDR resource development and installation in the stabilization phase of treatment of complex posttraumatic stress disorder. *Journal of Clinical Psychology*, 58(12), 1465–1487. https://doi.org/10.1002/jclp.10099

Logie, R., & De Jongh, A. (2014). The "Flashforward procedure": Confronting the catastrophe. *Journal of EMDR Practice and Research*, 8(1), 25–32. DOI: https://doi.org/10.1891/1933-3196.8.1.25

Parnell, L. (2013). *Attachment-focused EMDR: Healing relational trauma*. New York: WW Norton & Company.

Sessa, B., Higbed, L., & Nutt, D. (2019). A review of 3,4- methylenedioxymethamphetamine (MDMA)-Assisted Psychotherapy. *Front. Psychiatry* 10:138. https://doi.org/10.3389/fpsyt.2019.00138

Santos, I. (2019). EMDR case formulation tool. *Journal of EMDR Practice and Research*, 13(3), 221–231. https://psycnet.apa.org/doi/10.1891/1933-3196.13.3.221

Schmid, Y., Liechti, M. E. (2018). Long-lasting subjective effects of LSD in normal subjects. *Psychopharmacol (Berl)*,235, 535–545. https://doi.org/10.1007/s00213-017-4733-3

Schmidt, T. T., & Blankenburg, F. (2019). The somatotopy of mental tactile imagery. *Frontiers in Human Neuroscience*, 13, 10. https://doi.org/10.3389/fnhum.2019.00010

Shapiro F., (Ed.). (2002). *EMDR as an integrative approach: Experts of diverse orientations explore the paradigm prism*. Washington, DC: American Psychological Association. https://doi.org/10.1037/10512-000

Schwartz, R. (1997). *Internal Family Systems Therapy*. New York: Guilford Press.

Shapiro, R. (2016). *Easy ego state interventions: Strategies for working with parts*. New York: WW Norton & Company.

Shulgin, A. T., & Shulgin, A. (1991). *PIHKAL: A chemical love story* (Vol. 963009605). Berkeley, CA: Transform Press.

Thal, S. B., Wieberneit, M., Sharbanee, J. M., Skeffington, P. M., Baker, P., Bruno, R., & Bright, S. J. (2022). Therapeutic (Sub) stance: Current practice and therapeutic conduct in preparatory sessions in substance-assisted psychotherapy-A systematized review. *Journal of Psychopharmacology*, 36(11), 1191–1207. https://doi.org/10.1177/02698811221127954

Thompson, M. R., Callaghan, P. D., Hunt, G. E., Cornish, J. L., & McGregor, I. S. (2007). A role for oxytocin and 5-HT1A receptors in the prosocial effects of 3, 4 methylenedioxymethamphetamine ("ecstasy"). *Neuroscience*, 146(2), 509–514. https://doi.org/10.1016/j.neuroscience.2007.02.032

Winkelman, M. J. (2021). The evolved psychology of psychedelic set and setting: Inferences regarding the roles of shamanism and entheogenic ecopsychology. *Frontiers in Pharmacology*, 12, 619890. https://doi.org/10.3389/fphar.2021.619890

Winkelman M. J., & White, D. (1987). *A cross-cultural study of magico-religious practitioners and trance states: Database (HRAF Research Series in Quantitative Cross-Cultural Data III)*. New Haven, CT: Human Relations Area Files.

7 Psycholytic EMDR

Cannabis (THC)
Delta-9-tetrahydrocannabinol ($C_{21}H_{30}O_2$)

DOI: 10.4324/9781003431718-7

Cannabis sativa (marijuana) is a plant with psychoactive properties that has been cultivated by humans across the globe, with evidence of its use dating back to 4000 BC. It has been used for its fibre to make rope, as a high-nutrition food and as a medicine (Li, 1974). Its psychoactive properties have been used within various religious contexts as well as for recreational use. Currently, cannabis is legal in over 40 countries worldwide, with the US being one of the first countries to legalise medical marijuana. As a result, this is currently one of the few accessible entheogens that can be legally used to assist psychotherapy. Although there is awareness of its therapeutic value, adequate training and therapeutic techniques remain underdeveloped.

Interest in this medicinal plant was renewed in the 1990's upon the discovery of the endogenous cannabinoid system (eCB) in mammals, which is now regarded as a fundamental regulatory system involved in physiology and pathology. From a psychotherapeutic perspective, the eCB system is a key modulator of excitatory and inhibitory neurotransmission and is also involved in neuroplasticity (Kilaru & Chapman, 2020). It has also been implicated in the modulation of the hypothalamic–pituitary–adrenal (HPA) axis and the regulation of stress. However, research implicates the eCB system in the pathogenesis of many mental disorders (Parolaro et al., 2010).

Cannabis is made up of two compounds that target the eCB system differently, but both have consistently demonstrated antinociceptive properties (e.g. Rahn, 2007) which is relevant when considering the somatisation of trauma. Tetrahydrocannabinol (Δ9-THC) has an affinity for the cannabinoid-1 (CB1) receptors and is the component that remains illegal in many countries. THC has been shown to impact mood, sensation/pain and perception. The other component, cannabidiol (CBD), targets the CB1 and CB2 receptors indirectly and is also involved in other targets in the body. It has been shown to have antipsychotic, neuroprotective, anti-inflammatory, anxiolytic and antiemetic properties (Huestis, 2007). However, chronic cannabis use can have negative effects, particularly on younger populations because it has the potential to alter brain morphology, leading to poorer working memory and greater impulsivity (Crane et al., 2013).

Psycholytic therapy

High dose = psychedelic therapy
Low-medium dose = psycholytic therapy

Originally, there were two schools of psychedelic therapy. The American/ Canadian school preferentially utilised large doses of psychedelics over a short number of sessions in an attempt to induce a transcendental experience. In contrast to this, the European school of therapy developed the 'psycholytic' method that utilised the effects of low to medium doses of psychedelics combined with psychoanalytical therapy. Critics of the high-dose methods propose that it can lead to 'spiritual bypassing' (Masters, 2010) and avoids exploration of difficult biographical issues. The 'psychedelic' school of thought believes that high doses are required to induce the life-changing peak experiences that are believed to induce rapid positive change in one to three sessions and that focussing on biographical minutiae wastes time (Grof, 2019).

In the 1960s, Levine and Ludwig (1963, 1966) combined hypnosis with LSD in three-hour sessions where participants were administered 120–200 micrograms of LSD. A hypnotic induction was combined with trauma-focussed psychodynamic therapy, and the sessions concluded with hypnotic suggestions, similar to the use of the imaginal space re-scripting and positive cognitions in attachment-informed EMDR. Participants previously trained in hypnotic inductions were inducted into a hypnotic trance prior to acute effects of the LSD, then whilst under its effects, hypnotic suggestion was used to encourage them to let go and surrender to the experience. Hypnotic suggestion was also used to direct them to specific parts of their biography. This research had negative results with a very low overall remission rate for its participants, who were mainly being treated for alcoholism. This was thought to be partly due to the lack of sufficiently trained clinical staff (Levine & Ludwig, 1966).

In the 1960s, British psychoanalysts Pauline McCririck and Joyce Martin developed 'Fusion Therapy,' introducing the concept of 'nourishing physical contact' (McCririck,1966). This modality utilised medium doses of LSD in a low-lit room, where clients were held in 'warm embrace' like a 'good mother would do' (Martin, 1965). This regression therapy, where touch is proposed to act as an 'emotionally corrective experience' (Alexander & French, 1946), was experienced by Grof, who attended sessions with McCririck and Martin and was impressed by the ability of this approach to tend to emotional neglect in childhood. Grof then incorporated the use of touch in his work moving forward and is thought to be responsible for the inclusion of touch in many of the current psychedelic protocols (Grof & Grof, 2023). The introduction of touch inevitably divided opinion in the schools of therapy due to the perceived risks to the transferential relationship and remains a contentious issue in the field of PAP.

In response to his observations of psychedelic-assisted therapy, Grof also concluded that low doses, combined with more talking and reflection, 'diverted the process of vertical explorations' and slowed down the therapeutic progress because it served the avoidance of difficult issues (Grof, 2019). He therefore increased the dosages and introduced eyeshades and music to facilitate the internalisation of the process. These high-dose sessions, with minimal therapist intervention followed by integration sessions, are the predominant method currently used in the US and Canada.

Psychedelic doses and the EMDR toolkit

High doses of psychedelics are less tolerated by those with underlying physical health conditions and/or impaired self-regulation capacity. They may offer a glimpse into causal reality but, even in 'healthy normal' individuals, very high doses may lead to spiritual bypassing, hindering the exploration of the biographical content that is necessary to facilitate therapeutic change. Despite this, high doses may still be preferred, particularly in recreational settings or where previous psycholytic doses (in combination with therapy) have not given rise to the therapeutic outcome required.

Breathwork, mantras and resourcing techniques are traditional components of trauma therapy that are already being deployed to enhance the window of tolerance in psychedelic research settings. EMDR interventions can further increase this window and reduce the risk of ongoing adverse drug effects. Interventions from EMDR therapy can be intermittently deployed to support individuals navigating challenging moments during a high-dose experience. Techniques can be practised during the preparation phase, and then revisited during dosing if needed, or just deployed as harm-reduction interventions as and where required. The EMDR toolkit includes the following techniques:

- The PsyA-EMDR therapist encourages the participant to stay with their internal process whilst they stay out of the way, allowing the combination of psychedelics and BLS to stimulate the brain's innate healing mechanisms.
- During the acute phase, inner resourcing physical objects to represent members of the pre-established resource team can be used to give a multi-sensory supportive experience, without the need for visual or auditory input.
- Reminder of the mantras "in and through" and "trust, let go, be open" that were previously installed during preparation using BLS. Traditional

EMDR mantras such as "go with that" and "follow that" can also be used during dosing.

- **Accelerator:** BLS can be used intermittently to increase associative links during the reconsolidation process, especially during the descent from the peak of the experience.
- **Accelerator:** Connecting with an object or image that represents the participant's intention will activate the corresponding memory network.
- **Accelerator:** If the participant encounters a psychological defence that is blocking the reprocessing, BLS can be used to moderate the impact of the DMN by filling up the working memory.
- **Brake:** Pendulating material can help to maintain stability and optimal information processing.
- **Brake:** Hands on the floor or feet on the floor can enhance a sense of feeling grounded.
- **Brake:** Long slow exhalations support relaxation through parasympathetic activation. Bubble blowing using bubble mixture and a bubble wand can be a playful way of achieving this on psychedelics.
- **Brake:** Use of weighted blankets and handheld bean bags where physical containment would be beneficial.
- **Brake:** Distraction and delaying techniques can be used to support people to stay with the experience until the acute drug effects subside.
- **Brake:** BLS music that enhances the sense of safety can calm the nervous system until the drug effects subside.
- **Change gear:** If an individual starts to loop, BLS can be used to unstick the processing by activating other areas of the brain, allowing alternative connections to be made.
- **Change gear:** Changing the BLS modality/direction of eye movements can re-initiate stuck reprocessing.
- **Change gear:** Stuck processing can be explored using (previously installed) resourcing that utilises ego state interventions.
- **Change gear:** Gentle movement or stretching can unblock stuck processing.
- Encouraging the client to write down key experiences that can be added to the case conceptualisation later. The act of writing things down can help individuals to 'let go,' knowing that it can be revisited and explored during integration.

For more information see Chapter 5, 'Stabilisation.'

As previously mentioned, when integrating trauma with EMDR, it is possible to both integrate the memory and then utilise the imaginal space to create an embodied corrective emotional experience (Parnell, 2013). If there is chronic emotional neglect in childhood, 'empathogenic' compounds such as MDMA (Bedi et al., 2010), combined with the resourcing phases of AI-EMDR, can be used to create a felt sense of safety without the unnecessary additional risk of using touch as an intervention. See Chapter 4, 'Ethics.'

The musical soundscape

In psychedelic therapy, several environmental and psychological factors play a role in influencing the experience during drug administration. Music in PAP is sometimes referred to as 'the hidden therapist' (Kaelen et al., 2018), and some research participants have reported potent placebo effects, solely from their interactions with music in the psychedelic administration environment. Music appears as a standard feature in the clinical trials, although very little research has been done into the benefits (or pitfalls) of the music used during the psychedelic experience. Music appears to play a multifaceted role, supporting the process by serving as a catalyst for emotional exploration, and (especially when combined with noise-reducing headphones) reduces the impact of external stimuli. Neural correlates indicate that music increases asymmetric brain entropy, reflecting activation of the autonomic nervous system and indicating its role in modulating affect (Daly et al., 2019). The guidelines that were set out in early psychedelic research have meant that western classical music is still the standard genre used in trial settings. Although research suggests that mystical overtone sounds could be a marginally better alternative to western classical, albeit the difference between the two was not significant (Strickland et al., 2020).

In indigenous settings, traditional songs such as Amazonian icaros and musical instruments are offered as tools to facilitate emotional processing. When it comes to offering psychedelic therapy at scale, employing indigenous methods raises concerns of cultural misappropriation. Some also rightly question the appropriateness of universally using playlists solely created by European/American artists, particularly in settings where an individual's trauma might be linked to oppression through colonialism. Generic playlists may inadvertently trigger difficult experiences due to personal associations or activate individual preferences, disrupting a person's inward therapeutic process. One research participant suggested that their internal process became hijacked by the emotions of the composer, leading to the later removal of that track from the clinical trial's music set list. Experiential reports from those working in clinical trials have highlighted that where changes to the set list do occur, there can be a powerful impact on the sensitivity of the participants to the drug effects. Questions also remain around the use of silence and how the absence of sound might become meaningful within a therapeutic process. What is clear is that music can have a powerful effect on increasing the intensity and phenomenology of a psychedelic experience, that music is integral to attunement and that a failure of musical attunement can give rise to feelings of unsafety. This suggests that, if used, musical set lists need to be highly individualised to the person being dosed, to the substance that is being used and carefully matched to follow the arch of the drug experience. Crafting an appropriate playlist is a highly personal and time-consuming decision-making process that poses significant challenges to anyone who attempts it. Due to the powerful effects music can have on shaping a psychedelic experience, any music that is selected needs to reflect an intricate balance and be tailored to the delicate and nuanced needs of that current moment. If used at all, music needs to be highly individualised and extremely flexible.

While music can be incorporated into the preparation and stabilisation phases of PsyA-EMDR therapy (if desired), it is not integral to the process and might detract from the desired internalised effects of the bilateral stimulation. During the psychedelic medication session, silence or bilateral auditory clicks can help to maintain an internalised emotional focus, avoiding potential distractions evoked by a music soundscape or external noise. Whilst the potential of bilateral music set lists remains unexplored, sounds associated with the safe/calm place have been shown (through self-experimentation) to further amplify, strengthen, embody and then anchor resourcing experiences during a psychedelic treatment. To illustrate, the bilateral sound of waves or heartbeats can be used to replace the auditory clicks during resource development (phase 2) and reprocessing (phase 4). In PsyA-EMDR, safety remains paramount, and any sound introduces variability. By aligning the experience closely with an individual's internalised process and intentions, along with relational attunement to the individual's fluctuating needs, optimal therapeutic outcomes are generally achievable.

Variations in sensory perception, such as neurodiversity (e.g. ASD, ADHD or aphantasia), emphasise and compound the need for personalised approaches. Any sound used needs to mirror and add value to an individual, by matching their need for resourcing or embodiment at different times and in different ways throughout the different phases of the different treatments. It is also helpful to note that music (along with art, movement and exposure to nature) can be helpful with preparation and relaxation immediately before dosing and can also be helpful as a method of enhancing post-dose stabilisation.

Psycholytic EMDR

As previously discussed, EMDR is a comprehensive therapy with a number of different mechanisms of action that appear to target a range of functional

networks in the brain. High-dose psychedelic sessions are generally not conducive to concurrent psychotherapeutic interventions because the strength
of the compound can cause the participant to focus on their internal
process, meaning they are unable to engage with the therapist during the
acute phase of the treatment (which can last for hours).

Psycholytic EMDR offers an alternative paradigm, whereby low to medium
doses of psychedelic substances are administered to allow the participant to
engage with the therapist, in an attempt to enhance the psychotherapeutic
interventions by harnessing the effects of the psychedelic substance. Although
some posit that high doses are required to elicit perception-shifting 'mystical
experiences' that have been implicated in positive outcomes of PAPs (Barrett & Griffiths, 2017), the combination of low doses of psychedelics with
EMDR has the potential to elicit profound healing experiences, particularly
when paired with attachment-informed interventions that are skilfully used
in the imaginal space. Furthermore, lower doses of psychedelics might be
better tolerated by individuals with an impaired capacity to regulate affect,
allowing them to maintain a degree of control and avoid abreaction.

This chapter explores three psycholytic EMDR case studies through
interviews with practitioners working in training settings across the globe,
with the aim of encouraging more research in this area.

Psilocybin-assisted EMDR (psycholytic dose)

Therapists working in psychedelic training settings have been experimen-
tally combining EMDR with low doses of psilocybin (approximately half
a full dose), with encouraging results.

Method

During the period immediately following ingestion of a medium dose of
psilocybin, a pre-determined memory network that corresponded with the
participant's intention 'to learn to trust others' was deliberately activated.
This was done by discussing a current trigger linked to this intention in
the time after ingestion but before the acute effects began. A touchstone
memory naturally emerged in conversation during this latent phase.

As soon as the participant could feel the effects of the psilocybin, they
were administered auditory (headphones) and visual bilateral stimulation
(BLS) on a widescreen TV and were allowed to go into their process with
minimal interaction from the facilitator. The bilateral stimulation was then
on continuously for the remainder of the three-hour session. The diagram
below illustrates when the targeted memory network/ COEX was activated during the treatment.

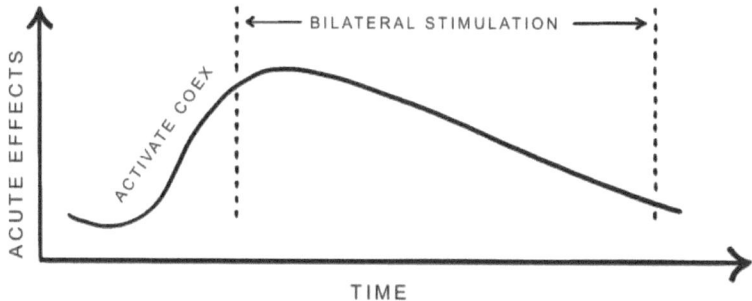

Figure 7.1 Graph illustrating that bilateral stimulation is administered when the acute effects begin.

Throughout the treatment, the participant was brought back to the 'touchstone' memory that had emerged at the beginning of the session, re-evaluating the target by assessing their somatic response to it (SUDs). This helped keep the work focused when the reprocessing wandered off into other networks. The touchstone memory acted as a portal back into the pre-determined memory network/COEX. Interestingly, when working with psilocybin, people are often drawn into transgenerational nodes outside of their biographical network. In this instance, the participant reported re-experiencing the very early developmental trauma of their mother. Experientially, this included hearing specific sounds and a deep sense of somatic overwhelm that soon dissipated as they followed the BLS dot on the screen. Content from a recent psychedelic experience that had induced a mild paranoid reaction also resurfaced. Reprocessing revealed how the content from that 'bad trip' correlated to the enduring narratives that were woven through the ancestral trauma of their mother and their grandmother. Later on in the experience, they connected to a somatic experience of danger and mistrust, which they interpreted as being the grandmother's trauma, specifically her experience of running away at the age of 15 and subsequently giving birth to a child (their mother).

Each time an ancestral or biographical 'memory' was processed (SUD reduced to a 0), that 'part' was taken to their peaceful place and tended to by a member of their resource team. By the end of the session, their grandmother, mother, three-year-old self and teenage self were all in their peaceful place around a fire. Below illustrates the order in which the psycholytic EMDR session unfolded:

Recent trigger	Approaching a group of people sat at a picnic table, panicked and had to leave the situation
Intention	'To learn to trust others'
Corresponding NCs	'I don't fit in' and 'I cannot trust others'
Initial memory	Feeling ostracised at secondary school
Biographical touchstone	Age 3, hiding under a table at playgroup
Transgenerational touchtone 1	Mother abandoned as a baby in children's home
Transgenerational touchtone 2	15-year-old grandmother running away and then giving birth to a baby alone under a table with no one there
Recent 'bad trip'	Feeling unsafe around people

From a Groffian perspective, the 'I don't fit in' and 'I cannot trust others' COEXs were activated at the beginning of the session and led back to transpersonal domains outside of their direct, biographical experience. Somatic memories emerged as if they had been passed down with all the sensory information intact. The startling difference here between standard EMDR and this session was the way that the participant's reprocessing was drawn to ancestral trauma that carried the same themes of 'I don't fit in' and 'I cannot trust others.' This was despite the facilitator repeatedly taking the participant back to the biographical touchstone memory from three-years-old. Expanding the concept of 'memory network' into transpersonal domains proves beneficial when working with psilocybin-assisted EMDR therapy in order to acknowledge the intergenerational nature of the work; the Groffian term COEX might be supplementary to and more fitting of this context. See Chapter 11 for more on transpersonal PsyA-EMDR.

eMDMAdr

MDMA is undergoing a gradual process of re-classification, from its former status as a restricted substance to its approval for use as a medicine in the treatment of PTSD. This worldwide initiative has been made possible through the persistent efforts of Rick Doblin and his team at MAPS. Reports suggest that attachment-informed EMDR and MDMA may be well matched, particularly because of their shared focus as a treatment for PTSD, along with evidence indicating that MDMA enhances memory reconsolidation (Schmidt et al, 2017; Feduccia & Mithoefer, 2018). To get a sense of the synergistic potential of combining these two modalities, we interviewed a clinician working in an underground setting who had used psycholytic eMDMAdr in their therapy practice. The clinician described in detail their experience of working with one client who had a complex trauma history and a predisposition to dissociate. The client had engaged in a considerable amount of self-development to integrate their past, including extensive EMDR therapy. They had used psychedelics therapeutically but had never used MDMA before, neither therapeutically nor recreationally. The AIP case conceptualisation highlighted that the focus of the work would be on utilising EMDR's resourcing elements to remediate their attachment deficits. MDMA was specifically chosen for this intervention because of the traumatic attachment history. EMDR aims to develop internal resources and adaptive information in the brain to aid the reconsolidation of traumatic memories. The case conceptualisation tool was used to identify the key attachment deficits and to guide the resourcing interventions using imaginal work during the preparation phase. MDMA then enhanced the sensory experience of the imaginal resources and created lasting memories of embodied positive affect. This holds particular potential when working with individuals with complex PTSD resulting from childhood abuse and/or neglect where positive resourcing experiences are limited.

Method

100 mg of MDMA was administered, although reports suggest that dose can be reduced. For context, the MAPS multi-site trials treating PTSD with MDMA have been using dosages between 120 and 180 mg (Mitchell et al., 2023). The bilateral stimulation used was a combination of auditory (headphones) and visual (on a widescreen TV). As the client began to feel the effects of the MDMA, they were guided through an extended version of connecting with their inner resource team. The visualisations focused on the sensory elements of direct eye-contact with the calm, grounded resource team in their pre-established safe/calm place. The client reported that they felt an embodied sense of safety that they had never allowed themselves to feel before. The resource team was utilised throughout the four-hour session. After installation of resources, the targeted memory network 'I am not worthy' and the pre-determined touchstone memory (from age two-years-old) were activated. The participant spent the majority of the session following a dot moving bilaterally on a screen, later stating that:

> "It was like watching my life on a TV, and I was not really aware of the dot…I followed the dot but my eyes could easily have been closed; I was completely absorbed."

One key point that was noted was the lack of any dissociation, which had previously been their experience during standard EMDR sessions. They reported:

> "My trance-like state on the moving ball helped shift the strong responses that emerged."

Another important point that was highlighted was how positive transferences with the facilitator were amplified. This has already been flagged as a risk factor in Chapter 4, 'Ethics.' Here is an excerpt from the individual's journal, written post-experience:

> *Am I trying to say things to be liked or accepted? Now that the drug effects have worn off, I am experiencing some paranoia and a bit of a vulnerability hangover. Have I shared too much? Or have I been too open? It is ok. I can trust my therapist. I can trust myself. I can trust the medicine. Sometimes being mistrustful has kept me safe. When is it right to be mistrustful? Having a good therapist helps me to know that I am safe to trust as she will tell me if I go wrong. I know that right now I am safe to mistrust the medicine. That is ok. Trust is so physical.*

This emphasises the importance of thorough integration following a psychedelic treatment to get the full benefit from the experience. In this example, the fears around trust and vulnerability that emerged in the aftermath were bridged from using the somatic bridge and reprocessed along with the biographical material that had been activated. Attachment-informed re-scripting with that part was then used to further stabilise the nervous system.

> *"What is also novel is that my projections were held by the eye movements. This allowed free associating with the content that emerged, rather than projecting it out onto our relationship. This feels safer and less messy. It allows me to stay with my own process."*

Cannabis-assisted EMDR

Cannabis is an underdog in the world of PAP and many disregard it as a psychedelic, but its proponents report that the use of the correct mix cannabis, in the right set and setting, can induce powerful psychedelic effects. Cannabis has been shown to be an effective treatment for a wide range of psychological and physiological issues including depression, anxiety and traumatic stress (Black et al., 2019), sleep disturbance (Choi et al., 2020), chronic pain (Stockings et al., 2018) and seizure disorders (Stockings et al., 2018b). Here it is used as a symptom management tool, but the effects of even small doses of cannabis on neuroplasticity (Casarejos et al., 2013; Campos et al., 2017) have the potential to be utilised in EMDR therapy to facilitate long-term positive change.

Medicinal cannabis has been de-restricted in many countries across the globe, but it has only been recognised as a potential tool for psychotherapy in the last decade. Despite its changing status back to a medicinal plant, it is still regarded by many therapists as an addictive drug. McQueen (2021) has developed a range of therapeutic techniques and practices that he calls cannabis-assisted therapy, with a focus on mindfulness and the aim of 'personal empowerment, healing and transformation.' McQueen administers strong doses of cannabis and encourages clients to go into their process using eyeshade in the appropriate setting. He refers to memory consolidation and fear extinction as potential mechanisms of action and refers to cannabis as a gentle but powerful tool (McQueen, 2021).

Psychedelic cannabis can be used to treat trauma and PTSD, and parallels have been drawn with MDMA therapy in the way that traumatic memories can be recalled and integrated. Cannabis has been shown to act on the amygdala and reduce the fear response in a similar way to MDMA (Phan et al., 2008). It is proposed that cannabis may serve as an accessible, more tolerable alternative to stronger psychedelic treatments that are yet to be de-restricted and has the potential to enhance phase 4 reprocessing even at low doses.

Pros

Cannabis-assisted psychotherapy puts less stress on the body than typical serotonergic psychedelics because its effects are milder and short lived with peak intensity and length that can be adjusted to last one to three hours. Psychedelic cannabis sessions are shorter with minimal recovery time and therefore more affordable and manageable for both busy people and clinical schedules. Its gentle effects, that have been shown to be neurogenerative, mean that it is likely safer for older populations than classic psychedelics. It can also be used to test tolerability for stronger psychedelic treatments like psilocybin or LSD.

It is possible to maintain a sense of agency on cannabis, which is important for individuals with trauma. They are able to choose how deep they want to go and even pause the experience and take a break by taking the eye shades off and coming out of their process (McQueen, 2021), which sets it apart from other serotonergic psychedelics.

Cons

Cannabis has retained much of the social stigma that was attached to it by Anslinger in the 1930s, where it was described as an 'addictive drug which produces in its users insanity, criminality and death' (Gasnier, 1936). Whilst heavy use has been shown to cause cognitive impairment, particularly in young people, there is some debate about the enduring effects after abstinence (Crane et al., 2013). There is also some evidence that cannabis can be addictive, particularly if people are using it to cope with trauma (Kevorkian et al., 2015). However, the physical and psychological symptoms of selective serotonin reuptake inhibitor (SSRI) withdrawal, reframed by the pharmaceutical industry as 'discontinuation syndrome' to avoid associating them with addiction, are driving people to look for natural alternatives. If clinicians are worried about a client's cannabis use, there is a questionnaire that's freely available online to assess their habits: 'the revised cannabis use disorder identification test' (CUDIT-R, Adamson et al., 2010).

McQueen states that intentional use is completely different to getting high and numbing your problems and that it has anti-addictive properties because, if used therapeutically, it reduces suffering and therefore people reduce their use (McQueen, 2021). There is a shortage of training and clear guidelines on this issue but there are a number of informative books on this topic that would be a good place for any inquisitive therapists to start. Cannabis is one of the only entheogens that is widely available on a prescription and can be legally combined with psychotherapy to harness its effects. Although it is becoming more accessible, medicinal cannabis on prescription is expensive and remains inaccessible to many.

Now that cannabis is being re-assigned its status as a medicinal plant, it is becoming more common to see clients who have a prescription for mental and/or physical health issues. The safety profile of cannabis as a medication has been rigorously investigated and its therapeutic effects appear to outweigh the potential adverse effects if taken according to guidelines (Pertwee, 2014). Currently, the FDA has only approved two medications for the treatment of PTSD: the SSRIs sertraline and paroxetine, with remission rates of less than 30% (Berger et al., 2009). Cognitive behavioural interventions such as exposure therapy and cognitive reprocessing therapy are favoured, despite their high attrition rates (20-40%) and low patient engagement (Cuijpers, et al, 2016). Whilst research is still in its infancy, the use of cannabis in the treatment of trauma, with a focus on its attenuation of dissociation, is beginning to be explored in the literature (Sarris et al., 2020; Ragnhildstveit et al., 2023).

Cannabis offers a novel strategy for targeting the dissociation caused by trauma through its relaxant and analgesic properties. Low doses have the potential to augment trauma-focussed psychotherapies such as EMDR because the subjective effects seem to encourage embodiment and facilitate the integration of overwhelming trauma memories (Ragnhildstveit et al., 2023). Below is subjective feedback from a client with a complex trauma history presenting with moderate amounts of structural dissociation caused by pre-verbal trauma. They had a medical cannabis prescription and would vape before and occasionally during EMDR reprocessing sessions because they said it helped them to stay connected with their body and engage with the reprocessing. The feeling from the cannabis is described as a 'warm hug inside that allows them to relax and sit with the somatic responses' that emerge:

"I have a tension in my torso, the muscles surrounding my core. A grip.
I then take an inhale and hold.

As I breathe out, the sides of my body start to uncoil and recede in their
grip of my core. Leaving a space. Spreading still further down my legs, my
body sinks back into the seat. If this could speak, it would say 'it's alright.'
I can let go enough, a feeling of reassurance.

A space to breathe and a moment of humour with you.
A different perspective.

I can do this, more trust to let go a little more now my body is not
gripping inside I can open my mind to the process."

Cannabis-assisted EMDR case study

Presenting issue: Treatment-resistant anxiety and depression

Case summary: 28-year-old Caucasian male. His family moved around throughout childhood for his father's work, creating a context of instability and emotional neglect that affected his ability to sustain interpersonal relationships throughout his childhood and adolescence. There was also a history of significant transgenerational trauma and attachment issues on both sides of the family.

Substance abuse history: He had serious issues with alcohol, cocaine and methamphetamine in his late teens and early 20s.

Prescription: Up to 30g of flower (bud) a month on prescription which also includes 20% CBD and 10% THC full-spectrum oil.

Reported effects: He feels that medicinal marijuana allows him to regulate because it allows him to identify and process his emotions; to "sit and think and process his thoughts and feelings." He describes being better able to "snap out and move on" from dips in mood more easily. Since starting prescription in March 2022, he has given up alcohol and drugs and feels that life is much better as a result. He has also doubled his salary and believes this is a byproduct of his prescription combined with EMDR therapy. He states that his prescription has saved his life because it helped him give up drinking and mitigate the risks of taking other harder drugs and impulsive behaviours.

Impact on sociability: He reports that cannabis helps him to socialise, especially if other people are drinking. A reduction in impulsivity.

Weight gain: He was very underweight before and is now consciously healthy and active. It has helped with inflammation and muscle pain.

Impact on REM: He remembers his dreams but is also aware of the potential negative impact that cannabis has on REM sleep. He takes regular tolerance breaks and, when on a break, he reports that he does not notice any REM rebound. He does not feel that his prescription negatively impacts his sleep. **Note:** He has a lower THC content in the afternoon to attenuate potential impact on sleep and does not take the medication after 5 pm.

Impact on EMDR sessions: He vapes cannabis approximately an hour before his EMDR session (at 9 am). He states that cannabis helps him to recognise the somatic elements of memories during the session and makes him feel more grounded. Cannabis improves his focus during the session and increases the intensity of feelings as they emerge. When he has not vaped before a session, he has reported that he has had 'difficulty getting out of his head' to connect with the emotional and somatic responses during reprocessing. He feels that cannabis supports trauma work and works well in tandem with EMDR.

Update: This client has now completely withdrawn from his cannabis prescription. He utilised its effects to navigate deep integration work with EMDR and now feels that he does not need the support of this medication. He has been free of all medication now for six months, and his mood remains stable.

Managing trauma-related sleep disturbance

It is well established in the literature that cannabis impacts sleep and one of its main medical applications is to manage sleep disorders (American Academy of Sleep Medicine, 2014). A potential issue that has been highlighted in the research is the impact of cannabis on REM sleep. REM sleep makes up 20–25% of human sleep time and begins approximately 90-minutes after the onset of sleep (Keenan and Hirshkowitz, 2011). Although cannabis promotes sleep, it suppresses REM, the stage in which we dream (Siclari et al., 2017), and research has revealed that it reduces dream recall but that there are many variables such as dosage, ratio of CBs and timing that influence this (Tringale & Jensen, 2011; Babson et al., 2017). The suppression of REM can lead to a phenomenon experienced during cannabis withdrawal called 'REM rebound' where heavy users can experience disruption to sleep in the form of intense dreaming. The sleep rhythm returns to normal once the REM debt has been made up, but this can take days or weeks depending on the amount of disruption caused by the cannabis use.

The link between nightmares and trauma is well documented and nightmares can disturb sleep, leaving individuals waking up feeling tired. This is thought to be because trauma impacts sleep architecture – one aspect of this being REM fragmentation (Colvonen et al., 2019). EEG data has shown the impact of cannabis on brain oscillations during REM sleep, and it has been hypothesised that the endocannabinoid system may modulate dream activity (Murillo-Rodriguez et al. 1998). Interestingly, synthetic cannabinoid receptor agonist Nabilone has been used to treat patients with PTSD, resulting in the cessation or significant reduction of nightmares (Cameron et al., 2014).

From an AIP perspective, nightmare disorder observed in PTSD is conceptualised as a memory disorder, whereby the brain is attempting to reconsolidate traumatic memories but is unable to do this because of the maladaptive encoding and high levels of cortisol that disrupt the reconsolidation of these memories. This can result in recurrent nightmares, with similar themed content to the original trauma. It is possible that cannabis could be used in conjunction with EMDR to minimise sleep disturbance for people who have PTSD. Cannabis could be used to reduce the immediate trauma-related nightmares and then EMDR reprocessing would act as a titrated version of REM/SWS whereby the trauma can be adaptively reprocessed in a controlled environment.

Summary

Subjective reports from experimental practice of psycholytic PsyA-EMDR indicate that large doses of psychedelics are not necessary to facilitate long-term positive change. This shows promise in expanding the treatment domain to make these treatments more inclusive. See Chapter 12, 'The future of PsyA-EMDR,' for expanding accessibility. Although there is some evidence that 'mystical experiences' increase the long-term benefits of psychedelic therapy, this is not always safe, possible or even necessary. Indeed, for some, even extremely high doses of psychedelics do not elicit any phenomenological response. Psycholytic doses have the potential to expand access, with comparatively lower risk factors and a reduction in the aftereffects (such as low mood or changes in suicidality) when compared to high-dose sessions. Compounds such as MDMA can be used synergistically with EMDR to enhance attachment-informed interventions by creating an embodied sense of love, safety and acceptance – affective states that this empathogen is renowned for and are unachievable for some. The use of psycholytic doses allows the participant to maintain some sense of agency, which can then be tempered using EMDR (like an accelerator and breaking system). This is particularly important for individuals with complex trauma histories, because the loss of control felt on full doses may cause too much dysregulation and, with the frontal lobe not online, could result in further retraumatisation/PTSD.

In light of contemporary research and the backdrop of an ever-increasing prevalence of cannabis prescriptions, it is imperative that clinicians stay up to date in their understanding of this ever-evolving area. To illustrate, cannabis-assisted EMDR therapy offers an accessible, legal treatment option that can already be used in many countries to facilitate trauma work with EMDR. It is likely that other psychedelic medications will soon follow suit, and professionals need to be adequately informed and trained in psychedelic-assisted therapies.

Although broadly anecdotal, the illustrative case material presented here provides a compelling glimpse into the psychotherapeutic possibilities of PsyA-EMDR. It is hoped that these reports will provide some traction for moving PsyA-EMDR into the research arena. The cost of research, the current legislative restrictions and the financial goals of companies funding current studies means that in the short term, innovative research design will be required to overcome these barriers. In the meantime, there is a rich untapped resource of practice-based evidence that could pave the way to more robust investigations to follow suit. EMDR is powerful as a stand-alone psychotherapy, but when combined with even low-dose psychedelics, the synergy between the two modalities indicates remarkable potential. We hope that others will soon share their work in this area and that this will help to reduce the risks and stigma associated with using EMDR alongside these powerful agents of change.

References

Adamson, S. J., Kay-Lambkin, F. J., Baker, A. L., Lewin, T. J., Thornton, L., Kelly, B. J., & Sellman, J. D. (2010). An improved brief measure of cannabis misuse: The cannabis use disorders identification test-revised (CUDIT-R). *Drug and Alcohol Dependence, 110*(1–2), 137–143. https://doi.org/10.1016/j.drugalcdep.2010.02.017

Alexander, F., & French, T. M. (1946). *Psychoanalytic therapy: Principles and application*. New York: Ronald Press.

Babson, K. A., Sottile, J., & Morabito, D. (2017). Cannabis, cannabinoids, and sleep: A review of the literature. *Current Psychiatry Reports, 19*(4), 1–12. https://doi.org/10.1007/s11920-017-0775-9

Barrett, F. S., & Griffiths, R. R. (2017). Classic hallucinogens and mystical experiences: phenomenology and neural correlates. *Behavioural Neurobiology of Psychedelic Drugs, 36*,393–430. https://doi.org/10.1007/7854_2017_474

Baudelaire, C. (1998). *Artificial Paradises: Baudelaire's masterpiece on hashish* (Kindle edn.). Secaucus, NJ: Citadel.

Bedi, G., Hyman, D., & de Wit, H. (2010). Is ecstasy an "empathogen"? Effects of±3, 4-methylenedioxymethamphetamine on prosocial feelings and identification of emotional states in others. *Biological Psychiatry, 68*(12), 1134–1140. https://doi.org/10.1016/j.biopsych.2010.08.003

Berger, W, Mendlowicz, M. V, Marques-Portella, C, Kinrys, G, Fontenelle, L. F., & Marmar, C. R. (2009). Pharmacologic alternatives to antidepressants in posttraumatic stress disorder: A systematic review. *Progress in Neuropsychopharmacology and Biological Psychiatry, 33*, 169–180. https://doi.org/10.1016/j.pnpbp.2008.12.004

Black, N., Stockings, E., Campbell, G., Tran, L. T., Zagic, D., & Hall, W. D. (2019). Cannabinoids for the treatment of mental disorders and symptoms of mental disorders: A systematic review and meta-analysis. *The Lancet Psychiatry, 6*(12), 995–1010. https://doi.org/10.1016/S2215-0366(19)30401-8

Cameron, C., Watson, D., & Robinson, J. (2014). Use of a synthetic cannabinoid in a correctional population for posttraumatic stress disorder-related insomnia and nightmares, chronic pain, harm reduction, and other indications: A retrospective evaluation. *Journal of Clinical Psychopharmacology, 34*(5), 559–564. https://doi.org/10.1097/JCP.0000000000000180

Campos, A. C., Fogaça, M. V., Scarante, F. F., Joca, S. R., Sales, A. J., Gomes, F. V., Sonego, A.B., Rodrigues, N. S., Galve-Roperh, I., & Guimarães, F. S. (2017). Plastic and neuroprotective mechanisms involved in the therapeutic effects of cannabidiol in psychiatric disorders. *Frontiers in Pharmacology, 8*,269. https://doi.org/10.3389/fphar.2017.00269

Casarejos, M. J., Perucho, J., Gomez, A., Munoz, M. P., Fernandez-Estevez, M., Sagredo, O., Fernandez Ruiz, J., Guzman, M., de Yebenes, J. G., & Mena, M. A. (2013). Natural cannabinoids improve dopamine neurotransmission and tau and amyloid pathology in a mouse model of tauopathy. *Journal of Alzheimer's Disease, 35*(3), 525–539. https://doi.org/10.3233/JAD-130050

Choi, S., Huang, B. C., & Gamaldo, C. E. (2020). Therapeutic uses of cannabis on sleep disorders and related conditions. *Journal of Clinical Neurophysiology, 37*(1), 39–49. https://doi.org/10.1097/WNP.0000000000000617

Colvonen, P. J., Straus, L. D., Acheson, D., & Gehrman, P. (2019). A review of the relationship between emotional learning and memory, sleep, and PTSD. *Current Psychiatry Reports, 21*, 1–11. https://doi.org/10.1007/s11920-019-0987-2

Crane, N. A., Schuster, R. M., Fusar-Poli, P., & Gonzalez, R. (2013). Effects of cannabis on neurocognitive functioning: Recent advances, neurodevelopmental influences, and sex differences. *Neuropsychology Review, 23*, 117–137. https://doi.org/10.1007/s11065-012-9222-1

Cuijpers, P., Karyotaki, E., Weitz, E., Andersson, G., & van Straten, A. (2016). The effects of psychotherapies for major depression in adults on the basis of randomized controlled trials: A meta-analytic study. *Journal of Affective Disorders, 202*, 511–521. https://doi.org/10.1016/j.jad.2016.03.063

Daly, I., Williams, D., Hwang, F., Kirke, A., Miranda, E. R., & Nasuto, S. J. (2019, July 1). Electroencephalography reflects the activity of sub-cortical brain regions during approach-withdrawal behaviour while listening to music. *Scientific Reports, 9*(1), 9415. https://doi.org/10.1038/s41598-019-45105-2

Di Marzo, V., & Petrosino, S. (2007). Endocannabinoids and the regulation of their levels in health and disease. *Current Opinion in Lipidology, 18*, 129–140. https://doi.org/10.1097/MOL.0b013e32803dbdec

Feduccia, A. A., & Mithoefer, M. C. (2018). MDMA-assisted psychotherapy for PTSD: are memory reconsolidation and fear extinction underlying mechanisms? *Progress in Neuro-Psychopharmacology and Biological Psychiatry, 84*, 221–228. https://doi.org/10.1016/j.pnpbp.2018.03.003

Gasnier, L. (1936). *Reefer madness [Motion picture].* Quebec: Madacy Entertainment.

Grof, S. (2019). *The Way of the Psychonaut Vol. 2, Encyclopedia for inner journeys* (1st edn.). Santa Cruz, CA: Multidisciplinary association for psychedelic studies.

Grof, S., & Grof, C. (2023). *Holotropic breathwork: A new approach to self-exploration and therapy.* Albany: State University of New York Press.

Huestis, M. A. (2007). Human cannabinoid pharmacokinetics. *Chemistry Biodiversity, 4,* 1770–1804. https://doi.org/10.1002/cbdv.200790152

Kaelen, M., Giribaldi, B., Raine, J., Evans, L., Timmerman, C., Rodriguez, N., Roseman, L., Feilding, A., Nutt, D., & Carhart-Harris, R. (2018). The hidden therapist: Evidence for a central role of music in psychedelic therapy. *Psychopharmacology (Berl). 235*(2), 505–519. https://doi.org/10.1007/s00213-017-4820-5

Keenan, S., & Hirshkowitz, M. (2011). Monitoring and staging human sleep. In: M. H. Kryger, T. Roth, and W. C. Dement (Eds.). *Principles and practices of sleep medicine* (pp. 1602–1609). Philadelphia: Elsevier-Saunders. https://doi.org/10.1016/B978-1-4160-6645-3.00141-9

Kevorkian, S., Bonn-Miller, M. O., Belendiuk, K., Carney, D. M., Roberson-Nay, R., & Berenz, E. C. (2015). Associations among trauma, posttraumatic stress disorder, cannabis use, and cannabis use disorder in a nationally representative epidemiologic sample. *Psychology of Addictive Behaviors, 29*(3), 633. https://doi.org/10.1037/adb0000110

Kilaru, A., & Chapman, K. D. (2020). The endocannabinoid system. *Essays in Biochemistry, 64*(3), 485–499. https://doi.org/10.1042/EBC20190086

Levine, J., & Ludwig, A. M. (1966). The hypnodelic treatment technique. *International Journal of Clinical Experimental Hypnosis, 14*(3), 207–213. https://doi.org/10.1080/00207146608412963

Levine, J., Ludwig, A. M., & Lyle Jr, W. H. (1963). The controlled psychedelic state. *America Journal of Clinical Hypnosis, 6,* 163–164. https://doi.org/10.1080/00029157.1963.10402334

Li, H. L., (1974). An archaeological and historical account of cannabis in China. *Economic Botony,28*(4),437–447. https://doi.org/10.1007/BF02862859

Martin, J. (1965). LSD analysis. Lecture and film presented at the second international conference on the use of LSD in psychotherapy held at south oaks hospital, May 8–12, Amityville, New York. Paper published in H. A. Abramson (ed.), *The Use of LSD in Psychotherapy and Alcoholism* (pp. 223–238). Indianapolis: Bobbs-Merrill.

Masters, R. A. (2010). *Spiritual bypassing: When spirituality disconnects us from what really matters.* Berkeley, CA: North Atlantic Books.

McCririck., P. (1966) The Importance of Fusion in Therapy and Maturation. (photocopy of unpublished manuscript), undated, box: 8, Folder: 4. Stanislav Grof papers, MSP 1. Purdue university archives and special collections. Found at https://archives.lib.purdue.edu/repositories/2/archival_objects/25584. Accessed 25.09.2023.

McQueen, D. (2021). *Psychedelic Cannabis: Therapeutic Methods and Unique Blends to Treat Trauma and Transform Consciousness.* Colorado: Inner Traditions Bear and Company,

Mitchell, J. M., Ot'alora, G. M., van der Kolk, B., Shannon, S., Bogenschutz, M., Gelfand, Y., Paleos, C., Nicholas, C. R., Quevedo, S., Balliett, B., & Hamilton, S. (2023). MDMA-assisted therapy for moderate to severe PTSD: A randomized, placebo-controlled phase 3 trial. *Nature Medicine, 29*(10), 2473–2480. https://doi.org/10.1038/s41591-023-02565-4

Murillo-Rodríguez, E., Sánchez-Alavez, M., Navarro, L., Martínez-González, D., Drucker-Colín, R., & Prospéro García, O. (1998). Anandamide modulates sleep and memory in rats. *Brain Research, 812*(1–2), 270–274. https://doi.org/10.1016/S0006-8993(98)00969-X

Parnell, L. (2013). *Attachment-focused EMDR: Healing relational trauma*. WW Norton & Company.

Parolaro, D., Realini, N., Vigano, D., Guidali, C., & Rubino, T. (2010). The endocannabinoid system and psychiatric disorders. *Experimental Neurology, 224*, 3–14. https://doi.org/10.1016/j.expneurol.2010.03.018

Pertwee, R. G. (Ed.). (2014). *Handbook of cannabis*. New York: Oxford University Press. https://doi.org/10.1093/acprof:oso/9780199662685.001.0001

Phan, K. L., Angstadt, M., Golden, J., Onyewuenyi, I., Popovska, A., & de Wit, H. (2008). Cannabinoid modulation of amygdala reactivity to social signals of threat in humans. *Journal of Neuroscience, 28*(10), 2313–2319. https://doi.org/10.1523/JNEUROSCI.5603-07.2008

Ragnhildstveit, A., Kaiyo, M., Snyder, M. B., Jackson, L. K., Lopez, A., Mayo, C., Miranda, A. C., August, R. J., Seli, P., Robison, R., & Averill, L. A. (2023). Cannabis-assisted psychotherapy for complex dissociative posttraumatic stress disorder: A case report. *Frontiers in Psychiatry, 14*, 1051542. https://doi.org/10.3389/fpsyt.2023.1051542

Rahn, E. J., Makriyannis, A., & Hohmann, A. G. (2007). Activation of cannabinoid CB1 and CB2 receptors suppresses neuropathic nociception evoked by the chemotherapeutic agent vincristine in rats. *British Journal of Pharmacology, 152*, 765–777. https://doi.org/10.1038/sj.bjp.0707333

Sarris, J., Sinclair, J., Karamacoska, D., Davidson, M., & Firth, J. (2020). Medicinal cannabis for psychiatric disorders: A clinically-focused systematic review. *BMC Psychiatry, 20*(1), 24. https://doi.org/10.1186/s12888-019-2409-8

Schmidt, S. D., Furini, C. R. G., Zinn, C. G., Cavalcante, L. E., Ferreira, F. F., & Behling, J. A. K. (2017). Modulation of the con- solidation and reconsolidation of fear memory by three different serotonin receptors in hip- pocampus. *Neurobiology of Learning and Memory, 142*(Pt. A), 48–54. https://doi.org/10.1016/j.nlm.2016.12.017

Siclari, F., Baird, B., Perogamvros, L., Bernardi, G., LaRocque, J. J., & Riedner, B. (2017). The neural correlates of dreaming. *Nature Neuroscience, 20*(6), 872–878. https://doi.org/10.1038/nn.4545

Stockings, E., Campbell, G., Hall, W. D., Nielsen, S., Zagic, D., & Rahman, R. (2018a). Cannabis and cannabinoids for the treatment of people with chronic noncancer pain conditions: A systematic review and meta-analysis of controlled and observational studies. *Pain, 159*(10), 1932–1954. https://doi.org/10.1097/j.pain.0000000000001293

Stockings, E., Zagic, D., Campbell, G., Weier, M., Hall, W. D., Nielsen, S., Herkes, G. K., Farrell, M., & Degenhardt, L. (2018b). Evidence for cannabis and cannabinoids for epilepsy: A systematic review of controlled and observational evidence. *Journal of Neurology, Neurosurgery & Psychiatry, 89*(7), 741–753. https://doi.org/10.1136/jnnp-2017-317168

Strickland, J. C., Garcia-Romeu, A., & Johnson, M. W. (2020). Set and setting: a randomized study of different musical genres in supporting psychedelic therapy. *ACS Pharmacology & Translational Science, 4*(2), 472–478. https://doi.org/10.1021/acsptsci.0c00187

Tringale, R., & Jensen, C. (2011). Cannabis and insomnia. *Depression, 4*, 0–68.

World Health Organization (WHO). (2018). Global status report on alcohol and health 2018. Geneva: WHO Press. Found at https://www.who.int/publications/i/item/9789241565639

8 Integration

Mescaline
3,4,5-trimethoxyphenethylamine ($C_{11}H_{17}NO_3$)

DOI: 10.4324/9781003431718-8

Mescaline or mescalin is a naturally occurring psychedelic alkaloid. It is found in several cactus species, most notably in the peyote cactus (*Lophophora williamsii*), San Pedro cactus (*Echinopsis pachanoi*) and Peruvian torch cactus (*Echinopsis peruviana*). It induces psychedelic effects akin to those of lysergic acid diethylamide (LSD) and psilocybin, altering perception, mood and thought processes, often resulting in vivid visual and auditory hallucinations.

Mescaline is one of the simplest phenethylamines compounds and remains the only naturally occurring phenethylamine hallucinogen. It has a low potency, requiring a dose of between 250 and 500 mg. Its effects last around eight to ten hours. The chemical structure of mescaline comprises of three methoxy groups attached to aromatic rings, resulting in a molecule that affects serotonin receptors in the brain, thus inducing its hallucinogenic effects. It also acts on dopaminergic and adrenergic receptors.

The traditional use of mescaline dates back thousands of years among certain Native American tribes, particularly in Mexico and the southwestern United States. The Native American Church was established in the late 19th century and regards peyote as sacred, using it as a ceremonial sacrament. The religious rituals involving mescaline are seen as a means of spiritual communion, healing and obtaining guidance from the divine. The ceremonies often include chanting, prayer and other rituals that have been passed down through generations. The use of peyote in these ceremonies is often referred to as the "peyote way" and is considered integral to the religious practices of the NAC. The use of peyote in ceremonies by the NAC is protected by law in the United States. In Central and South America, shamans use mescaline in healing and divination rituals. It is used as a tool to connect with the spiritual realm, gain insights and address physical or psychological ailments. It is also used in rites of passage ceremonies to mark significant milestones such as initiation into adulthood. Here, the psychedelic experience is thought to bring personal transformation and spiritual growth.

Although mescaline has no recognised medical application, it has been investigated for the treatment of alcohol-dependency disorder, as well as several other psychiatric conditions, including depression (Vamvakopoulou et al., 2023).

The first wave

Indigenous cultures across the globe still practise traditional plant medicine with entheogenic substances to create altered states of consciousness in ritual or religious contexts (Wexler, 2018). For example, the current NAC and its ceremonial use of peyote cactus dates back 5,700–10,000 years (Bruhn, et al., 2002). Ibogaine has been used in West African tribal rituals for centuries (Modir et al., 2018), and there is evidence in South America of ceremonial use of *Banisteriopsis caapi*, the main ingredient in ayahuasca, dating back at least 1,000 years (Naranjo, 1979). In these traditions, the mind, body and spirit are often viewed as one entity – the focus of the work is to re-address imbalance or disconnection. A natural drive towards connection is deeply rooted in a cultural view that is holistic and strives towards balancing the physical, emotional and spiritual aspects of the human experience. The centrality of spiritual belief, ritual, tradition and community reflects this and stands in stark contrast to the dualistic conceptualisation of mental and physical wellbeing used in the West (Sue et al., 2019).

It has been suggested that indigenous cultures do not require formal integration in the same way the West does, because psychedelics are integrated into their daily lives and culture. In contrast, Western culture has lost its connection with the natural world and does not possess adequate cultural references to assimilate the experience (Loizaga-Velder & Pazzi, 2014; Aixalà, 2022). In indigenous communities, integration is often an ongoing practice that is woven into the general functioning of the group and illustrates the centrality of a worldview that orients towards balance. In these settings, herbalism is a cornerstone of life which is used to support mental, physical and spiritual health with a holistic approach that encourages a balancing of the systems, rather than symptom management as in Western medicine. The use of sacred plant medicine in these traditions encompasses gathering and interacting with the plants on a deep level and connecting with them as living beings with a spiritual context in the world (Tedlock, 2005). Our innate drive towards self-actualisation has indeed been obstructed by Western culture (Maslow, 1968) and lessons can be learnt from the centrality of the holistic approach to mental and physical wellbeing in indigenous communities.

Traditional integration rituals can take place before, during and/or after the use of entheogens. The practice of fasting prior to, or in conjunction with, herbal remedies to prepare the body for entheogens and cleanse the system is common, and participants may abstain from sex, alcohol and sweet, spicy, salty or rich foods prior to a ceremony. Techniques such as hypnotic inductions into trance-like states with drumming and chanting, all within a communal context, bear some resemblance to reprocessing in

EMDR because of the combination of bilateral stimulation (drumming/BLS) and induced altered states (Winkelman, 2021). Dreamwork is another practice found in many indigenous cultures. Dream incubation is achieved through the induction of a purposeful dream state, followed by communal interpretation which is often intertwined with plant medicine because negative dreams are thought to be closely linked to illness (Tedlock, 2005). See Chapter 11, 'Transpersonal Healing,' for dreamwork with EMDR.

A dark side to the psychedelic renaissance has emerged, in which the explosion of psychedelic tourism has resulted in the exploitation of indigenous communities. The disruptive influence of the power imbalance between Western health tourism and indigenous communities has led to negative impacts on these communities and has been referred to as a continuation of colonialism. For example, the rapid depletion of peyote, the main sacrament used by the Native American Church, through high-demand and illegal poaching. Another example of this is the exploitation of the Bufo Alvarius toad, from which 5-MeO-DMT is collected when the toad comes out of hibernation. Conservationists have warned that the exploitation of this animal – through what has been described as an 'international toad venom smoking phenomenon' – could lead to the extinction of this sacred toad (Villa, 2020). However, alternatives are available; 5-MeO-DMT was first synthesised in 1936, and current versions of this compound have been shown to be 99.86% pure. This more ethical and pharmacologically stable version is being used in the ongoing trials in the UK.

Unfortunately, this book does not have the scope to cover this important area in sufficient depth to fully explore the ancient relationship that humans have with entheogens and the pivotal role they have played in the fabric of society and consciousness. Whilst acknowledging that the roots of many integration activities lie in traditional use of entheogens, this chapter focusses on modern models of integration being employed in Western psychedelic therapy and research.

The second wave

In 1938, Swiss chemist Albert Hoffman created the first synthetic hallucinogen, LSD, whilst attempting to make a chemical compound that would stimulate the respiratory and circulatory systems from ergot derivatives. He accidentally dosed himself during work in the lab on 19 April 1943 – a date now celebrated as 'Bicycle Day'. He experienced what he later described as a 'voyage into chemically induced psychosis' (Hoffman, 1983). This intriguing substance was then marketed by the pharmaceutical company Sandoz as an adjunctive psychotherapy medication and a compound for the study of psychoses (Hoffmann, 1983).

Early research in the field of psychedelic-assisted psychotherapy focused on 'psycholytic' therapy, which utilised moderate doses of psychedelic substances such as LSD to facilitate the therapeutic process (Sandison 1957; Grof, 1980). The term 'psycholytic' refers to the concept of 'psyche-dissolving' or loosening the grip of psychological defences, allowing for deeper exploration of the unconscious and emotional experience. The objective was to promote emotional healing and self-exploration by enhancing introspection, emotional release and insight during the therapy sessions. Psycholytic therapy emerged during the 1950s and has theoretical roots in psychoanalysis, the dominant psychotherapy at that time. A broad spectrum of newly discovered psychoactive substances was utilised to facilitate psychotherapeutic interventions such as 'free association' and 're-enactment' (Freud, 1913) by reducing the strength of psychological defences. Material that emerged was then analysed through the lens of the therapist, which would generally be Jungian, Freudian or similar. See Chapter 7, 'Psycholytic EMDR.'

It was around this time that the concept of integration began to emerge, when it was suggested that some patients might require additional support after a psycholytic session. One of the earliest references to integration is seen in the psycholytic work of Sandison (1954) where he refers to the need for 'rehabilitation' after a course of LSD-assisted psycholytic psychotherapy. He also noted the need for exploration of the psychedelic experience. The researcher and therapist Sydney Cohen discussed issues around integration in his work that include the inability to integrate trauma that emerges during psychedelic treatments, as well as issues around re-integrating with the everyday and the depression that can follow destabilisation caused by the shift in perspective that can be precipitated by psychedelics (Cohen, 1965). The psycholytic methodology was used up until President Nixon's 'war on drugs' which pushed this work underground for 40 years until its resurgence in the early 2000s, when restrictions on research were finally lifted (Nicolas, 2016). In response to this, Stanislav Grof developed Holotropic Breathwork™ as a method to legally create altered states of consciousness that resemble psychedelics. This type of breathing practice, based on Eastern breathing practices, can also be used as an adjunct to psychedelic and other psychotherapies therapy to facilitate integration of trauma.

The term 'integration' became a part of treatment protocols in the 1960s at the Maryland Psychiatric Treatment Centre, where the Spring Grove team were beginning to systematise working with psychedelic substances. This team included some of the grandfathers of psychedelic research: Stanislav Grof, Bill Richards, Walter Pahnke and Albert Kurland. They developed guidelines that are still used today within the large studies at Multidisciplinary Association of Psychedelic Studies (MAPS) (Mithoefer, 2017). Early on, integration was summarised as working through – and integrating – the psychedelic experience by relaying the subjective account of the experience (Grof et al., 1973). Later, Grof further defined a number of integration activities that are familiar in the field today, such as rest, connection with nature, meditation and artistic expression (drawing, poetry, dance, etc.). He also encouraged clients to pay attention to dreams and analysis of the psychedelic experience, paying particular attention to aspects that hold negative emotional charge.

The third wave

In the field of modern psychedelic therapy research, the concept of integration is broad and illusive but loosely refers to the process of making sense of the insights and emotions that arise during a psychedelic session and incorporating them into one's daily life (Gorman et al., 2021). This often involves reflection and exploration of the psychedelic experience with a therapist or trusted individual, with the aim of gaining insights. It can take place in a group session with peers, such as the integration groups run voluntarily by members of psychedelic societies, or one to one with a therapist, coach or peer. See Chapter 12, the future of PsyA-EMDR, for more information on working with groups.

The general consensus is that integration is an ongoing process that takes significant time and effort and that any insights gained are likely to fade without active engagement (Richards, 2017). The broad approach to therapeutic support during psychedelic dosing sessions is non-directive and the therapist's (or sitter's/facilitator's) role is to support the individual through whatever emerges, in a person-centred manner (Rogers, 1951). The main exception is the MAPS approach to treating PTSD, which is discussed later in this chapter.

There is a distinct lack of clarity across modalities as to what goes on during the integration/debriefing phase following a psychedelic treatment. These sessions often involve the participant re-telling the session with the therapist facilitating reflection in a non-directive manner (e.g., Johnson et al., 2014). During the following integration sessions, studies have utilised more directive modalities such as Internal Family Systems (Schwartz, 2001; Mithoefer, 2015) or Acceptance and Commitment Therapy (ACT; Hayes, 2004). Cognitive-behavioural approaches (ACT, DBT, MBCT, etc.) have become the default adjunct psychotherapy, particularly in the UK, despite having no previous empirical evidence of efficacy in the psychedelic field. The reason given for this by its proponents is the existing evidence base and that these protocols can easily be manualised for use in a research context for a broad range of psychological presentations. These standardised approaches are combined with the traditional debriefing/integration sessions that accompany psychotherapy. Participants are encouraged to make connections between the intention they set (goals for therapy) and what unfolded during the psychedelic experience and consider how 'take away messages' can be implemented in their daily lives. In practice, clients are reporting that therapists can put too much emphasis on the behavioural interventions and skip over the exploration of the psychedelic experience. This appears to be a shortcoming, especially when we consider the transformative power of the 'mystical experience' and healing potential of transpersonal work in psychotherapy (Ko et al., 2022).

The Yale Manual for Psilocybin-Assisted Treatment of Depression states that integration is "a means of both making sense and meaning out of the experience, and helping positive changes and insights carry forth into day-today life" (Guss et al., 2020, p. 10). There is a general assumption that if insight is gained and then applied to everyday life, sustained positive change will follow. However, this cognitive approach to behavioural change is at odds with the core tenets of the AIP model. Namely, for sustained change to happen, the corresponding pathogenic memories need to be reprocessed and stored in an adaptive manner to eliminate maladaptive behaviours in the present (Hase et al., 2017). In contrast to the cognitive-behavioural approaches, EMDR therapy is fundamentally a somatic integration approach that also includes the cognitive and behavioural elements of traumatic memory during reconsolidation.

Treating PTSD in psychedelic research

Founded in 1986, MAPS has developed a model for working psychotherapeutically with 3,4-methylenedioxymethamphetamine (MDMA). Its founder Rick Doblin has worked tirelessly over the last 35 years, playing a pivotal role in the re-classification of psychedelic compounds in the US and across the globe. He chose to focus their research on the treatment of PTSD with MDMA because he anticipated that this was the most likely treatment to get approved by the Food and Drug Administration (FDA; Doblin, 2023). They were able to secure funding for the research because the early clinical populations were US soldiers with PTSD, and funding for military-based research is more available than other populations because of the profits involved in the military-industrial complex (Cox, 2014).

MAPS focused on utilising the acute mood-enhancing effects of the 'empathogen' MDMA to enhance trauma processing when used in conjunction with psychotherapy. Their research has shown that MDMA can attenuate the fear response and allow access to previously overwhelming memories in order to reconsolidate them. They reference trauma research, demonstrating a deficit in the extinction of fear conditioning causes chronic hyperarousal in PTSD. MAPS research has shown that MDMA reduces the stress-induced activation of the amygdala and that accompanying psychotherapy can use this change in physiological state to access and integrate previously overwhelming memories (Metzner & Anderson, 2001; Bedi et al., 2009). MAPS state that:

> This combination of drug effects should support the participant in overcoming the emotional numbing of PTSD and allow her/him to be more fully open to experiencing the full range of emotions (grief, fear, rage, as well as joy, happiness, love, comfort) without the subjective feeling of being overwhelmed.
>
> (Mithoefer et al, 2013, p. 30)

The participant is encouraged to lie down and use eye shades and headphones to invite focus on the inner experience. The guidelines suggest a 50:50 balance between interaction with the therapists and intrapsychic focus. The participant is encouraged to "breathe into the process and trust [their] own inner healing intelligence with the help of the medicine" (p. 31). Participants often re-experience traumas which can go on for prolonged periods of time. During this time, the therapist sits with them and has minimal input, unless the client becomes overwhelmed and requires help grounding. Mithoefer states that:

> It is common for participants to make connections spontaneously between their feelings about specific traumatic events and earlier childhood experiences. Often, they arrive at insights about how earlier experiences may have left them more vulnerable to being traumatised later or may have affected their response to subsequent trauma.
>
> (p. 32)

The foundations of the MAPS approach were developed by a team led by Stanislav and Christina Grof, Leo Zeff, George Greer, Requa Tolbert and Ralph Metzner. The protocol is designed for therapists across modalities but a person-centred to the integration of trauma is encouraged. The manual mentions the use of internal family systems (Schwartz, 2001), sensorimotor psychotherapy (Ogden et al., 2006) and the work of Peter Levine but this is mainly in reference to working with complex clients who require extra input/stabilisation from the therapist. MAPS advocate for:

> A nondirective approach to therapy based on empathetic rapport and empathetic presence should be used to support the participant's own unfolding experience and the body's own healing process. A non-directive approach emphasizes invitation rather than direction.
>
> (Mithoefer et al., 2013, p. 6)

MAPS offer one of the more detailed accounts of the method of integration compared to other studies and list valuable insights, alternative perspectives, development of emotional resilience, emotional language and improved interpersonal skills as the outcomes if the treatment is integrated successfully into the client's daily life. The manual highlights the need for flexibility from the integrative therapist because the level of input required to support the client's integration can vary dramatically. This protocol has a 90-minute integration session the morning following an MDMA treatment. MAPS state that:

> The ultimate goal of MDMA-assisted psychotherapy is to eliminate symptoms and attain an improved level of wellbeing and functioning.
> (Mithoefer et al., 2013 p. 44)

The therapists are permitted to offer minimal interpretations of the participant's experience but a supportive, person-centred to the exploration of the treatment is encouraged above all. Here we see a distinct move away from the analytical roots of PAP. The MAPS manual states that all integration sessions should be client led to:

> [..]ensure that the participant's experience rather than the therapists' agenda will direct the session
> (Mithoefer et al., 2013, p. 45)

The MAPS protocol only introduces focused bodywork if the client is in emotional or somatic distress that they are unable 'to move through spontaneously.' If there is continued dysregulation following a dosing session, they encourage clients to set time aside to experience the thoughts, feelings and emotions 'fully.' They also suggest teaching relaxation techniques such as slow breathing. If this fails, they suggest medications such as benzodiazepines (p. 46), which is a common intervention for adverse reactions cross across PAP settings.

EMDR is mentioned in the MAPS literature in reference to empirically validated treatments for PTSD, but MAPS and the majority of other PAPs do not utilise EMDR to work with this. Instead, MAPS opt for interventions that have minimal empirical evidence such as IFS and somatic experiencing as adjunct therapies. They state that:

> CBT, EMDR, and psychodynamic therapy may bring attention to somatic experiences, but do not include working directly with the body through movement or physical touch.
> (p. 69)

We would argue that physical touch is not necessary to integrate trauma and given the prevalence of physical boundary intrusions in the field of trauma (e.g. rape, sexual violence, physical abuse), the use of touch is potentially harmful and an unnecessary risk. There is also limited evidence to suggest that physical movement is necessary to integrate traumatic memories and clients often spontaneously shake, abreact or tick during reprocessing. EMDR is at its core a somatic therapy, in which levels of disturbance in the body are constantly tracked throughout the process. It also includes the visual, auditory, cognitive and emotional aspects of the material being targeted, in acknowledgement of the key components of memory encoding and the fundamental importance of meaning making in brain development. Perhaps MAPS protocols are referring to the somewhat unsophisticated version of EMDR that is taught as part of its basic training, which is not powered by an in-depth knowledge of the AIP model and its ability to conceptualise frameworks for working with the wide range of complex presentations.

Non-directive integration vs EMDR

The non-directive approach to integration seen across PAPs suggests that the core conditions alone are sufficient to facilitate sustained change (Rogers, 1957). This default to the person-centred is even observed in ACT models where, aside from the directive behavioural change interventions (which are the focus of the work), the integration of the actual psychedelic experience relies on reflective talking therapy. We propose that this approach is not always sufficient to integrate psychedelic material that has emerged, because it is often representative of maladaptively encoded information in the brain that is dissociated (disconnected) from the main memory networks. The targeting of specific memory networks linked thematically to the intention/treatment goal, combined with bilateral stimulation of the brain, facilitates the re-integration of this information which can occur naturally and spontaneously during reprocessing.

A common misconception about EMDR therapy is that it is directive in nature. This is perhaps caused by people's awareness of the structured format of the preliminary stages, prior to reprocessing. As in psychedelic therapy, the preparation phases of EMDR consist of thorough history taking, case conceptualisation and treatment planning. These preparatory stages are important for harm reduction as they prepare the individual for any possible destabilisation. EMDR differs from other modalities because its practitioners do not profess to being an expert in the client's experience, just experts in the structure of the therapy. This is reflected in Shapiro's notion of the client's innate information processing system (Shapiro, 2001). Once the EMDR scaffold is in place, the therapist is encouraged to stay out of the way and the intervention becomes non-directive. Therapists are required to be sensitive to the client's process and react promptly if a problem arises, whilst not being intrusive. Encouraging words are used by the therapist during reprocessing, with care to not get in the way of the client's process (Hase and Brisch, 2022).

For clients with more adaptive experiences in their early childhood, it is sufficient for the therapist to be more 'hands off' and allow the reprocessing to happen with BLS. But when working with clients with limited adaptive information in their memory networks, the therapist is required to take a more active stance to facilitate co-regulation, particularly during reprocessing. Secure bonding with the therapist is essential for this (Hase and Brisch, 2022) and Shapiro highlights that the therapeutic relationship forms part of the client's adaptive memory networks, suggesting that attunement in the psychotherapeutic dyad can lead to the creation of new adaptive memories of a healthy attachment relationship. This adaptive information can be actively used for co-regulation during reprocessing, creating a 'corrective emotional experience' (Alexander and French, 1946) whilst the client is actively reconsolidating interpersonal trauma from the past, adding an additional reparative layer to the work.

The three-pronged approach to psychedelic integration

Integration = to integrate the past into the present to achieve a happier and energetically sustainable future

If we define psychedelic therapy in terms of memory reconsolidation, a successful outcome can mean the difference between PTSD and post-traumatic growth (Tedeschi & Calhoun, 1996). The three-pronged approach of EMDR conceptualises the impact of past traumatic events on both present and future functioning. As EMDR therapists, we work under the AIP hypothesis that psychological difficulties are often the result of maladaptively stored material in the memory networks. Psychological and physiological energy is wasted, being reactive rather than receptive to our surroundings, and our past experiences influence the way that we interact with the world when pockets of dissociated memories reactivate in the present.

When the AIP model is applied to the psychedelic space, it can be used in conjunction with EMDR to facilitate the integration of maladaptive material to achieve a less reactive stance by calming the nervous system. The three-pronged approach in EMDR addresses past trauma, present triggers and perception of the future. If the subjective units of distress scale (SUDS; Wolpe, 1969) is used to assess all domains, this is a belt-and-braces method to ensure the material that emerges is fully integrated and no longer holds emotional charge, therefore eliminating its impact in the present. For example, a client encountered a vision during a psychedelic treatment that had no obvious autobiographical links but left them shaken with sustained dysregulation after the acute effects of the psychedelics had worn off. The somatic bridge can be used to identify the corresponding material in the memory networks that had been reactivated by the psychedelics. After EMDR reprocessing of the corresponding psychological material, the image from the psychedelic experience no longer held any somatic charge.

The prevalence of mystical experiences during altered states of consciousness, and the way that insights and adaptive information surface in response to psychedelics, demonstrates the need for an additional domain in the 3-pronged approach. Reflective clinical practice with PsyA-EMDR has led to the emergence of a fourth 'transpersonal' prong that encompasses the past, present and future domains of EMDR reprocessing. The practical application of this is demonstrated in Chapters 10 and 11 where the expansion of EMDR and the AIP model into this domain from a theoretical perspective is explored with case material to illustrate.

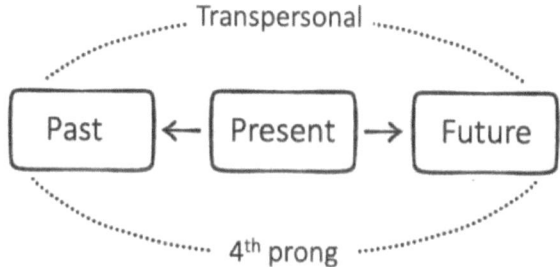

Figure 8.1 The transpersonal prong encompasses the past, present and future.

Measuring integration

A key issue in PAP is the current lack of a direct measure for integration, which may be a result of the vague nature of the concept being measured. The scales used to monitor change in ACT-based PAP track psychological flexibility in the six core areas of the model: acceptance (of thoughts and feelings), cognitive fusion (with thoughts and feelings), being present, self as concept (meta-cognition), values and committed action – all of which have their own empirically validated questionnaires. The MAPS manual for treating PTSD with MDMA sites the following outcomes as indirect indicators of successful integration:

- Valuable insights.
- The development of emotional resilience and emotional language.
- Improved interpersonal skills.

Other psychometric tools are being used in research such as the Integration Engagement Scale (IES) that attempts to measure 'positive behavioural engagement with integration' and the Experienced Integration Scale (EIS) that assesses internal aspects of feeling integrated (Frymann et al., 2022). Neither of these scales target the emergent psychedelic material directly; instead, they use vague statements such as 'I feel harmony between my inner being' and 'I've spent time in nature to nurture my experience' that the participant rates using a Likert scale.

If we conceptualise the healing effects of psychedelic therapy through the lens of memory consolidation theory, the client's somatic response in the present to a) the memory of the psychedelic experience and/or b) the corresponding biographical material could be used to measure levels of integration. This is based on the theory that maladaptively encoded memories retain their original somatic/emotional charge. Therefore, if something (memory or experience) is fully integrated, there should be no maladaptive somatic response. It is the information stored in the memory networks that we want to be adaptively integrated through the reconsolidation process which is started off by psychedelics but completed using BLS in the reprocessing phase of EMDR.

During EMDR therapy, clinicians constantly track the levels of integration of specific stimuli (traumatic memories or current triggers/stressors) using the SUDS, which is a self-rated measure of anxiety, developed for clinicians to track changes in client's affect. It was incorporated into the EMDR protocol by Francine Shapiro and expanded to measure any emotional disturbance. It is used as a measure to track the progress of memory reconsolidation during the reprocessing phase of EMDR therapy as quantitative measure of integration. The SUDS scale has been empirically validated as a global measure of both physical and emotional discomfort (e.g. Kim et al., 2008; Tanner et al., 2012).

PsyA-EMDR integration tools

At its core, EMDR therapy is an integration therapy. Originally designed to integrate unprocessed trauma that causes PTSD, it has now been adapted for use with many psychological presentations based on the AIP framework. The psychodynamic nature of the somatic bridge intervention – that is used to identify key attachment experiences – is aligned with the psychoanalytical roots of psychedelic therapy. However, it re-addresses the power imbalance by putting the client in the role of expert of their own experience. Here we explore some of the ways that reprocessing can be used in the PsyA-EMDR protocol to facilitate integration.

The debrief (short-term integration intervention)

Some definitions of integration focus on the short-term, post-session support that is also referred to as 'aftercare' (Coder, 2017). The PsyA-EMDR protocol combines both long-term and short-term integration to maximise the treatment effects of the psychedelic because it is suggested that the first integration session is within the window of neuroplastic effects for that particular substance. The onset of neuroplasticity for many psychedelics is thought to be from when the acute psychoactive effects start (approx. 30 mins–1.5 hours) and can last for days.

Integration Phase 1: In the first session of post-psychedelic treatment, the client can debrief the experience whilst eliciting BLS (Shapiro & Laub, 2015). The 'Google search' technique and other elements from the RTEP protocol can be helpful if there is not yet a coherent narrative of the experience. Background auditory BLS played quietly through headphones is ideal for this, although tactile or visual BLS can also be used. During this debrief, the clinician notes down key items that hold emotional charge and/or link with core schemas in the client's case conceptualisation. Allow a limited amount of free association to happen to start making connections to biographical content but bring the client back to the debrief of the experience if they go off track.

> **Tip:** When they relay specific scenes/encounters from the psychedelic treatment, ask them to define the accompanying **thought (NC/PC), feeling, somatic response and SUD** to add to the case conceptualisation.

Post dose Phase 2: Once the client has debriefed the event, encourage reflection through an AIP lens, considering their intentions (goals) and how the thoughts, feelings and images that have emerged may fit with their past experiences.

Post dose Phase 3: Together select the target to reprocess first. A general rule of thumb is to go with the item that holds the most charge (has highest SUDS rating) whether that is positive or negative affect.

Choice point: Use the somatic bridge to identify corresponding material in the memory networks or reprocess and re-script the psychedelic material directly in a similar way to working with nightmares (Luber, 2010).

Post dose Phases 4–7: Use the standard protocol with attachment-informed interventions to reprocess the maladaptively stored memories that have been identified by the somatic bridge.

Post dose Phase 8: Re-evaluate the material from the psychedelic treatment phase. If the experience is fully integrated, the SUDs should be 0/1. If higher, repeat the process again (i.e. bridge somatically to remaining unintegrated material) until the SUDs in response to the psychedelic material is 0/1.

Mid/long-term integration

Although a lot can be achieved in just one session of EMDR following a psychedelic treatment, extending the work over a number of sessions, utilising the 4-pronged approach, allows for a more thorough integration of the psychedelic experience and the corresponding memory network. It is suggested that a minimum of six integration sessions using EMDR allows for enough time to identify and integrate the core memory networks that have been reactivated. This is because there is often more than one maladaptive memory converging at the point at which a trauma occurs, which increases the somatic response to the stressor.

Note: If the client has had an adverse reaction to the psychedelics and/or has a complex trauma history, it is likely that more than six sessions will be required.

Unintegrated content

A common mantra in the world of psychedelics is 'there's no such thing as a bad trip.' On the surface, this adheres to the AIP model of the psychedelic space, i.e. a strong negative experience on psychedelics generally correlates with unprocessed trauma. The emergence of trauma in response to the neuroplasticity elicited by psychedelics creates an opportunity to integrate it and heal. However, there is a sense that the phenomenon of adverse experiences is minimised in the psychedelic therapy literature because it undermines the current attempts to de-regulate these substances (Breeksema et al., 2022).

When psychedelics are experienced in an unsafe setting, a 'bad trip' can become dangerous and cause current and/or ongoing intense physical and psychological distress (Barrett et al., 2016). Grof states that difficult psychedelic experiences have the tendency to re-emerge in later trips because the brain is trying to resolve the unprocessed content (Grof, 1980). Through an AIP lens, this is because the somatic response to the emerging material dysregulates the nervous system sufficiently to disrupt the reconsolidation process. Every 'bad trip' will add more material (and somatic charge) to that particular memory network until it is adaptively integrated.

In the past, patients would be given another dose of psychedelics to facilitate the completion of the integration process, and whilst this practice still continues in some settings, this would be considered unsafe and/or unethical in medicalised contexts.

In the wake of the psychedelic renaissance, many trauma therapists are seeing an influx of clients suffering from PTSD/complex PTSD caused by unsafe use of psychedelics. The eight phases of EMDR have been developed to stabilise activated clients, and therapists who understand the clinical application of the AIP model have the tools to support these clients to process what has emerged. Again, this highlights the need for trauma-informed harm-reduction interventions such as screening and psychoeducation, so people understand the risks and can make informed choices about embarking upon psychedelic therapy. See Chapter 5, 'Stabilisation and Risk Reduction.'

Hallucinogen persisting perception disorder

Hallucinogen persisting perception disorder (HPPD) is described as a cognitive disorder which causes an individual to experience a reoccurrence of visual disturbance following intoxication that is reminiscent of acute hallucinogen intoxication (HPPD; American Psychiatric Association, 2013). These can include derealisation, flashbacks, altered motion perception, pareidolia, micropsia, macropsia, troboscopic perception of moving objects and visual snow. There is limited research on this topic, and the treatment recommendations are mood stabilisers and tranquilisers.

Although HPPD is considered a 'rare disorder,' we are seeing an increasing number of referrals into private practice with this presentation. Clinical work with this client group often reveals an impaired ability to self-regulate dating back to early childhood. Clients often describe complex attachment/trauma histories (or intergenerational trauma) and a predisposition to dissociate that predates the damage from the psychedelics. From an AIP perspective, this presentation appears to be similar to PTSD in that it is the result of dysregulation to the nervous system whilst intoxicated, caused by maladaptive encoding of the psychedelic experience. The resulting visual distortions are then accentuated by their individual's inability to self-regulate, increasing the strength/frequency of the symptoms. The symptomology is similar to dissociation with the addition of visual interference (possibly the visual fragment of the maladaptively encoded psychedelic memory).

We have found that these clients often benefit from an attachment-informed EMDR that focusses on stabilisation and grounding techniques. These clients should be encouraged to develop their own breathing and self-regulation practices outside of therapy to help expand their window of tolerance. HPPD can be treated successfully, but individual differences mean that outcomes are varied. It is important to manage expectations and make it clear from the outset that clients will need to develop a mindfulness-based practice outside of the therapy room for the best chance of recovery.

IMPORTANT: When working with HPPD, developing a self-care regime outside of the EMDR sessions is essential. Yoga, breathing, meditation, neurofeedback and heart rate variability training are all useful self-regulation skills that can be supported through psychoeducation.

Breathwork

For incomplete integration during psychedelic treatments, Grof developed breathing techniques based on ancient Eastern practices combined with Western psychology that induce what he coined 'holotropic' states (Grof & Grof, 2023). Translated from Greek to mean 'moving toward wholeness,' these breathing exercises were designed to reactivate psychedelic material and facilitate the integration of any remaining unprocessed content. Controlled breathing practices called pranayama ("prana" = life energy and "yama" = control in Sanskrit) have been shown to increase neuroplasticity (Tolahunase, 2018), and studies of hyperventilation have shown substantial increases in delta (up to 4 Hz) and theta (4–8 Hz) activity, which are the frequencies associated with slow wave and REM sleep (Terekhin, 1996). The expanded states experienced during controlled breathing practices are caused by a reduction in CO_2 levels in the brain, creating a transient hyperplastic state. Breathwork is now being used in clinical trial settings for the purposes of staff training to better prepare research therapists to work with the subjective experiences of a participant's psychedelic journey.

Breathwork-assisted EMDR vignette

'Tom', a 30-year-old man, had attended EMDR therapy in the past and had experience of attending breathwork sessions. Prior to starting this batch of EMDR, a memory emerged during a breathwork session of an abusive relationship from when he was 19 years old.

Case summary

Tom's father was an alcoholic and absent for most of his childhood. His mother had difficulty regulating her emotions and experienced prolonged periods of depression which caused her to be bed-bound throughout Tom's childhood. Tom's sister had been sexually abused by their paternal grandfather when they were children, although Tom was unaware of this at the time.

EMDR session 1

The memory that became the main target of reprocessing was of his partner locking him out of the flat during a domestic violence incident. He initially recalled this scene from a third-person perspective, potentially because he was dissociated due to the stress at that time.

Image: Tom hiding under the public staircase in a block of flats.
NC: 'I am shameful'
Emotion: Shame
SUD: 5

The somatic bridge technique was used to identify the following memories in the network, with the aim of identifying the touchstone memory to allow the network to integrate:

Age	Memory
9	Under stairs locked out during DV **fear + shame**
7	Under stairs at grandparent's **fear + shame** of getting told off
5	Under mum's bed **fear + shame** of getting told off
3	In dark cupboard (v. vague memory) **no emotion – TOUCHSTONE**

During the EMDR session, Tom was unable to identify enough detail of the touchstone memory to fully reprocess it. There was just a dark cupboard with no SUDs and he was viewing it from a third-person perspective (implying dissociation at the time of encoding). Instead, we focused on the memory of hiding under the bed away from mum at age five, which unlocked a whole network of memories of hiding under things whilst afraid.

Interim breathwork

Tom attended two separate one-hour online breathwork sessions during the week between his EMDR sessions. Tom set an intention 'to forgive all the people who have hurt me.'

Breathwork session 1: More detail from age three memory emerged. The cupboard doors were in a 1930s-style house. He gleaned from this that he was at his paternal grandparents' flat. His sister had been molested during this time and Tom realised that the memory was of him hiding whilst his sister was abused. He utilised his resource team from EMDR to calm down his three-year-old self in the breathwork session.

Breathwork session 2: In this breathwork session, the shame and pain about the DV relationship at age 19 emerged which took him by surprise because it 'felt really strong.' He reconnected with the dissociated feelings of **shame** and **fear** under the stairs that he had initially remembered from a third-person perspective. He cried uncontrollably for most of the hour-long session.

EMDR session 2

When he re-evaluated the age 19 memory, the SUD was 3, and he was now able to remember it in first person. It seemed that the breathwork had integrated the majority of the somatic affect, but the residual SUDS scored at a 3 and would not reduce further, indicating that there was an earlier memory blocking it from being fully reprocessed and integrated (demonstrated by a SUD 0 or 1).

The **somatic graft** technique (see Chapter 9) was used to implant the residual feelings from the age 19 memory into the scene in the dark cupboard at age three. He was now able to access a first-person perspective and reprocess the memory. This allowed more detail to come through of being taken out of the cupboard and reunited with his sister. In recalling this moment, he felt a rush to his stomach and saw an echo of being let back into the flat in the age 19 memory and shame about not challenging his partner about their behaviour. He then remembered his sister being 'despondent and floppy' what he now recognises as a trauma response.

He then used Grace Jones and Miss Honey from his resource team to re-script the memory, and he took himself and his sister to the safety of the peaceful place. By this point he felt calm. When he re-evaluated the DV memory at age 19, his perspective had shifted into first person and he experienced a moment of strong emotion, at which point the SUDs immediately reduced to 0. Adaptive information spontaneously emerged of the good times after he left his abusive partner, further confirming the adaptive integration of the trauma network.

Summary

This vignette highlights the potential use of breathwork to enhance trauma integration in EMDR therapy. By inducing an altered state of consciousness, breathwork facilitated the emergence of dissociated emotions and helped complete the reprocessing of the targeted memory. The altered state, coupled with a focused intention to activate the memory network, allowed for deeper emotional release. Breathwork offers a unique advantage over psychedelics, as it is both more accessible and controllable, with effects that are transient and quickly dissipate once the breathing pattern is stopped. Additionally, its legality makes it a practical and accessible option for individuals seeking transformative experiences without legal barriers.

Warning

Breathwork practices can cause dysregulation to the nervous system (albeit at a much lower level than psychedelics) due to the way that the increased brain connectivity reactivates unprocessed trauma. This can activate more material than is possible to integrate, which can overwhelm the nervous system and lead to emotional flooding. If this happens, it is important to pause the breathwork sessions or psychedelic medication. EMDR can be applied along with the stabilisation tool kit until the nervous system has calmed. **See Chapter 5 'Stabilisation and Risk Reduction.'**

References

Aixalà, M. (2022). *Psychedelic integration: Psychotherapy for non-ordinary states of consciousness*. London: Synergetic Press.

Alexander, F., & French, T. M. (1946). *Psychoanalytic therapy: Principles and application*. New York: Ronald Press.

American Psychiatric Association (APS). (2013). *Diagnostic and statistical manual of mental diseases (DSM-V)* (5th ed.). Washington, DC: American Psychiatric Association Press. https://doi.org/10.1176/appi.books.9780890425596

Barrett, F. S., Bradstreet, M. P., Leoutsakos, J. M. S., Johnson, M. W., & Griffiths, R. R. (2016). The challenging experience questionnaire: Characterization of challenging experiences with psilocybin mushrooms. *Journal of Psychopharmacology, 30*(12), 1279–1295. https://doi.org/10.1177/0269881116678781

Breeksema, J. J., Kuin, B. W., Kamphuis, J., van den Brink, W., Vermetten, E., & Schoevers, R. A. (2022). Adverse events in clinical treatments with serotonergic psychedelics and MDMA: A mixed-methods systematic review. *Journal of Psychopharmacology, 36*(10), 1100–1117. https://doi.org/10.1177/02698811221116926

Cohen, S. (1965). The beyond within. The LSD story. *Psychosomatic Medicine, 27*(4), 397–398. https://doi.org/10.1097/00006842-196507000-00016

Cox, R. W. (2014). The Military-Industrial complex and US military spending after 9/11. *Class, Race and Corporate Power, 2*(2), 1–20. https://doi.org/10.25148/CRCP.2.2.6092117

Doblin. (2023). 'MDMA-assisted therapy for PTSD', closing speech at breaking convention 2023. Found at: https://www.youtube.com/watch?v=ymSumKJvxn4&list=PLG6lerAb0Hitk8QwzLm2mPrI2pJTHXimA&index=111

Freud, S. (1913). *On the beginning of treatment* (Standard edition of complete works Vol. XII). London: Hogarth Press.

Gorman, I., Nielson, E. M., Molinar, A., Cassidy, K., & Sabbagh, J. (2021). Psychedelic harm reduction and integration: A transtheoretical model for clinical practice. *Frontiers in Psychology, 12*, 645246. https://doi.org/10.3389/fpsyg.2021.645246

Grof, S. (1980). *LSD psychotherapy*. Alameda, CA: Hunter House

Grof, S., & Grof, C. (2023). *Holotropic breathwork: A new approach to self-exploration and therapy*. Albany: State University of New York Press.

Guss, J., Krause, R., & Sloshower, J. (2020). The yale manual for psilocybin-assisted therapy of depression (using acceptance and commitment therapy as a therapeutic frame). Connecticut, Yale Psychiatry Department. https://doi.org/10.31234/osf.io/u6v9y

Hase, M., & Brisch, K. H. (2022). The therapeutic relationship in EMDR therapy. *Frontiers in Psychology, 13*, 835470. https://doi.org/10.3389/fpsyg.2022.835470

Hayes, S. (2004). Acceptance and commitment therapy, relational frame theory, and the third wave of behavior therapy. *Behavior Therapy, 35*, 639–665. https://doi.org/10.1016/S0005-7894(04)80013-3

Kim, D., Bae, H., & Park, Y. C. (2008). Validity of the subjective units of disturbance scale in EMDR. *Journal of EMDR Practice and Research, 2*(1), 57–62. https://doi.org/10.1891/1933-3196.2.1.57

Luber. M. (2010). *Eye movement desensitization and reprocessing (EMDR) scripted protocols: Special populations*. New York: Springer Publishing. https://doi.org/10.1891/9780826122452

Maslow, A. H. (1968). *Toward a Psychology of Being* (2nd ed.). New York: Van Nostrand Reinhold.

Metzner, R., & Adamson, S. (2001). Using MDMA in healing, psychotherapy and spiritual practice, In J. Holland (ed.), *Ecstasy, A complete guide: A comprehensive look at the risks and benefits of MDMA* (pp. 182–207). Rochester: Inner Traditions. https://doi.org/10.1046/j.1360-0443.2002.t01-3-00202.x

Mithoefer, A., Jerome, L., Ruse, J., Doblin, R., Gibson, E., & Marcela Ot'alora, G. (2013). *A manual for MDMA-assisted psychotherapy in the treatment of post-traumatic stress disorder*. Santa Cruz, CA: Multidisciplinary Association for Psychedelic Studies.

Naranjo, P. (1979). Hallucinogenic plant use and related indigenous belief systems in the Ecuadorian Amazon. *Journal of Ethnopharmacology, 1*(2), 121–145. https://doi.org/10.1016/0378-8741(79)90003-5

Rogers, C. R. (1957). The necessary and sufficient conditions for therapeutic personality change. *Journal of Counselling Psychology, 21*, 95–103. https://doi.org/10.1037/h0045357

Sandison, R. A. (1957). The contribution of LSD therapy to analytic theory and practice. *Bulletin of the British Psychological Society, 33*, 24.

Shapiro, F. (2001). *Eye movement desensitization and reprocessing (EMDR): Basic principles, protocols, and procedures*. New York: Guilford Press.

Shapiro, E., & Laub, B. (2015). Early EMDR intervention following a community critical incident: A randomized clinical trial. *Journal of EMDR Practice and Research, 9*(1), 17. https://doi.org/10.1891/1933-3196.9.1.17

Sue, D. W., Sue, D., Neville, H. A., & Smith, L. (2019). *Counseling the culturally diverse: Theory and practice* (8th ed.). New York, NY: John Wiley and Sons.

Tedeschi, R. G., & Calhoun, L. G. (1996). The posttraumatic growth inventory: Measuring the positive legacy of trauma. *Journal of Traumatic Stress, 9*, 455–471. https://doi.org/10.1002/jts.2490090305

Terekhin, P. (1996). The role of hypocapnia in inducing altered states of consciousness. *Human Physiology*, 22(6), 100–105.

Tolahunase, M. R., Sagar, R., Faiq, M., & Dada, R. (2018). Yoga-and meditation-based lifestyle intervention increases neuroplasticity and reduces severity of major depressive disorder: A randomized controlled trial. *Restorative Neurology and Neuroscience, 36*(3), 423–442. https://doi.org/10.3233/RNN-170810

Vamvakopoulou, I. A., Narine, K. A., Campbell, I., Dyck, J. R., & Nutt, D. J. (2023). Mescaline: The forgotten psychedelic. *Neuropharmacology, 222*, 109294. https://doi.org/10.1016/j.neuropharm.2022.109294

Villa, R. (2020). Toad smoke: (Un)Natural history of the sonoran desert toad. Found at https://tucsonherpsociety.org/2020/09/28/online-presentation-september-28-2020-7pm-pst-robert-a-villa-toad-smoke-unnatural-history-of-the-sonoran-desert-toad/. Accessed 9.2.24

Wexler, P. (2018). *Toxicology in Antiquity*. London: Academic Press.

Wolpe, J. (1969). Subjective units of distress scale. *Journal of EMDR Practice and Research*. https://doi.org/10.1037/t05183-000

9   Bridging to the matrix

Iboga
Ibogaine hydrochloride ($C_{20}H_{25}N_3O$)

DOI: 10.4324/9781003431718-9

Ibogaine hydrochloride known colloquially as 'Iboga' is a powerful psychedelic made from the root bark of the *Tabernanthe iboga* shrub, commonly found across Central Africa. Ibogaine is a mild stimulant in small doses. In large doses, the strong psychedelic effects induce transcendent experiences and users describe a deep dreamlike state with long-lasting effects. Ibogaine was first isolated in 1905 by Édouard Landrin, and in 1970 it was classified as an FDA Schedule I drug (Drugs Enforcement Agency, n.d.). It is not listed under the Misuse of Drugs Act in the UK and so is legal to possess, but not supply (UK Government, 1971). Due to its revered status in the Bwiti tradition, it is legal in its homeland of Gabon in Central Africa.

The indigenous Bwiti spiritual tradition is centred around the sacrament of ibogaine, which is treated as a medicine and teacher. Bwiti is roughly translated as 'School of Life' and ibogaine is at the core of their rituals and beliefs. It is used as a path to gnosis and allows direct communion with spirt or God. Weekly ibogaine ceremonies called 'ngoze' are conducted by the community, which also include feasting and dancing in colourful costumes to induce a state of communal energy, referred to as 'nlem myore' or 'one heart only' (Bekale & Alagidede, 2021).

Psychotherapeutically, ibogaine has been linked to a loss of desire for addictive substances such as heroin and cocaine, and research has been carried out to investigate its properties as a 'chemical dependence interrupter' (dos Santos et al., 2017). There is a notable dearth of research into the effects of this substance, with the publication of only one RCT investigating its effects on substance dependence (Apler et al., 1999). Although contemporary research is now ongoing, evidence suggests that Iboga, and pharmaceutically produced Ibogaine, can cause cardiotoxicity in those with underlying health conditions (Koenig & Hilber, 2015) which highlights ethical considerations and causes regulatory restrictions.

Worldwide it is estimated that 0.7 percent of the population (range: 0.4 to 1.0 percent) suffer from drug misuse disorder (this does not include alcohol). Furthermore, it is reported that 1.04% of Africa and 1.9% of West Africa's combined 1.3 billion population are addicted to opioids, Tramadol in particular. There are also significant issues with stimulants such as methamphetamine across the continent (UNDOC, 2020). Despite growing evidence that Ibogaine could be an effective treatment for substance misuse disorder, it is still illegal in many countries which cause significant barriers to carrying out further research.

The impact of trauma reverberates across a lifespan; the echoes of which are evident in an individual's subjective experience of psychedelics. Psychedelic medications frequently take individuals directly to the root node (touchstone) of a themed memory network and the content is often symbolic in nature, indicating pre-verbal and perinatal material that has been encoded by an immature brain (Grof, 2016; Gaensbauer, 2004). Psychedelics can spontaneously remediate early attachment trauma, the symbolism of which may manifest as an omnipotent care-receiving experience. For example, it may no longer matter that our caregivers failed us, if we discover that we were being cradled by the entire universe all along. This powerful adaptive information can over-ride prior held beliefs and facilitate dramatic, instantaneous shifts in perception. When psychedelics are combined with the somatic bridge in EMDR, it is possible to identify the most appropriate developmental deficit to target and reprocess. Psychedelic medications enhance the power of EMDR therapy as a means of identifying and addressing the most salient aspect of a person's trauma experiences and attachment-informed EMDR can be used to build and fortify adaptive capacity. This chapter frames the practical applications that underpin the PsyA-EMDR framework and unpacks the unique value of this intervention as a trauma-focused approach to psychedelic healing.

The overarching aim of integration in psychedelic-assisted therapy is to assimilate insights gained from altered states of consciousness into daily life. As discussed in Chapter 8, Integration, in the field of PAP this insight is currently gained through person-centred exploration, with perhaps the addition of CBT or psychodynamic analysis. In contrast, PsyA-EMDR integration is achieved by first identifying and then reprocessing the information in the memory networks that corresponds with the psychedelic experience. This is based on the hypothesis that transient hyperplastic states caused by serotonergic psychedelics allow maladaptively encoded information to emerge. The EMDR technique – the somatic bridge – is a useful intervention to facilitate this process because it is designed to identify the unconscious material linked to sensory information that has been reactivated in the present and can easily be adapted to work with psychedelic experiences.

This example illustrates how similar sensory information emerges in two separate altered states of consciousness experiences (psychedelics and breathwork). Both bridged to the same root memory, demonstrating the hypothesis that trauma can re-emerge during transient hyperplastic states.

Psilocybin imagery

Breathwork imagery

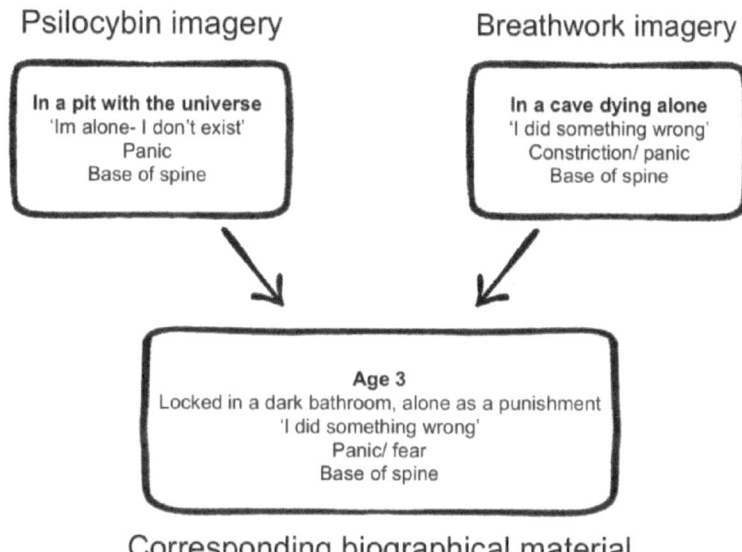

In a pit with the universe
'Im alone- I don't exist'
Panic
Base of spine

In a cave dying alone
'I did something wrong'
Constriction/ panic
Base of spine

Age 3
Locked in a dark bathroom, alone as a punishment
'I did something wrong'
Panic/ fear
Base of spine

Corresponding biographical material

Figure 9.1 Illustration of a somatic bridge being used from targets from two altered states of consciousness: Psilocybin and breathwork, landing on the same trauma in childhood.

History

The 'affect bridge,' referred to as the somatic bridge or floatback in EMDR therapy, was originally developed as a hypnoanalytic technique to move a client experientially from a presenting symptom in the present to a past event. In so doing, revealing the unconscious link between the two (Watkins, 1971). Watkins presented this technique as an alternative to traditional 'free association.' Free association is a fundamental tool of psychoanalytic therapy, whereby chaining thought processes during streams of consciousness are used to identify unconscious material (Freud, 1913). Although free association can work, the cognitive nature of the approach means that, at times, psychological defences obscure/block connection with traumatic material, in an attempt to avoid overwhelm. Watkins states that the failure of psychoanalytic therapy is often due to the 'over intellectualisation of the therapy' and that it overlooks the integration of emotional content. He believed that in order to integrate a 'pathogenic experience,' and for insights to be genuinely therapeutic, the impact of the experience must be a 'felt as well as known' response (1971, p 22). He highlighted the tendency for traditional psychoanalytic therapy to become 'emotionally flat and sterile' and does not achieve what Alexander and French (1946) referred to as the 'emotionally corrective experience' required to achieve sustained change. Watkins developed the affect bridge in response to this to encourage chaining of affect (associated emotional responses) rather than the cognitive chaining of ideas. It is perhaps best described as the physiological version of free association, with a focus on the emotional response. This avoids the cognitive processing areas of the brain being activated, thereby bypassing any cognitive defences.

Bridging in EMDR

The somatic bridge in EMDR therapy develops the affect bridge one step further. The somatic bridge focusses specifically on the body's somatic response to a stressor in the present. This somatic response is then paired with the emotional response in the present, and these are used as the bridging point, diverting the thought processes around the intellectual 'chaining' of events, and straight to the emotional (somatic) core of an experience. The importance of the cognitive element of experience is also taken into account, when the negative cognition (NC) or self-referencing belief is identified to summarise how they feel in that moment. This is based on memory consolidation theory which posits that memory encoding is a process where sensory input is processed and stored via the neocortex, an area of the brain involved in cognitive processing (Huitt, 2003; Brown et al., 2014). This information is assimilated into networks of association in the brain known as schemas (Tse et al., 2007), although these are referred to as memory networks in EMDR.

AIP case conceptualisation uses the NC combined with the emotional response to group memories together in their networks of association (see Shapiro & Laliotis, 2011). During reprocessing, the phenomenon of 'chaining' demonstrates the themed connections between memories in the same network (generally linked by thought, feeling and sensation), which can be viewed as a somatic version of free association as used in psychoanalysis. During bridging, the addition of the NC facilitates the reactivation of the maladaptively encoded material that is being targeted and directs the somatic bridge to the corresponding memory network. See Chapter 11 'Transpersonal Healing' for an exploration of memory networks in the context of psychedelic therapy.

Note: Even though the client labels the experience with an NC, they are encouraged to focus on their body's somatic response whilst bridging, because this diverts around their cognitive defences.

The somatic imprint of trauma

Adapting the traditional psychoanalytic bridging technique to focus on the somatic response to a stressor has been validated by recent neuroscientific research into the somatic imprint of trauma (e.g. Van der Kolk, 2014). As previously mentioned, disruption to memory encoding systems under stress can result in information being stored in a maladaptive, state-specific format, retaining its emotional and somatic charge, rather than being consolidated adaptively into long-term semantic memory (Panksepp, 1998; Hase et al., 2017). The resulting 'engram' of fear or threat is encoded in the neural circuits and can be reactivated by internal or external stressors, therefore becoming the basis for the persisting somatic and psychological effects of the traumatic event (Maddox et al., 2019). In a bid to maintain stability of the nervous system, the psyche creates conscious and unconscious psychological defences to avoid reconnection with the trauma. If there are high levels of dissociated material/unprocessed trauma, this can lead to intrusions that impact daily functioning (Spiegel & Cardeña, 1991).

It is hypothesised that the resulting compartmentalised trauma memories, accompanied by their state-specific sensory information, re-emerge during psychedelic treatments, which is why these powerful treatments can cause destabilisation of the nervous system. The somatic bridge specifically targets the somatic fragment of pathologically encoded memories that have been reactivated and traces the associative network back to the root node (touchstone) in the memory network.

Pre-verbal memory

Many traditional trauma therapies focus on declarative memories that have been encoded since the individual was consciously aware of their surroundings (beginning around 2–3 years; Peterson, 2021), but it has been shown that implicit (non-declarative) memories do not require conscious awareness for encoding (Squire, 1992) and that perinatal stimuli such as sound is encoded in the womb and can be recalled by the infant once born (Pino, 2016). Deceleration in neonatal heart rate in response to stimuli previously encountered in the womb is thought to demonstrate 'habituation,' which is a basic form of learning known as the 'cardiac version of the orienting response' (Kreuger & Garvan, 2014). It is thought that the foetus's autonomic nervous system (ANS) and central nervous system (CNS) need to be mature enough to encode this information – approximately 28–32 weeks, three weeks after the cochlea and peripheral sensory organs are structurally complete (Granier-Deferre et al., 2011).

Psychedelics offer a unique window into the abstract pre-verbal encoding of memory that has been shown to take place in the womb. Psychiatrist Stanislav Grof's theory, 'Systems of Condensed Experience' (COEX), is a theoretical framework that includes these perinatal experiences. His case conceptualisation of this process was created by gathering data from participants on his LSD trials in the 1970s (Grof, 2016). There are parallels between Grof's COEX concept and the themed grouping of memory networks (NC, somatic response and emotion) in EMDR therapy. See

Chapter 11 'Transpersonal Healing' discussing the expansion of the AIP model into the perinatal and transpersonal using Grof's research.

Using the psychodynamic approach in PsyA-EMDR

The somatic bridge is a bottom-up (body-up) technique that diverts around the cognitive defences in the brain. Facilitating access to implicit memory and EMDR therapy has co-opted this intervention as an alternative way to identify memories that correspond with presenting symptoms. In contrast to the standard protocol method of creating a list of memories with the client based on their history – which relies on declarative memory recall – the somatic bridge is a psychodynamic method that organically identifies biographical material that corresponds to the presenting symptom or emotional stressor (commonly called a 'trigger' or trauma stressor). When executed successfully, it is possible to demonstrate the link between the symptom and the maladaptively encoded memory by reassessing the presenting symptom (the original bridging point) using the subjective unit of distress (SUD) scale. Once reprocessed, there is often a significant quantifiable reduction in somatic response to a current stressor. This is experientially valuable as a psychoeducation tool for clients because it clearly illustrates the AIP model, verifying the link between the past and the present by rapidly reducing their somatic response to an emotional stressor.

Another key benefit of the use of the somatic bridge is that it organically identifies formative developmental experiences or deficits that can often be overlooked during the history-taking/case conceptualisation phase.

The adaption of the somatic bridge for PsyA-EMDR

Using memory consolidation theory and the AIP model as a guide, the somatic bridge combined with reprocessing with BLS has been used successfully in clinical practice to reprocess and integrate material that has emerged during psychedelic therapy (Rose & Raine-Smith, 2023). The clearest demonstration of the efficacy of this technique in the context of PAP is when treating PTSD-like intrusions that have manifested as a result of the administration of a psychedelic. If a client is experiencing flashbacks and/or intrusions after the acute drug effects have worn off, the symptoms can be bridged from, to identify the corresponding material in the memory networks. Reprocessing (integrating) this sensory information using BLS will attenuate the unwanted symptoms in the present (this can be biographical, perinatal or transpersonal – see Chapter 11 'Transpersonal Healing'). From an AIP perspective, the psychedelic experience allows traumatic material in the memory networks to emerge and be reprocessed using EMDR to integrate the sensory material sufficiently, so that it no longer reactivates in the present, demonstrated by a SUD rating of 0/1 (out of 10).

Case material: the application of the somatic bridge in PsyA-EMDR therapy

Thirty-year-old male client attending private psychotherapy with the aim of integrating material that emerged during a legal psilocybin treatment in the Netherlands a year prior. There had been limited improvement, despite attending talking therapy for the past five months. Themes that had emerged of **loneliness, shame, dread, isolation and rage** were still causing emotional flashbacks and heightened anxiety.

The client referred to his mother as a "textbook narcissist" who was regularly violent and emotionally abusive towards him and his twin brother. He also reported that his father was an alcoholic. Both parents appeared to have experienced severe attachment deficits and trauma throughout their childhoods and adolescence. The client stated that his parents should not have had children because they appeared uninterested in their emotional wellbeing.

PsyA-EMDR intervention

This treatment was given via an online platform designed specifically for EMDR therapy. The BLS was a combination of concurrent audio (metronome clicks through headphones) and eye movements (following a ball on the screen). One set of BLS for this particular client was approximately 20 seconds at 1.46 Hertz (88 beats/min).

During the preparation phase, the client created a peaceful place visualisation and set up a team of resource figures consisting of nurturers, protectors, and a wise figure (Parnell, 2013). See Chapter 6 'Preparation.'

The client was initially phobic of connecting with or discussing the material from the psilocybin treatment because they found it destabilising to think about (SUD 10). To counteract this, two preliminary sessions of reprocessing were used to get him used to the concept of memory work with BLS. When he was comfortable with reprocessing and the therapeutic relationship was strong enough, the therapy moved on to integrating the material that emerged from the psilocybin treatment.

Psychedelic imagery: Everything is dark, there is a "shadowy figure who is a metamorphosis of all his previous partners."
NC: 'You're not worthy of love, you'll always be alone' (He heard these words during the psychedelic treatment).
Emotion: Fear and abandonment
SUD: 10
Location: Chest

The following account is of the psychedelic material that was integrated one 60-minute session:

Somatic Bridge 1

The somatic bridge was used to identify the corresponding maladaptively stored content and he landed on the memory of a recent break-up. The image was his partners' hurt face and the feeling he experienced was **guilt/shame** (SUD 8). When BLS was applied, the SUD reduced to 4 within a few sets but stayed at this level – which according to the AIP model implies that there is an earlier memory in the network blocking integration of the targeted memory. This needed to be reprocessed in order to proceed.

Somatic Bridge 2

The client bridged again to an earlier memory of suddenly breaking up with a girlfriend and the **guilt** (SUD 8) that he felt at their shock and pain. With the BLS running, he spontaneously began to make links between their feelings during the psychedelic session and biographical material from the break-up. In the session, he was saying "I'm sorry, I'm sorry, I'm sorry!." The SUD reduced to 4.5 within 4 sets of BLS, but then stayed at this level, indicating that was once again, earlier content was blocking the integration of the targeted memory.

Somatic Bridge 3

He then bridged back to the "earliest version of this feeling" and landed on what appeared to be a root node in this memory network (touchstone memory) from age ten:

> **Touchstone memory:** His parents, sat in the dark in the kitchen smoking cigarettes
> He says to his mother "I am really sad"
> Mum says "No you're not, you just need to be happy"
> **NC:** 'No one cares about me, I'm alone'

He continued to connect with later memories of "flings and one-night stands" in the same memory network. He then returned to the touchstone memory (age ten) and reported "getting in touch with his child self" (NC:

"No one cares about me). You don't see or hear me. I'm alone." He then jumped to age eleven where his mother was "antagonising him through the bedroom door" when he was trying to get to sleep.

He then re-evaluated the touchstone memory and reported feeling **anger**. This reduced from a SUD 5 to a 0 within 4 sets of BLS. His nurturer was then sent into the imaginal space to validate his feelings and co-regulate his ten-year-old self by inviting him to share how he was feeling and validating the feelings that came up. The positive cognition "I am worthy, I am worthwhile" was installed.

When he re-evaluated the material from the psychedelic treatment, he reported it feeling "much less intense." Another "bubble of feeling" was spontaneously experienced when he remembered the fear of looping during his psychedelic session. When BLS was added the SUDs reduced quickly. We re-evaluated the psychedelic material again and he reported SUD 0.

One final part of the psilocybin trauma was after he removed his blindfold and the sitters attempted to ground him unsuccessfully, which left him feeling like they "weren't doing anything to help him" (mirroring his mother's behaviour in the touchstone memory). BLS was applied and the SUD reduced to 0 in two sets. The nurturer was used to re-script the final part of the psilocybin treatment trauma and to support him in the imaginal space. In the following session, we re-evaluated the psychedelic experience (SUD 0).

Discussion

From an AIP perspective, it appeared that the psilocybin treatment dislodged some previously compartmentalised attachment trauma. The network that was triggered had themes of self-defectiveness/responsibility, with an over-arching emotion of guilt/shame. As described by Brayne's illustration of the somatic bridge technique in EMDR therapy, it is often necessary to bridge back more than once to arrive at the formative developmental memory, although sometimes clients can bridge all the way to their early years during the first attempt (Brayne, 2022). This appears to be mediated by the complexity of their trauma history and their overall ability to self-regulate. For example, their overall window of tolerance (Siegel, 2020) needs to be increased by first attending to more recent, less overwhelming memories so as to allow the brain's defences to be relaxed enough to attempt reprocessing of the earlier, more overwhelming memories from childhood.

The more complex the history → the less capacity for self-regulation → meaning psychological stressors throughout their life have a deeper impact → therefore there is a need to attend to lower SUDs incidents first. The impaired ability to self-regulate means it is necessary to reprocess lesser traumas in the network first to stabilise the system enough to then process early overwhelming experiences.

Once the touchstone was reprocessed, this generalised to later memories in the network, illustrated by his brain bouncing around later experiences of the same theme. After one set of BLS, where he allowed his mind to wander and allow the generalisation to happen, he re-evaluated the touchstone, his perspective of the memory had shifted to third-person, and his guilt and shame had changed to anger. This change in his response to the memory implied a shift from re-experiencing the state-specific childhood emotions of guilt and shame that were encoded maladaptively to a narrative (episodic) encoding (Bernsten & Reuben, 2006) format from his adult perspective, which allowed him to see the injustice of his experience.

In the field of trauma, shame is thought to be a conditioned survival response linked to the dissociative freeze response of the parasympathetic nervous system (Schore, 2009). Following the shock of activation of the fight or flight system, Porges (2011) describes shame as the 'dorsal vagal drop' as a rapid regulation of arousal in the absence of a caregiver. It is the shift from hyper- to hypo-arousal through the activation of the vagal brake. From a polyvagal perspective, his anger is conceptualised as an activation of his sympathetic nervous system to get him from the dorsal vagal state of shutdown associated with shame towards the ventral vagal state of homeostasis (Porges, 2011).

Dysregulation (activation) → Shame (shutdown) → Anger (activation)

This conditioned pattern of response to emotional dysregulation was deeply engrained for this client, highlighting the importance of reparative work to re-script his attachment experience and calm the emotions of his traumatised inner child. Once the touchstone had been fully reprocessed (SUD 0), the imaginal space was utilised to heal some of the deficit on his attachment relationship with his mother. He was encouraged to imagine an embodied sense of co-regulation with his nurturing imaginal character, where she held him and validated his emotions. Here, we used a version of the 'Loving Eyes Protocol' (Knipe, 2018) with added sensory attunement to the nurturer's warmth, noticing their slow heartbeat, and slow, calm breathing, recreating the co-regulation of the 'good enough' caregiver (Winnicott, 1986; Schore & Schore, 2008). See Chapter 6 'Preparation' for more resourcing techniques.

Note: In this example, the psychedelic therapy provider had inadvertently re-enacted a childhood dynamic with his mother by being unable to help him ground himself adequately at the end of the treatment. This highlights the need for trauma-informed wraparound care delivered by trained clinicians to support the integration of anything that may emerge and access to AIP-informed harm reduction techniques to process any such shortcomings.

The somatic graft technique

This intervention has been developed to activate and reprocess pre-verbal and/or perinatal trauma (see Chapter 11 for application with transpersonal material). If there is information about a pre-verbal trauma, the somatic graft technique utilises the somatic memory that is stored in the body, combined with the concept of repeating themes of trauma in the memory. Sandra Paulsen, a specialist in treating dissociative identity disorder with EMDR, suggests that EMDR acts like a 'divining rod' for dissociated material, referring to the associative nature of the process (Paulsen, 1995). The associations that are observed during reprocessing can be used to create a picture of dissociated or pre-verbal experience because, as mentioned previously, the memory networks are grouped together in themes of association. Using information that is gleaned from a psychedelic treatment, combined with any autobiographical information from family members, the somatic graft technique can be used to reactivate and then reprocess pre-verbal memory.

Using the pre-verbal memory as the starting point, the AIP model is used to create a case conceptualisation by integrating information from the client's history, current symptoms, and patterns of biographical or transgenerational trauma. A declarative memory of a later trauma in the same associative memory network as the pre-verbal memory is chosen, for example, an accident that occurred at age seven with the NC 'I'm in danger' is re-activated triggering the accompanying fear response. The somatic component of the declarative memory from age seven, is then grafted on to an imagined image of the pre-verbal memory (created with information from family members, etc.). If the conceptualisation is accurate and the somatic response is matched to the correct memory network, the application of BLS to this 'imagined' scene can activate any additional maladaptively processed, state-specific information linked to the pre-verbal trauma. Further application of BLS with the standard protocol (ideally with attachment-informed re-scripting) will reprocess and integrate this memory.

Case material: the Somatic graft vignette

A client had an experience during a psychedelic treatment that completely overwhelmed them and left them in a shutdown state of hypo-arousal after the acute effects of the psychedelics had worn off.

> **Psychedelic imagery:** "A dark void of nothingness, then suddenly
> an unbearably loud sound with flashes of white light"
> **NC:** "I'm in danger," I can't escape'
> **Emotion:** Fear and overwhelm
> **SUD:** 10

From his assessment we knew that he had been left on his own in his cot as a toddler during a thunderstorm and that his mother had come in to find him staring up at the window. The client had no conscious recollection of this incident because he was approximately one year old at the time. His mother's family story of this incident was that he was "staring up in wonder" at the lightening outside his window, but the information that had emerged during the treatment appeared to contradict this narrative.

The AIP conceptualisation of this event/network was that he had in fact been terrified by the storm and his mother had observed frozen terror rather than wonder. There were other symptoms around sleep and darkness that also validated this case conceptualisation. Given that he did not remember the incident from childhood, we used the somatic graft technique to reactive the memory by:

1 Initially reconnecting with the somatic affect experienced during the psychedelic treatment by closing his eyes and remembering the image, cognition and feeling.
2 This reactivated the somatic memory of what had emerged in the psychedelic experience.
3 Moving from the psychedelic experience to a visualisation of the created scene in the cot during a thunderstorm.
4 Adding BLS.
5 Reprocessing using an attachment-informed standard protocol.

If the somatic echo of the original trauma that emerged during the psychedelic treatment is activated sufficiently, this will – with the help of BLS – reactivate any corresponding maladaptive information in the memory network.

In this case, he first experienced the memory from a third-person perspective, implying that rather than "staring in wonder" he was in fact dissociated in an attempt to self-regulate. After a couple of sets of BLS, he got into a first-person perspective and briefly experienced the terror that his one-year-old self experienced in response to the storm. It then shifted to a third-person perspective and the somatic response, along with the detail of the imagery, faded until he was no longer able to connect with the scene.

We used a nurturing figure to come in and calm him down before finishing. When we re-evaluated the memory of the psychedelic treatment, the SUD was 0, implying that the maladaptive information that had emerged had been integrated.

Note: The client had visual and auditory BLS which helped to keep him regulated and reduced the overwhelm quickly by reprocessing efficiently.

Summary

The somatic bridge is well aligned to be used in PAP because of its roots in the field of psychoanalysis – a modality that is still drawn upon heavily in the field of psychedelics. The ability of this intervention to identify maladaptively stored memories that correspond with presenting symptoms, by diverting around the cognitive defences, means that it provides client-led individualised care which is a key aim in PAP. When used alongside the AIP model to identify appropriate targets and integrate them using BLS, this approach delivers a comprehensive treatment to explore and integrate the meaning of phenomenon experienced during psychedelic treatments.

References

Alexander, F., & French, T. M. (1946). *Psychoanalytic therapy: Principles and application*. New York: Ronald Press.

Bekale, A. N., & Alagidede, I. P. (2021). The holy spirit of Iboga and a contemporary perspective on Africa's spiritual renaissance: Focus on Gabonese Bwiti tradition. *Journal of Indigenous and Shamanic Studies*, 2(1), 1–32.

Berntsen, D., & Rubin, D. (2006). Emotion and vantage point in autobiographical memory. *Cognition and Emotion*, 20(8), 1193–1215. https://doi.org/10.1080/02699930500371190

Brayne, M. (2022). *Unleash your EMDR: Release the magic: A guidebook for attachment-informed, integrative, transpersonal EMDR*. Seattle: Amazon Media.

Brown, A. D., Addis, D. R., Romano, T. A., Marmar, C. R., Bryant, R. A., Hirst, W., & Schacter, D. L. (2014). Episodic and semantic components of autobiographical memories and imagined future events in post-traumatic stress disorder. *Memory*, 22, 595–604. https://doi.org/10.1080/09658211.2013.807842

dos Santos, R., Bouso, J., & Hallak, J. (2017). The antiaddictive effects of ibogaine: A systematic literature review of human studies. *Journal of Psychedelic Studies*, 1, 20–28. https://doi.org/10.1556/2054.01.2016.001

Drugs Enforcement Agency. (n.d.). Drug scheduling. Found at: https://www.dea.gov/drug-information/drug-scheduling. Accessed 01.08.2023

Freud, S. (1913). *On the beginning of treatment. Standard edition of complete works* (vol. 12). London: Hogarth Press.

Gaensbauer, T. (2004). Telling their stories: Representations and re-enactment of traumatic experiences occurring the first year of life. *Zero to Three*, 25, 25–31.

Granier-Deferre, C., Ribeiro, A., Jacquet, A. Y., & Bassereau, S. (2011). Near-term fetuses process temporal features of speech. *Developmental Science, 14*(2), 336–352. https://doi.org/10.1111/j.1467-7687.2010.00978.x

Grof, S. (2016). *Realms of the human unconscious: Observations from LSD research*. London: Souvenir Press.

Hase, M., Balmaceda, U. M., Ostacoli, L., Liebermann, P., & Hofmann, A. (2017). The AIP model of EMDR therapy and pathogenic memories. *Frontiers in Psychology, 8*, 1578. https://doi.org/10.3389/fpsyg.2017.01578

Huitt, W. (2003). The information processing approach to cognition. *Educational Psychology Interactive, 3*(2), 53.

Knipe, J. (2018). *EMDR toolbox: Theory and treatment of complex PTSD and dissociation*. New York: Springer Publishing Company. https://doi.org/10.1891/9780826172563

Koenig, X., & Hilber, K. (2015). The anti-addition drug Ibogaine and the heart: A delicate relation. *Molecules, 20*(2), 2208–2228. https://doi.org/10.3390/molecules20022208

Krueger, C., & Garvan, C. (2014). Emergence and retention of learning in early fetal development. *Infant Behavior and Development, 37*(2), 162–173. https://doi.org/10.1016/j.infbeh.2013.12.007

Landrin, A. (1905). *De l'iboga et de l'ibogaïne*. Imp. levé.

Maddox, S. A., Hartmann, J., Ross, R. A., & Ressler, K. J. (2019). deconstructing the gestalt: mechanisms of fear, threat, and trauma memory encoding. *Neuron, 102*, 60–74. https://doi.org/10.1016/j.neuron.2019.03.017

Panksepp, J. (1998). The periconscious substrates of consciousness: Affective states and the evolutionary origins of the self. *Journal of Consciousness Studies, 5* (5–6), 566–582.

Panksepp, J. (2005). *Affective neuroscience: The foundations of human and animal emotions*, New York: Oxford University Press.

Paulsen, S. (1995). Eye Movement Desensitization and Reprocessing: Its cautious use in the dissociative disorders. *Dissociation: Progress in the Dissociative Disorders*. 8(1), 32–44.

Parnell, L. (2013). *Attachment-focused EMDR: Healing relational trauma*. WW Norton & Company.

Peterson, C. (2021). What is your earliest memory? It depends. *Memory, 29*(6), 811–822. https://doi.org/10.1080/09658211.2021.1918174

Pino, O. (2016). Fetal memory: The effects of prenatal auditory experience on human development. *BAOJ Medical and Nursing, 2*(4), 2. https://doi.org/10.24947/baojmn/2/2/120

Porges, S. W. (2011). *The polyvagal theory: Neurophysiological foundations of emotions, attachment, communication, and self-regulation* (Norton series on interpersonal neurobiology). New York: W. W. Norton & Company.

Raine-Smith, H., & Rose, J. (2023). Psychedelic-assisted EMDR therapy (PsyA-EMDR): A memory consolidation approach to psychedelic healing. *EMDR Therapy Quarterly, 4*, 1. https://doi.org/10.13140/RG.2.2.24683.35366

Rose, J. C. & Raine-Smith, H. (2023). EMDR as a preparation and integration tool in psychedelic-assisted therapy: a collaborative case study. *EMDR Therapy*

Quarterly, Vol 5 Issue 1, EMDR Association UK. https://doi.org/ 10.13140/ RG.2.2.22717.27369Schore, A. N. (2009). Right-brain affect regulation: An essential mechanism of development, trauma, dissociation, and psychotherapy. In D. Fosha, D. J. Siegel, & M. F. Solomon (Eds.), *The healing power of emotion: Affective neuroscience, development & clinical practice* (pp. 112–144). New York: W. W. Norton & Company. DOI: https://doi.org/10.1037/e60892 2012-004

Schore, J. R., & Schore, A. N. (2008). Modern attachment theory: The central role of affect regulation in development and treatment. *Clinical Social Work Journal, 36*(1), 9–20. https://doi.org/10.1007/s10615-007-0111-7

Shapiro, F., & Laliotis, D. (2011). EMDR and the adaptive information processing model: Integrative treatment and case conceptualization. *Clinical Social Work Journal, 39*(2), 191–200. https://doi.org/10.1007/s10615-010-0300-7

Siegel, D. J. (2020). *The developing mind: How relationships and the brain interact to shape who we are.* New York: Guilford Publications.

Spiegel, D., & Cardeña, E. (1991). Disintegrated experience: The dissociative disorders revisited. *Journal of Abnormal Psychology, 100*(3), 366. https://doi.org/10.1037/0021-843X.100.3.366

Squire, L. R. (1992). Declarative and nondeclarative memory: Multiple brain systems supporting learning and memory. *Journal of Cognitive Neuroscience, 4*(3), 232–243. https://doi.org/10.1162/jocn.1992.4.3.232

Tse, D., Langston, R. F., Kakeyama, M., Bethus, I., Spooner, P. A., Wood, E. R., Witter, M. P., & Morris, R. G. M. (2007). Schemas and memory consolidation. *Science, 316*(5821), 76–82. https://doi.org/10.1126/science.1135935

Van der Kolk, B. (2014). *The body keeps the score: Brain, mind, and body in the healing of trauma.* New York: Penguin Books.

Watkins, J. (1971). The affect bridge: A hypnoanalytic technique. *International Journal of Clinical and Experimental Hypnosis, 19*(1), 21–27. https://doi.org/10.1080/00207147108407148

Winnicott, D. W. (1986). The theory of the parent-infant relationship. In P. Buckley (Ed.), Essential papers on object relations (pp. 233–253). New York University Press. (Reprinted from the "International Journal of Psycho-Analysis," Vol. 50, pp. 711–717)

United Nations Office on Drugs and Crime (UNDOC). (2020). Drug use and health consequences – World drug report. Vienna: United Nations publication. Found at https://wdr.unodc.org/wdr2020/field/WDR20_Booklet_2.pdf. Accessed 26.02.2023

UK Government. (1971). Misuse of drugs act 1971. Found at https://www.legislation.gov.uk/ukpga/1971/38/contents. Accessed 18.07.2023

10 Working with historic psychedelic content

LSD
Lysergic acid diethylamide ($C_{20}H_{25}N_3$)

DOI: 10.4324/9781003431718-10

Lysergic acid diethylamide (LSD) known colloquially as "Acid" is a potent psychedelic drug. Effects typically include intensified sensory perception, thoughts and emotions. At sufficiently high dosages, LSD manifests as mental, visual and auditory hallucinations. LSD is a Class A (Schedule I) restricted substance.

Derived from ergot fungus, evidence of its use has been found on 3000-year-old Greek pottery depicting the Greek god Demeter receiving ergot in the context of the Eleusinian mysteries, a great celebration of art and culture that took place from 1600 BC to 392 CE. It is thought that the ritualistic ingestion of ergot during this time is responsible for the emergence of culture, mathematics, philosophy and democracy in ancient Greece, which forms the foundation of Western culture (Wasson et al., 2008).

The therapeutic effects of LSD underwent a comprehensive exploration from the time of its accidental rediscovery by Swiss chemist Albert Hoffman in 1943, until its classification as a controlled substance by President Nixon in 1971. Indications from these early investigations suggested its potential use as a powerful agent of therapeutic change across a variety of mental health presentations, including anxiety, depression, alcohol dependency disorder and anxiety in terminal illness.

During the 40-year hiatus, very little research was conducted into the therapeutic potential of LSD. Researchers such as Stanislav Grof, who had once pioneered LSD Assisted Therapy research, turned to Holotropic breathwork as a therapeutic alternative (Grof, 1980).

Whilst its therapeutic potential remains, the profile of LSD has been tainted by negative media portrayal and earlier recreational misadventures. Consequently, it is unlikely that LSD will be one of the first psychedelics approved for contemporary therapeutic use. However, its efficacy as an agent of change, particularly in treating alcoholism, is likely to open new doors in the not-too-distant future. And with time, and the growing body of evidence-based applications, the therapeutic value of LSD to reduce psychiatric symptomology is expected to become more widely accepted (Fuentes et al., 2020).

Described in the Lancet in 1955 as "experiences more than 24 hours after administration of LSD..." (Cooper, 1955) and later defined as flashbacks (Horowitz, 1969), post-substance flashbacks are a complex phenomenon of hallucinogen-induced experiences. There is wide variation in experience; typically occurring after drug-free periods, varying in length and echoing experiences from the acute administration phase. Studies have shown that between 5% and 50% of hallucinogen users are reported to have experienced at least one flashback (Alarcon et al., 1982; McGee, 1984). For those struggling with the post-substance effects of hallucinogens, identification and classification of these symptom clusters facilitates access to medicalised treatments.

In the International Classification of Diseases, 11th revision (ICD-11), disorders due to the use of hallucinogens are listed under 6C49. ICD-11 acknowledges that "Among the mental disorders related to hallucinogen use, Hallucinogen-Induced Psychotic Disorder is the most frequently seen, although worldwide it is still fairly uncommon." The DSM-5 (American Psychiatric Association [APA], 2013) describes several hallucinogen-related disorders. Hallucinogen persisting perception disorder (HPPD) is one such condition in which "a person, after the cessation of intake of hallucinogens, re-experiences certain disturbing visuals which were experienced while intoxicated with the hallucinogen." In contrast to classical psychotic disorders, patients with HPPD recognise the unreal nature of their visual disturbances which qualifies them as pseudohallucinations. DSM-5 suggests that whilst the exact prevalence of HPPD is unknown, initial estimates of the disorder among individuals who use hallucinogens is approximately 4.2% (DSM V, 2013). Some question whether pathologising these perceptual experiences is helpful (Prideaux, 2021). The clinical relevance of such psychological sequelae remains unclear (Hermle et al., 1992; Hermle et al., 2008) but, for most, the therapeutic value of working with the content from these aftereffects has been left largely unexplored.

LSD therapy pioneer Stanislav Grof wrote that "[L]ong after the pharmacological effect of the drug has subsided, the patient may still report anomalies in color-perception, blurred vision, after-images, spontaneous imagery, alterations in body image, intensification of hearing, ringing in the ears, or various strange physical feelings" and "sometimes, various combinations of the above and emotional, psychosomatic, ideational and perceptual changes constitute completely new clinical syndromes which the subject has never experienced before. The occurrence of new forms of psychopathology can be understood as a result of activation and exteriorisation of the content of previously latent unconscious matrices. These symptoms usually disappear instantly when the underlying material is fully experienced and integrated" (Grof, 1980). Herein, realigning with contemporary trauma-informed terminology, we redefine flashback as a reactivation.

The question remains, how best to address this underlying material so that it can be psychologically integrated? Sophisticated, trauma-informed therapeutic tools need to be developed and robustly tested to ascertain the efficacy of any such psychological interventions. Until legislative changes enable the testing of therapeutic interventions, working with and learning from the successes and challenges of the entheogenic past, as well as from problematic reactions to recreational drug use, may offer crucial insights into the most effective treatments for a wide range of symptoms. These insights would also help to build an understanding of how to integrate material from the most treatment-resistant presentations.

Specifically, therapeutic integration of problematic reactions emerging from the counterculture drug scene in 1950–1970s merits further exploration. Research and wide cultural use of psychedelics peaked in the 1960s. This era produced more than 1,000 clinical papers covering 40,000 patients and six international conferences on psychedelic drug therapy (Grinspoon and Bakalar, 1979). Moreover, the controversial use of psychedelics by the CIA and ethically questionable research were hidden from public scrutiny. Some people still carry these unintegrated psychedelic experiences. Pushing the psychedelic frontiers whilst ignoring the fallout and casualties of the past could be perilous. A thorough and exhaustive analysis of what can be learned from challenges faced is at the heart of the reflective practice process (Gibbs, 1998; Kolb, 1984). In this population, trauma-informed, measurable and reliable therapeutic approaches were not available and unprocessed content was largely left to conventional medical and psychological treatments. A focused approach to exploring the psychedelic discourse; adverse events, problematic reactions and ethically questionable practice need to be part of the learning which cultivates and shapes the unfolding of the psychedelic renaissance. Without addressing these problems, the therapeutic potential may be lost to scapegoating organisations and individuals, as was the case with Timothy Leary (Lee & Shlaim, 1992). Much can be learned from these trailblazing psychedelic pioneers, and the cultural and ethical discourse that ensued. Delving into and processing the pitfalls will glean new insights and propel contemporary legislative and therapeutic advancement.

The cultural 'set and setting' has also moved on since the post-war era. These cultural shifts may indicate (or result in) changes to the phenomenological experiences of modern psychedelic drug users. In the post-war era, the delusional state triggered for many may well have been activated by cPTSD reactions to Adverse Childhood Experiences (Felitti, 1998; Hill, 2013) mapped out by the political situation in Europe, the Middle East and the Far East at that time (Maté, & Maté, 2022). Whilst these socio-political-geographic issues persist globally, added to that mix is, amongst other things, the impact of climate change on the collective psyche. This perceived existential threat and the anticipatory grief associated with it will likely frame the early-years experiences of generations to come. The development of robust preparatory frameworks for dealing with the fallout of this culturally and temporally relative phenomena and the impact that this issue will play on regressed early experiences needs further exploration. If 'Set and Setting' are fundamentals in psychedelic therapy, a meta-awareness for formulating treatment interventions based on predictions of emergent cultural issues needs to be an established part of the therapeutic framework. Reliably resourcing individuals for material that relates to these issues could be a predictor of a successful psychedelic therapy outcome. Developed for working with cPTSD presentations, EMDR provides a robust and reliable framework and focused resourcing for individuals addressing challenging content. PsyA-EMDR cultivates an applied, rigorous approach to holding the therapeutic 'set and setting.' For more information on preparation and on designing resources related to specific individual and cultural issues, see Preparation Chapter 6. If we are to optimise the healing potential of psychedelics, we cannot ignore the cultural milieu. The link between individual healing and planetary healing, and how healthcare systems respond to the climate emergency, requires further investigation and will be explored later in this chapter and also in Chapter 4, Ethics. There is a growing body of evidence that EMDR therapy is a safe and feasible intervention for people with psychosis (Adams et al., 2020; Varese et al., 2021). Currently, the evidence base is insufficient to determine the effectiveness and acceptability of the intervention specifically for drug-induced psychotic reactions. Larger confirmative trials are required to form more robust conclusions about acceptability and tolerability in this population (Adams et al., 2020; Raine-Smith & Rose, 2023).

Case material

The material presented emerged from a series of difficult LSD trips that Scott Hill experienced in 1967. These encounters precipitated a delusional state with varying degrees of paranoia which perpetuated intermittently as reactivations for many years. Generally, his symptoms presented as ideological and emotional flashbacks, i.e. Scott had no HPPD/perceptual symptoms. Initially, these reactivations could last for several hours; later diluting into uncountable reactivations, usually lasting only a few minutes. From 1970, Scott primarily took an intellectual approach to integrating this material, beginning with dream work and personal journaling and continuing with conventional academic degrees in psychology. In 2002, Scott returned to graduate school to study with experts in psychedelic studies such as Ralph

Bridging from the reactivation symptom

Flashbacks, physical sensations, perceptual distortions (e.g. micropsia, macropsia, floaters, monochromatic vision), somatic reactions (e.g. tics, synaesthesia and repetitions), dreams and emotions can all be used as the starting point for the somatic bridge technique (Watkins, 1971) – see Chapter 9. Alternatively, the somatic bridge technique can be used to identify the maladaptively stored content directly from the psychedelic experience, following the PsyA-EMDR protocol – see Chapter 3.

Troubleshooting

Processing historic content presents EMDR practitioners with several challenges. For example, the narrative around the psychedelic content can be entrenched in the person's identity. Over time, this generalises out into other aspects in the formation of the Self. Blocking Beliefs (Knipe, 1998), Secondary Gains (Davidhizar, 1994) and Systemic Conditions (Seikkula & Olson, 2003) may also undermine efforts to integrate the psychedelic content.

When working with historic treatment-resistant material, the following tools might be useful:

- Client-led interventions that promote patient empowerment.
- Full assessment of secondary gains and systemic blocks during Phase 2 Preparation.
- Working holistically and systemically following the Open Dialogue Approach (Seikkula & Olson, 2003).
- Multimodal integrative approach combining family therapy with EMDR (Silvestre & Tarquinio, 2022).
- EMDR for psychosis-adapted protocol EMDRp (Varese et al., 2021).

Metzner and Stanislav Grof. In 2009, upon publication of his doctoral dissertation, Scott recognised that the process of writing and talking to others about his experiences led to a significant decrease in the number and intensity of reactivations. Scott published 'Confrontation with the Unconscious: Jungian Depth Psychology and Psychedelic Experience' in 2013, and he began giving presentations at Jungian and psychedelic workshops and conventions. Over the years, long-term individual therapy, group work therapy, Holotropic breathwork and three underground psychedelic medicine sessions (each of which elicited the same delusional state) were accessed and described as being 'helpful.' Fifty-five years on, the reactivations still persist, but he now describes them as very brief and rare.

Initially, 6 sessions of PsyA-EMDR therapy were proposed. The material offered relates to 55+-year–old psychedelic content and demonstrates the application of the protocol and its efficacy. Such material is rare to present in a clinical setting. Consequently, this case material was contracted for as a collaboration piece between Scott Hill and Jocelyn Rose, to explore the potential of PsyA-EMDR when working to integrate historic psychedelic content. Given the unblinding, it is important to note that this was a collaboration piece and not a therapeutic relationship. Generous thanks to Scott for sharing his experiences so generously for the purposes of educating and training others.

Course of intervention

Phase 1: History taking

During the detailed history taking, the following adverse experiences were reported:

- 1947 – Birth. Forceps delivery to a depressed, narcissistic mother and an absent, workaholic father.
- Age 2 – No contact with other children for first few years of his life.
- Age 2 – Sustained significant third-degree burns.
- Age 15 – Family home in Kansas – culture of heavy drinking from young age.
- Age 16 – Family moved to California. First significant allies are formed in high-school and in college.
- Age 19 – Discovered marijuana and stopped drinking.
- Age 19 – Psychedelics become a significant influence until the spring of 1967 with the fourth, and final, difficult psychedelic trip.
- Age 23 – Gave up all drug use and started reading and writing extensively about his experiences. Lived in Europe for two years and attended art school.
- Age 26 – Returned to college and earned a B.A. and M.A. in Psychology.
- Age 55 – Returned to graduate study, earning a Ph.D. in Philosophy and Religion.

Scott dedicated himself to recovering from these challenging formative experiences. Even before EMDR, Scott reported the benefits of what he had gone through, expressing gratitude for all that he had learned from integrating the challenging content. He values the therapeutic potential of his psychedelic experiences and continues to work with expanded states through breathwork. Breathwork involves hyperventilation which can evoke challenging cognitive content, heightened emotions, and intense somatic reactions. Engaging in breathwork can indicate a capacity for tolerating other body-orientated psychotherapies such as EMDR. Additionally, research indicates that EMDR is well tolerated by older adults, proving effective in reducing the burden of disease (Gielkens et al., 2022; Gielkens et al., 2023).

Scott now recognises that his confrontation with the numinous content that first emerged during his traumatic psychedelic experiences in 1967 is an integral part of his identity. An academic career and a book have emerged because of his experiences. He recognises that these constitute benefits, and there may well be other such secondary gains that have come about because of his work with psychedelics. Scott states that he has no benefit in holding on to what is still difficult from those experiences. During preparation, blocking beliefs, looping, systemic blocks and resistance to reprocessing the traumatic experiences were explored as potential hurdles to a successful therapeutic outcome.

Pre-intervention psychometric assessment put his GAD7 score at a 15 and on the PHQ9 he scored a 3. He reported some ongoing health issues which were not contraindicatory to EMDR treatment.

Following the clinical interview, a treatment plan was agreed on:

- Ongoing issues of collaborative consent explored.
- Health issues and contraindicators explored.
- Psychometric assessment using GAD7 and PHQ9.
- Development of the therapeutic container/collaborative alliance.
- Psychoeducation – trauma-informed practice and EMDR therapy.
- Secondary gain/systemic blocks explored.
- Resource development and recourse enhancement installed.
- Establishing target – first/worst of the psychedelic material.
- Bridging from the Psychedelic Matrix – image, emotion, body, belief.
- Radical acceptance (Linehan, 2015) of the emergent content reprocessed using BLS.
- Cognitive interweaves (if necessary).
- Use BLS to clear the NC for past, present and future prongs.
- Support for resilience linked to the NC based on future content.
- Psychometrics taken at final processing, +2 weeks and +2 months.

Phase 2: Preparation – risk minimalisation and resource development

Treatment goals

Scott's primary goal was "to go back into that psychedelic-induced delusional state I first experienced in 1967." He wanted to re-experience what emerges during reactivations to gain further insight into the content from his deep psyche. He hoped to "re-experience the sense of being terrified at finding myself in the wrong world" as a tool for healing.

When asked "How would you know if PsyA-EMDR therapy is successful" he described that he would have the sense that "wow I have been brought back," "back to die again," "feeling the fear," "feeling crazy," but also indicated his desire to "remain able to keep my mind to report this to you." We (that is Scott and I, Jocelyn) discussed the notion of looping, and what it might look like to fully reprocess this traumatic event (Shapiro, 2018). Scott reported that he would "probably continue to have these experiences" and described a sense of "stuckness." We talked about how we might be able to work through and come out of that state and I asked him how we would "notice that he had come out of it." He reported that he was still "developing an ability to come out of it." Given the nature of delusional material that occasionally emerged during his altered states, we discussed that mistrusting the therapist in the present might be a part of this process and discussed how we would work through such delusional feelings of not being safe if they emerged in during our work together.

Being mindful of his delusional reaction to the psychedelic content, and the potential for destabilisation, resourcing was an integral part of our first preparation session. A safe/calm place was established. Protective figures, nurturing figures and a wise figure were installed using BLS (Parnell, 2013). These were tested for effectiveness and tolerance. Self-regulation and re-stabilisation into the window of tolerance were established to be effective. Resourcing experiences of letting go and bravery were installed using BLS. The popular EMDR metaphor of 'the tunnel' was used to remind Scott that the 'fastest way to get through difficult content is to put your foot on the accelerator to get to the other side.' Journaling, which supports adaptive information processing (AIP), was used as an adjunct to therapy. He was encouraged to journal throughout the course of treatment and note any new material that emerged between sessions. This information was then used in re-evaluation (Phase 8). Helpfully this, along with dream content, was shared ahead of each subsequent session.

Case conceptualisation

In his book, *Confrontation with the Unconscious: Jungian Depth Psychology and Psychedelic Experience* (Hill, 2013), Scott occasionally refers to his psychedelic experiences with adverse reactions to illustrate the concepts he discusses. The intensity of his psychological response suggests that several memory networks, with converging themes, could have been activated by these psychedelic experiences. In this piece of work, two predominant themes (trust and safety) were explored; both of which are in the EMDR cognition category of safety/vulnerability.

The traumatic event of being burnt by boiling water at the age of 2 appeared to be the touchtone memory (or root node) in the network. The pain of the third-degree burns sustained at such a young age disrupted his sense of safety in the world. From an AIP perspective, the psychedelics caused a delusional reaction because they reactivated a delusional historic belief of 'I am not safe,' and feelings of safety/vulnerability that had been maladaptively stored in his memory networks. This was identified/confirmed by somatically bridging from the feelings that had emerged in his psychedelic experiences, into the thematically corresponding childhood trauma memory stored in the memory network.

Once reprocessed, another underlying network was revealed; memories and features of abandonment were reported. The accident at the age of two occurred in the context of suboptimal attachment relationships with his primary caregivers. Having a mother who displayed narcissistic traits and symptoms of depression, coupled to an emotionally absent father, indicates that there was an absence of sufficient co-regulation in the parent-child dyad. Hereby, to avoid the feelings of abandonment, the infant developed an ability to deny his dependence on others. Whilst this worked for a while, ultimately it is a hollow solution. Although in this state, briefly, he is all he needs, his dependence on others is denied, leaving an internalised message around not trusting others to remain available to meet his needs. It is conceptualised that the theme of abandonment resulted in a maladaptive network response (dissociative) as an attempt to compensate and calm his nervous system. The impaired or insufficient co-regulation from his caregivers resulted in traits of self-reliance and mistrust.

Combined, these outcomes create a perfect storm. The insufficient attachment experiences lead to chronic dysregulation in an infant's developing brain. When an acute trauma like a burn occurs, the infant anticipates inadequate emotional containment, and the resultant dysregulation fragments the overwhelmed psyche. This fragmentation is likely to be caused by rapid fluctuations in 5HTP levels, resulting in a transient hyperplastic state facilitating rapid learning effects (Carhart-Harris et al., 2017). The dissociation of this overwhelming sensory information allows for re-establishment of homeostasis and prepares the body for a rapid response if a similar experience reoccurs in later life. The cognitive and emotional sensitivity contained in that dissociated fragment primes the brain for specific sensory experiences in later life which will give rise to 'not safe' delusional symptoms. That is, later in life, Scott's psychedelic-induced disturbed states of mind (along with the subsequent reactivations) appear to be rooted in his early relational and physical traumas. During EMDR, BLS prevents these neural pathways from being overwhelmed by stress, whilst increases in entropic brain activity disrupt the pervasive thought processes. This allows consolidation of the dissociated fragments in the memory networks and, in so doing, clears the way for Scott's innate healing processes to unfold.

Working with historic trauma is a core tenet of EMDR therapy. Crucially, EMDR therapy is flexible, addressing various causative historical factors with systematic and procedural EMDR techniques. First developed as a psychological treatment for Vietnam veterans, it now seems that representatives from both sides of the cultural divide, both Veterans and counterculture rebels, could stand to benefit from a memory consolidation approach to psychological healing.

Despite the lack of any previous religious inclination, Scott suffered the delusional vision that God was demanding that he sacrifice his life in this world as an act of spiritual redemption by jumping from the Bixby Creek Bridge (California) into the canyon below, where he first felt he had come into the "Wrong World."

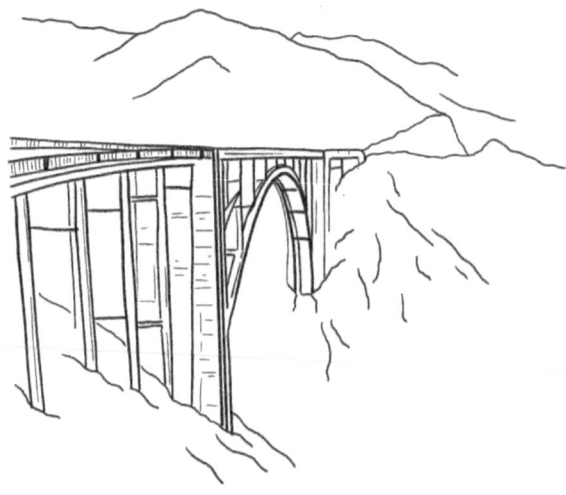

Figure 10.1 Illustration of Bixby Creek Bridge (California) where Scott had intended to end his life during an adverse reaction to LSD.

Phases 3–8

Assessment

A collaborative discussion exploring the content that had come from Scott's psychedelic experiences in 1967 enabled target identification. As is customary in target selection, the worst of Scott's four reported difficult psychedelic experiences was selected. In this image, during his second difficult LSD trip, aged 19, Scott was on a beach in the middle of the night with two friends. He suddenly realised that existence in this world was pervaded by absurdity; and he simultaneously felt himself being "pulled into the ocean to die" – and to a world free of all absurdity, madness and evil. But he was terrified of dying, so he begged his two friends to help him back up the dunes above the beach. As he crawled terrified on his hands and knees up these dunes and away from death, he knew he was crawling back into the wrong world. The NC was "I am not safe." The SUDS was a 7, with a strong sense of fear in the chest and upper abdomen. Scott described a wish to cultivate an ability to overcome his fear and mistrust for the sake of working through his reactions and Scott's positive cognition (PC) was "I am open to the experience of dying, letting go, ego death." Scott scored this validity of cognition scale (VOC) at a 6. At this point, the PC would have merited further exploration as ego death and acceptance might be viewed as an intellectual defence (Freud, 1987) or as a spiritual bypass of a faulty schema (Wellwood, 2011). This was later verified as the PC was later refined to "I Survived" and then on to "I thrived." On some level, it was possible that Scott believed that he had died, which fits with an occasional fear that has remained with him; that maybe "I did die from my suicide attempt on the way to the bridge, and that all my life since then is only a vision that some day will come to a sudden and violent end." This defence would not have benefitted being unpacked at this point (PC and VOC). Therefore, we went with the PC that was offered.

Somatic bridge

The thoughts and somatic sensations triggered by the LSD were used as the starting point for the somatic bridge technique (Watkins, 1971) to identify the corresponding maladaptively stored material that had emerged (Browning, 1999).

Image: Age 19. "On the beach with friends." "Being pulled into the ocean to die." "Begging his friends to help him away from the ocean shore and back up the sand dunes."
Emotion: Fear / Terror.
Body: Chest / Abdomen.
Belief: I am going to die.

The somatic bridge landed on a memory of the touchstone memory or 'root node' of the safety/control memory network that we were targeting (Shapiro, 2001a).

Image: Age 2 ½ "In the kitchen," "before the accident," "seeing the kettle cord" and that "no one else was there" (Being on his own indicates an attachment wound).
Emotion: Fear / Anxiety.
Body: Chest / Stomach.
Belief: I am not safe.

Reprocessing

BLS was applied to commence reprocessing. The memories chained from the kitchen to the hospital bed; a memory of him insisting that his mother lie beside him so that he lay between her and a wall at his back. At times, the BLS modality (butterfly hugs/tapping) looked arduous for this 75-year-old man. On occasion, he was encouraged to "tap firmly on his collar bones" but the taps soon descended back into circular rubs. We went with it. A spontaneous bridge emerged where he was reminded of his mother teaching him to rub Nivea cream into one of the scarred areas of his body that had been most severely injured by the burns. He paused to show me the scarring on his upper chest and shoulders. It appeared that the circular movements during the BLS were an integral part of the somatic memory (Van Der Kolk, 2014). The nurturing image of him rubbing in the nourishing cream as his mother must have done when he was younger appeared to be a reparative act. This ameliorative enactment addressed an attachment wound that predated the burns and could be harnessed as a psychological resource to bolster the adaptive information in his memory networks, supporting him to reprocess the pre-verbal content. Once this network was sufficiently reprocessed using BLS, subsequent themes of safety were revealed, which were then reprocessed accordingly. Throughout this process, all the main traumas identified during the history-taking phases were addressed, either directly with BLS or indirectly with imaginal re-scripting of touchstone attachment experiences.

"I walked into the kitchen and was carried out" soon gave way to phrases such as "I made it," "so much beauty," "so much joy," "so much good fortune" and "goodness and gratitude." These comments show the adaptive information emerging as the memory was reprocessed and the SUDs subsequently reduced (Shapiro, 2001a). He finished the session with the words "I fucking made it" which was installed using BLS. The SUDS was reported as a 2; however, this was later followed up by an email reporting that, upon reflection, the SUDS should have been reported at a 0. He reported an "afterglow" from the session. In the following session, the SUDS were checked (phase eight re-evaluation) and continued to score a 0. The VOC had changed to "I fucking made it" and scored a 7. The body scan is clear.

With the past target cleared, we then revisited the difficult psychedelic experience at age 19. The SUDS had generalised and was now also at a zero with reports of "warmth and gratitude" for the experience. A realisation that he had been "touched to think of how meaningful it has all become." That this was "rich ground" and that "I thrived." I thrived became the new PC and the VOC scored a 7. The phrase "you (I) made good use of it, kid" was installed using BLS. The body scan was also clear.

Informed by the EMDR standard protocol (Shapiro, 2001b) and transpersonal theory (See Chapter 11), PsyA-EMDR therapy follows the 4-pronged approach to follow the memory network across the lifetime. Tentatively, we looked at some sensitive content that had been shared about Scott's present scenario. Scott's wife had recently been diagnosed with dementia. This was set as the target in the present. The worst image was of a recent moment of "anticipatory grief" (Allen, 2008) where they were together in the garden when his wife had experienced some difficulty remembering a recent conversation. Upon realising this, she had "tears in her eyes" and had described the experience to him as "I feel like I'm going into a mist." He described himself as "disturbed by her cognitive decline" and "frightened." The emotion was a "soft sadness," and the NC reported was "I am not safe" verifying that it formed part of the same memory network initially identified. The SUDS scored as a 2, with a sensation again reported in the upper chest. He said, "it's not unbearable," and that "it just is." BLS was applied.

Images of his mother's end of life emerged. One meaningful experience came to mind, where, together with his wife, they had witnessed his mother's cremation. Scott suggested that the difficulty he experienced in momentarily witnessing his mother's partially consumed body during cremation might be linked to his childhood experience of being burned as a little boy. He spontaneously bridged from this to his climate activism. Referring to climate change and the responsibility to take action, he contemplated that, akin to his past suicide attempt where he faced the challenge of sacrificing his life to demonstrate spiritual integrity, this situation "is a test," and that "maybe, I will be able to do what is needed" and finally this generalised to "I will show up." Encouraged to "not edit and not judge," he linked the anticipatory grief for his wife's cognitive decline to the anticipatory grief of ecological destruction. Little boy being burned, mother being burned, planet being burned. Entering into what he described as "the outer edges of the psychotic state," he held the full weight of the burden of not feeling safe or in control with the "pending climate catastrophe." A cognitive interweave was applied to knit in his pre-established resource team, and with his protective, nurturing and wise figures beside him, he was able to turn and face the full enormity of what is yet to come with the realisation that "There are things that you can do, even in the worst of times," "We are all in this together, aren't we?" With the attachment wound repaired, he was able to bear the full weight of this shared anticipatory grief and to simply witness what needs to be seen. The session ended with the target incomplete.

In our sixth and final session, the future template was applied, and issues connected to the impending climate emergency remerged. A tragic image from an event in 2018 during which a fire storm decimated the city of Paradise, California. The image of people burned alive in their cars as they tried to escape the fire was chosen as a representation of the environmental crisis. The NC continued to be 'I am not safe.' BLS was applied. Themes outlining the complexity of the global situation emerged; the complex realisation that climate change deniers are also impacted by such events. That ineffective local politicians are also decent people. Art used as a form of expression for the riches of the human condition were woven into the tragic reality of ecological disaster. Lyrics from Joni Mitchell's iconic environmentalist 1970 protest song emerged; "they paved paradise and put up a parking lot." So too did Leonard Cohen's 1984 lyrics of a "broken halleluiah." Art from his wife's portfolio including images of witches being burned and of biblical paradises lost. The SUDS spontaneously split into the SUDS of the individual's experience and the SUDS of collective experience. Individually, adaptive thoughts emerged such as "we will survive what we need to go through." The SUDS reduced to a 0, indicating target completion.

However, the 'Collective SUDS' did not reduce for this tragic image of a paradise lost. SUDS remained at a 7 for the collective. This appeared to be an appropriate degree of disturbance given the enormity of all that is lost and threatened by ecological devastation. This raises a potential transpersonal variance to the AIP model, or forth prong, differentiating individual and collective healing.

Outcomes

Scott's baseline scores were 15 for GAD-7 and 3 for PHQ-9. On the final day of EMDR, reprocessing a post-intervention psychometric assessment put Scott's GAD-7 score at a 3 and on the PHQ-9 he scored a 2. At the 14-day follow-up, he scored 3 on GAD-7 and 2 on PHQ-9. Two months after the PsyA-EMDR intervention, Scott's final psychometric assessment placed his GAD-7 at 0 and PHQ-9 at 1.

As a collaboration, this piece of work might not be a genuine representation of a PsyA-EMDR therapy session, and we must therefore consider the results to be contrived. It is likely that Scott is more emotionally grounded and has a greater level of psychological awareness than a client, patient or research participant. However, the opportunity to work in the public domain with content of this nature is rare and, as such, this illustrative case material opened the possibilities of sharing PsyA-EMDR for the purposes of demonstration and training. More extensive research on the outcomes and longevity of PsyA-EMDR when working with historic psychedelic content is needed.

References

Adams, R., Ohlsen, S., & Wood, E. (2020). Eye movement desensitization and reprocessing for the treatment of psychosis – A systematic review. *European Journal of Psychotraumatology, 11*(1), 1711349. https://doi.org/10.1080/2000 8198.2019.1711349

Alarcon, R., Dickinson, W., & Dohn, H. (1982). Flashback phenomena: Clinical and diagnostic dilemmas. *The Journal of Nervous and Mental Disease, 170*, 217–223.

Allen, J. (2008). The long road: An article on anticipatory grief. Found at https://www.jenniferallenbooks.com/grief/pdf/longroad.pdf (https://web.archive.org/web/20120222111722/). Accessed 11.11.2024.

American Psychiatric Association, DSM-5 Task Force. (2013). *Diagnostic and statistical manual of mental disorders: DSM-5™* (5th ed.). Washington, DC: American Psychiatric Publishing, Inc. https://doi.org/10.1176/appi.books.9780890425596

Carhart-Harris, R., & Nutt, D. (2017). Serotonin and brain function: A tale of two receptors. *Journal of Psychopharmacology, 31*(9), 1091–1120. https://doi.org/10.1177/0269881117725915

Cohen, L. (1984). *Hallelujah.* New York: Various positions, Columbia Records.

Cooper, H. (1955). Hallucinogenic drugs. *Lancet 1*, 1078–1079. https://doi.org/10.1016/s0140-6736(55)91156-9

Davidhizar, D. (1994, Sep). The pursuit of illness for secondary gain. *Healthcare Supervision, 13*(1), 10–5. PMID: 10172109.

Felitti, V. J., Anda, R. F., Nordenberg, D., Williamson, D. F., Spitz, A. M., Edwards, V., Koss, M. P., & Marks, J. S. (1998, May). Relationship of childhood abuse and household dysfunction to many of the leading causes of death in adults. The adverse childhood experiences (ACE) study. *American Journal of Preventive Medicine, 14*(4), 245–258. https://doi.org/10.1016/s0749-3797(98)00017-8

Freud, S. (1987). *On metapsychology. The theory of psychoanalysis: Beyond the pleasure principle, ego and the ID.* London: Penguin Library.

Fuentes, J. J., Fonseca, F., Elices, M., Farre, M., & Torrens, M. (2020, Jan 21). Therapeutic use of LSD in Psychiatry: A systematic review of randomised controlled clinical trials. *Frontiers in Psychiatry: Sec. Psychopharmacology, 10*, 943. https://doi.org/10.3389/fpsyt.2019.00943

Gibbs, G. (1998). *Learning by doing a guide to teaching and learning methods.* Oxford: Oxford Brooks University.

Gielkens, E., Rossi, G., & Sobcazak, S. (2023). A first exploration: Can eye movement desensitization and reprocessing improve cognition in older adults with posttraumatic stress disorder? *Journal of Geriatric Psychiatry and Neurology, 37*(3), 206–221. https://doi.org/10.1177/089198872312076

Gielkens, E., Turksna, K., Kranenburg, L. Stas, L., Sobczak, S., Lphen, S., & Rossi, G. (2022). Feasibility of EMDR in older adults with PTSD to reduce frailty and improve quality of life. *Clinical Gerontologist, 4*,1–11. https://doi.org/10.1080/07317115.2022.2114397

Grinspoon, L., & Bakalar, J. B. (1979). *Psychedelic Drugs Reconsidered.* New York: Basic Books.

Grof, S. (1980). *LSD psychotherapy.* Alameda, CA: Hunter House.

Grof, S. (2009). *LSD: Doorway to the numinous: The ground breaking psychedelic research into realms of the human unconscious*. New York: Simon and Schuster.

Hermle, L., Funfgeld, M., Oepen, G., Botsch, H., Borchardt, D., Gouzoulis, E., Fehrenbach, R. A., & Spitzer, M. (1992). Mescaline-induced psychopathological, neuropsychological, and neurometabolic effects in normal subjects: Experimental psychosis as a tool for psychiatric research. *Biological Psychiatry, 32*(11), 976–991. https://doi.org/1016/0006-3223(92)90059-9

Hermle L., Kovar K., Hewer W., & Ruchsow M. (2008). Hallucinogen-induced psychological disorders. *Fortschr Neurol Psychiatry, 76*, 334–342. https://doi.org/10.1055/s-2008-1038191

Hill, S. (2013). *Confrontation with the unconscious: Jungian depth psychology and psychedelic experience*. London: Muswell Hill Press.

Horowitz, M. J. (1969). Flashbacks: Recurrent intrusive images after the use of LSD. *American Journal of Psychiatry, 126*, 565–569. https://doi.org/10.1176/ajp.126.4.565

Knipe, J. (1998). Blocking beliefs questionnaire. EMDRIA newsletter. Found at https://emdrtherapyvolusia.com/wp-content/uploads/2016/12/Blocking_Beliefs_Questionnaire.pdf. Accessed 27.01.2024

Kolb, D. A. (1984). *Experiential learning: Experience as the source of learning and development*. Englewood Cliffs, NJ: Prentice-Hall.

Lee, M., & Shlain, B. (1992). *Acid dreams: The complete social history of LSD: The CIA, the sixties, and beyond*. New York: Grove Weidenfeld.

Linehan, M. (2015). DBT *skills training manual* (2nd ed.). New York: The Guilford Press.

Mackenzie, D. L., Browning, K., Skroban, S. B., & Smith, D. A. (1999). The impact of probation on the criminal activities of offenders. *Journal of Research in Crime and Delinquency, 36*, 423–453. https://doi.org/10.1177/0022427899036004004

Maté, G., & Maté, D. (2022). *The myth of normal: Trauma, illness & healing in a toxic culture*. London: Vermilion.

McGee, R. (1984). Flashbacks and memory phenomena. A comment on flashback phenomena – clinical and diagnostic dilemmas. *The Journal of Nervous and Mental Disease, 172*, 273–278. https://doi.org/10.1097/00005053-198405000-00004

Mitchel, J. (1970). *Big yellow taxi. Ladies of the canyon*. Burbank, CA: Reprise Records.

Parnell, L. (2013). *Attachment-focused EMDR: Healing relational trauma*. W. W. Norton & Company.

Prideaux. (2021). *Mad in America*. Found at https://www.madinamerica.com/2021/12/psychedelic-medicine-flashbacks/. *Accessed on* 27.01.2024

Raine-Smith, H., & Rose, J. (2023). Psychedelic-assisted EMDR therapy (PsyA-EMDR): A memory consolidation approach to psychedelic healing. *ETQ, 4*, 1. https://doi.org/10.13140/RG.2.2.24683.35366

Rucker, J., Ko, K., Knught, G., & Cleare, A. (2022). Psychedelics, mystical experience, and therapeutic efficacy: A systematic review. *Frontiers in Psychiatry, 13*, 917199. https://doi.org/10.3389/fpsyt.2022.917199

Seikkula, J., & Olson, M. (2003). The Open Dialogue Approach to Acute Psychosis: Its Poetics and Micropolitics. *Family Process, 42*(3), 403–418. https://doi.org/10.1111/j.1545-5300.2003.00403.x

Shapiro, F. (2001a). *Eye movement desensitization and repro- cessing: Basic principles, protocols and procedures* (2nd ed.). New York: Guilford Press.

Shapiro, F. (2001b). Trauma and adaptive information-processing: EMDR's dynamic and behavioural interface, In M. Alpert, D. Malan, L. McCullough, R. J. Neborsky, F. Shapiro, & M. Solomon (Eds.), *Short-term therapy for long-term change* (pp. 112–129). New York: Norton.

Shapiro, F. (2018). The role of eye movement desensitization and reprocessing (EMDR) therapy in medicine: Addressing the psychological and physical symptoms stemming from adverse life experiences. *Permian Journal, 18*(1), 71–77. https://doi.org/10.7812/TPP/13-098

Silvestre, M. l., & Tarquinio, C. L. (2022) Systemic family therapy and EMDR therapy: An integrative approach. *European Journal of Trauma & Dissociation, 6*(4), 100291. https://doi.org/10.1016/j.ejtd.2022.100291

Varese, F., Sellwood, W., Aseem, A., Awenat, Y., Bird, L., Bhutani, G., Carter, L. A., Davies, L., Davis, C., Horne, G., Keane, D., Logie, R., Malkin, D., Potter, F., Van Den Berge, D., Zia, S., & Bentall, R. (2021). Eye movement desensitization and reprocessing therapy for psychosis (EMDRp): Protocol of a feasibility randomized controlled trial with early intervention service users. *Early Interventions in Psychiatry, 15*(5), 1224–1233. https://doi.org/10.1111/eip.13071

Wasson, R. G., Hofmann, A., & Ruck, C. A. (2008). *The road to Eleusis: Unveiling the secret of the mysteries.* Berkeley, CA: North Atlantic Books.

Watkins, J. G. (1971). The affect bridge: A hypnoanalytic technique. *International Journal of Clinical and Experimental Hypnosis, 19*(1), 21–27. https://doi.org/10.1080/00207147108407148

11 Transpersonal healing

DMT
N, N-Dimethyltryptamine ($C_{12}H_{16}N$)

DOI: 10.4324/9781003431718-11

When administered, DMT produces an intense, short-lived psychedelic experience. It can be smoked, vaporised, injected or consumed orally as one component in a psychoactive brew called ayahuasca, traditionally used by indigenous people in the Amazon rainforest for spiritual and healing purposes.

DMT has been coined the 'spirit molecule' (Strassman, 2000) because the experiences induced by it are often described as otherworldly, featuring vivid and colourful visual hallucinations, altered perceptions of time and space and encounters with entities or beings. Users commonly report experiencing profound insights, introspection and a sense of connectedness to metaphysical realms. The duration of a DMT trip is very short, typically lasting around 10 to 15 minutes when smoked, which makes it distinct from other hallucinogens like lysergic acid diethylamide (LSD) or psilocybin mushrooms. Research into the process of dying has indicated that DMT is one of the neurochemicals associated with death and near-death-like experiences. It was originally thought to be produced in the pineal gland, but recent studies have shown that it is produced in several regions including the neocortex and hippocampus (Borjigin et al., 2013).

Because of its potent effects and potential for inducing intense experiences, DMT is considered a Schedule I controlled substance in many countries, meaning it is illegal to possess, distribute or use recreationally. However, research into its potential therapeutic applications and its effects on consciousness continues as scientists seek to understand the brain mechanisms underlying its effects and its potential for treating conditions such as depression, anxiety and addiction.

N,N-Dimethyltryptamine (DMT) is a powerful serotonergic psychedelic that naturally occurs in some plants and animals and can also be synthesised. Production of endogenous DMT has been confirmed in the mammalian brain and is thought to contribute to high order brain functions such as information processing and memory. It belongs to the tryptamine family of chemicals and is structurally similar to serotonin, a neurotransmitter that plays a role in mood regulation and other physiological processes.

To many psychonauts and researchers, the mystical layer of the psychedelic experience is fundamental to its healing potential, though this territory is still referred to by some as 'woo.' There is a mounting body of evidence to suggest that there is more to our perceived reality than meets the eye, from the imprint of ancestral trauma that is passed down epigenetically through the generations (Crew, 2008) to the release of previously confidential government reports confirming the existence of extra-terrestrials (Greenewald, 2021). In light of the strange world we find ourselves living in, it seemed fitting to include a chapter on this contentious aspect of psychedelic research.

The term 'transpersonal' literally means 'transcending the personal,' a term that encourages an unbiased viewpoint free from the burden of spiritual or religious dogma. Here, the concept of 'spirit' is not deemed supernatural but is instead treated as another aspect of human nature; an extension of our current understanding of physics. It is part of a spectrum of reality where physical reality is the one that is most familiar, but if one changes frequency and shifts to another channel, encounters with what is called 'non-physical reality' or the 'spirit realm' also become possible. This fluid transition from one reality to the next is an extension of current understanding of the nature of subjective experience and this is beginning to be explored in the field of quantum mechanics.

Science is always eager to remove emotion and consciousness from experiments, but so much of physical reality depends on our perception and state of consciousness in the moment of observation. This reductionist approach to science, in search of a universal theory for everything by reducing phenomena down to find a single principle, has the potential to distort the view of complex systems by discounting the synergy of all the parts combined. It is becoming clear that until consciousness is included in the equation, progress will be limited in our understanding of reality. This is demonstrated by the 'observer effect,' an established fact in quantum mechanics, whereby the act of observation has been shown to influence the phenomenon being observed (Heisenberg, 1930).

Psychedelic states frequently include experiences of psychological death and rebirth, together with spiritual or mystical components. They have the power to evoke a wide range of transpersonal experiences, including a sense of oneness with others, nature, the universe and God. Psychonauts routinely report contacts with archetypal entities, past life sequences from different cultures, flying saucers and extra-terrestrial abduction experiences (Davis et al., 2020). These reports occur with such regularity that they merit additional research and a further exploration herein.

Multidimensional memory networks

Stanislav Grof was one of the original founders of transpersonal psychology along with Abraham Maslow and 'the Stephen Hawking of psychology,' Anthony Sutch. Also known as a spiritual depth psychology, the transpersonal approach integrates Eastern and Western approaches and studies all states of consciousness in an inclusive, integrative manner that bridges the gap between ancient spiritual traditions and the pragmatism of modern science. Grof asserts that the Freudian concept of unconscious experience being limited to postnatal biography is insufficient to explain the varied transpersonal phenomena that occur during psychedelic experiences. Furthermore, he proposed that the classification of altered states of consciousness as pathological products of the brain, referred to "endogenous psychoses," demonstrated a lack of understanding of the aetiology of mental disorder in the field of psychiatry.

Grof was heavily influenced by the work of Carl Jung, specifically his theory of 'complexes.' Jung proposed that individuals develop a complex (belief system) in response to early trauma as a means of diminishing overwhelming negative affect (Jung, 1960). Grof utilised psycholytic therapy (low-medium dose LSD combined with psychoanalytic therapy) and controlled breathing protocols to explore the various layers of the human subconscious (Grof, 2016). According to Grof, the procedure is similar to peeling back the layers of an onion, with each layer representing a 'system of condensed experience' or COEX system. He defines these as 'a specific constellation of memories (and associated fantasies) from different life periods of the individual' (p.46). The memories that belong to a particular COEX system have a similar basic theme or contain similar elements and are accompanied by a strong emotional charge of the same quality.

This conceptualisation bears a striking resemblance to the concept of memory networks in EMDR, the main difference being that Grof places less emphasis on specific memories and instead focusses on the affective state associated with each network. He describes the formation of themed COEXs in declarative memory that are formed in early childhood, in the same way the AIP model conceptualises this process, but Grof expands the networks back to perinatal experience and goes even further to explore transpersonal domains of ancestral trauma and past life experiences. Grof states that these memories are dissociated over time via procedural learning and classical conditioning, whereas the AIP model proposes that they are dissociated in the moment of initial encoding due to a fault in the memory encoding system.

Grof preferentially targets the feeling rather than a specific memory because he conceptualises four other domains outside of biographical memory and views the affective response as the consistent element to be targeted. EMDR is also an affect-based model, but the standard protocol limits this by subscribing to the idea that a memory is the main focus, where the preferred target is a specific moment anchored in time with accompanying sensory and cognitive elements. Cornil and Van Limbergen (2024) question whether it is the memory or affect that is being processed during EMDR, stating that the memory is just one entry point to process the 'core affect.' They refer to Shapiro's less well-known affect/valence hypothesis which states that it is the intensity of the negative affect that is the binding aspect of the trauma memory in a dissociated memory network (2001, p.37). She posits that it is not dysfunctionally stored memories, but dysfunctional information stored in the neural networks *around the affect*. The stronger the valence of affect, the stronger the binding of the information in the network surrounding it. This applies to both positive and negative networks of information.

> "Thus, while a person's beliefs, stated via language, are clinically useful distillations of experience, it is the affect feeding them that is the pivotal element in the pathology."
>
> (Shapiro, 2001, p. 41)

This is why affect could be considered more important than the negative cognition, particularly when it comes to early trauma where there are no words to express what has happened. Van Limbergen has developed a progressive version of EMDR that targets the 'core affect' with the aim of activating the associated memory network. Reducing the affect weakens the binding of that network allowing the therapy to happen (Shapiro, 2001). There are many other examples of EMDR protocols that only target the affect and achieve sustained results without targeting a specific memory: Flashforward (Logie and De Jong, 2014), Desensitising to Triggers (DeTur; Popkey, 2005) and the Flash Technique (Manfield et al., 2017). The approach of accessing the core affect in order to reprocess it and facilitate change offers further illumination on the motivation behind Grof targeting affect to activate and then integrate the COEX.

During his LSD research, Grof observed a continuity in the content that emerged, and that a COEX was revisited in consecutive sessions, each time at a deeper level until eventually 'the resolution of the matrix [the COEX] occurs when the unconscious content is experienced consciously in original form and full intensity' (1980, p. 169). As in EMDR, this resolution results in the disappearance of the COEX system and the accompanying dysfunctional behaviours diminish and often disappear completely. Grof highlights that this integration takes a number of psychedelic sessions and that clients can be left feeling dysregulated in between treatments. The approach advocates for the use of breathwork sessions or additional psychedelic treatments to resolve difficult experiences (Grof & Grof, 2017).

We posit that if there is sustained dysregulation following a psychedelic experience, EMDR could be a safer, more ethical way to carry on the work and stabilise the nervous system than offering repeated doses. Only after the material has been reprocessed and the nervous system stabilised, and only then, should further psychedelic treatments be undertaken.

Fractals in the chaos

The AIP model asserts that the themes of maladaptively encoded adverse life experiences re-occur in response to subsequent trauma across a life-time. Self-similarity is observed in the repeating patterns of a client's relational dynamics, and EMDR practitioners look out for overarching themes and track the network back to touchstone or root node memories in early childhood. Self-similarity is a key aspect of fractal geometry, where the large-scale pattern of the whole is repeated at multiple scales within its parts (see the cover image to illustrate). 'The universal meta-pattern' or 'prime substrate' that underlies this interaction between subjective and objective reality (Mark-Tarlow & Shapiro, 2021) correlates with the concept of themed memory networks in EMDR. The clients presenting issues or symptomology, and interpersonal dynamics manifesting in the therapeutic dyad, are a microcosm of the overarching themes of the macrocosm (the memory network or COEX), defined by the thought (NC), feeling and somatic response. This trauma imprint is repeated transgenerationally and self-similar forms of interpersonal dysfunction are passed down from one generation to the next as repeated patterns of disturbance.

> "What occurs within us bears fractal correspondence to what is happening in a wider world because the inner and outer domains are in a self-similar relationship with each other. "
>
> (Marks-Tarlow & Shapiro, 2021, p. 47S7)

The 'fractal geometry of nature' offers a mathematical framework to describe aspects of nature that were previously considered too complex and irregular to model successfully (Mandelbrot, 1977). Since its inception, fractal geometry has been used to model everything from the pattern of galaxy clusters all the way down to nanoscopic particles. Clinical psychologist Dr. Terry Marks-Tarlow has written extensively on this subject and believes that fractal geometry offers a flexible meta-framework capable of mapping complex interpersonal systems (Marks-Tarlow, 1999, 2020). The fractal view of interpersonal consciousness posits that there is not a rigid Cartesian split between internal and external reality or between the body and the mind (Marks-Tarlow, 2020). Mental and physical processes interpenetrate, producing self-similar patterns manifesting as synchronicities that are ignored by the reductive clinical sciences. Jung observed that synchronicities often emerge during emotionally charged moments in therapy (Jung, 1952). Marks-Tarlow posits this is because these moments are arousal states that are close to the edge of chaos, revealing 'fractal seams' at the relational edges between people and the world at large. She states that fractals develop in the porous, observer-dependent boundaries between self and other, and synchronicities indicate this because self-similar patterns emerge at the interface between subjective and objective levels of reality. Therapists work at the point of 'optimal frustration' (Kohut, 1971) for the stress to activate a pivotal mental state and clinicians hone their 'fractal consciousness' in an attempt to facilitate change at the edge of chaos.

This model of semi-permeable boundaries between the self and other can be integrated with the AIP model in PsyA-EMDR to begin to explain the quantum phenomena that have thus far been largely ignored by the scientific community. For example, the psychophysical phenomena observed when at the fractal seams, such as synchronicities, clinician intuition and shared somatic responses, are currently labelled as non-scientific. However, in an age of validated proof of quantum entanglement, a nonreductive model that challenges the Cartesian dualism of mind and physical reality is long overdue.

Psychedelics, psychosis and EMDR

Large doses of psychedelics have been shown to induce a 'mystical' state, but this can also manifest as a more challenging psychotic-like experience, characterised by fear of loss of control/autonomy, impaired reasoning, delusions of grandeur or anxiety and panic (Vollenweider & Smallridge, 2022). Grof highlights the lack of distinction between mystical states and mental illness in modern psychiatry, often labelling people who experience spiritual phenomena as psychotic (Grof, 1998). He calls this diagnosis into question and views these experiences as 'spiritual emergencies,' believing that they can be used as vehicle for psychological healing if supported in the appropriate way, rather than suppressing growth with psychopharmacological interventions (Grof & Grof, 1989). This conceptualisation of psychotic symptomology aligns with the emerging view that childhood trauma plays a pivotal role in the pathogenesis and maintenance of psychotic symptoms (Matheson et al., 2013). There is also increasing evidence that intrusions experienced during psychosis have a direct link to the individual's trauma history (Varese et al., 2012). A number of models of psychosis have been developed based on the transient states elicited by psychedelics. But instead of adopting a holistic approach, many of these models focus on the minutia of neurotransmitter malfunction (Murray et al., 2013), which is perhaps a reflection of the lucrative medicalised approach to treating psychosis. In clinical settings, extra-pharmacological factors such as 'set' and 'setting' are implicated in influencing the quality of acute psychedelic experiences. However, trauma is often discounted as a reason for adverse reactions, perhaps because 'little t' attachment trauma (trauma of omission) and its impact on memory encoding is not considered significant (Evans et al., 2023).

According to the National Institute of Clinical Excellence, PTSD symptoms are present in 30% of patients with psychosis (NICE, 2014), and EMDR performed well in several trials that evaluated the use of trauma-focussed therapies to treat PTSD in this population (Sin & Spain, 2017). Recent research has also validated the use of EMDR to treat first-episode psychosis in a study of NHS patients attending an early psychosis service in the UK (EMDRp, Varese et al., 2023). Here, participants attended 16 sessions over six months in a design that utilised standard protocol EMDR with adaptions to address the needs of the participants. The results of the feasibility study indicated that EMDR is a suitable early intervention to stabilise individuals with psychosis (within three years of onset) when compared to treatment as usual. The use of the AIP model to guide interventions by conceptualising the presenting symptoms as the product of pathological memories further corroborates the trauma-focussed conceptualisation of psychotic symptomology. The next phase is a multi-site trial of the intervention, and it is hoped that a secondary data set can be gleaned from the multi-site trial to demonstrate that EMDR can be used to stabilise drug-induced psychosis (specifically psychedelics). The findings of this study are still some way off, but so too are the legislation and licences required for the therapeutic use of psychedelic drugs. The findings of the EMDRp RCT will likely be published within a similar timeframe to some psychedelic compounds being brought to market, evidence which may pave the way for EMDR to be used as a scalable stabilisation intervention in PAP.

An expanded AIP model

As previously mentioned, Grof expanded the dimensions of the human psyche beyond the reductive realms of Freudian postnatal biography into the perinatal domain and beyond. Through his work with LSD, he defined a number of groups of psychedelic experience that he linked to the psychological imprint left on the psyche from the following domains of adverse experience:

Biographical – the focus of traditional psychiatry.
Perinatal – pre-verbal memories of in utero and the birth experience.
Transpersonal – experience that transcends the usual boundaries and limitations of body, ego, three-dimensional space and linear time.

Many EMDR therapists already work with pre-verbal trauma (see Paulsen, 2017), and there is potential benefit in expanding the realms of the AIP model based on Grof's observations of holotropic states. This could provide a more coherent framework to work with perinatal and transpersonal material, particularly in the field of PAP. Equally, Grof's COEX framework could benefit from defining the COEXs using the thought (NC), feeling and somatic response to describe the 'basic theme that permeates all its [the COEX's] layers and represents their common denominator' (Grof, 1998, p. 346).

Grof (2016) asserts that each COEX is anchored in a particular aspect of birth trauma that he has divided into different birth 'matrices' depending upon which part of the birth was traumatic. The three stages of birth according to Grof, the first perinatal matrix, BPM I, corresponding with the stage in utero, before birth, and BPM II-IV cover the three clinical stages of the birthing process. He conceptualised that each of the stages correspond with particular imagery and affect that emerge on psychedelics. This book does not have the scope to go into detail about the different themes that emerge but here is a summary:

BPM I – Primal union with mother. In utero. If undisturbed, a vast region, boundaryless, limitless. If a "bad womb" experience – menacing, poisoned, polluted, demonic figures. Apocalyptic.
BPM II – Antagonism with mother. Swallowed by a beast, sucked into a whirlpool. Devoured, entangled. Descending into hell. Cervix is contracting but is not yet open. A claustrophobic nightmare. Helplessness. The dark night of the soul.
BPM III – Synergism with mother. Propelled down the birth canal. Dynamic battles and bloody violence. Problematic sexual energy linked to the erotic nature of oxygen deprivation. A mixture of sexual arousal and panic.
BPM IV – Separation from mother. Emergence into the world. Enormous fear and struggle to survive. Symbolised by fire. Cleansing (purgatory) and emergence (phoenix).

Annihilation → Rebirth → Resurrection

Grof hypothesises that an individual's experience in utero and of birth sets them up for a lifetime of repetition: that the same beliefs, behaviours, attitudes and somatic responses repeat again and again. From an

AIP perspective, it could be conceptualised that the prenatal experience is the root node (touchstone) of the maladaptive memory networks. It is likely that the memory of birth is encoded maladaptively because of the amount of physiological stress experienced during this process. Developmental neuroscience has now shown prenates record and recall memory from as early as the third trimester of pregnancy (Movalled et al., 2023), so even for the clinicians who do not resonate with the transpersonal domain of this discussion it is feasible that maladaptive material is encoded prenatally.

> **Tip:** It can be useful to ask the client about their birth experience in the initial session. Was it a natural birth? Were there any complications? Did they receive skin-to-skin contact immediately after birth? What else was going on in the family system at that time? Any notable intergenerational or ancestral traumas? etc.

Multidimensional reprocessing

If transpersonal or abstract material emerges during a psychedelic session, it can be worked with in a number of ways:

- Reprocess the material as if it is a trauma memory.
- Bridge somatically from the experience to identify corresponding biographical material.
- Construct and reprocess birth trauma based on imagery that has emerged.
- Construct and reprocess past-life/ancestral trauma based on imagery that has emerged.
- Utilise the experience as a psychological resource (if positive).

The key to this type of reprocessing is radical acceptance of whatever emerges (images, thoughts and feelings) because **everything is an expression of the self** and wherever the focus of the work, a microcosm of the whole can be revealed. If the manifestation of dysfunctional behaviours is conceptualised as a response to unresolved trauma, information can be gleaned from the client's descriptions of presenting issues and cross-reference this with their trauma history to ascertain which targets might be early enough in the memory network to reconsolidate enough material to resolve the symptom. If practitioners are inclined to go a step further and consider the concepts of past life or ancestral trauma, the same information can be used to construct an event in the imaginal space, using somatic responses from more recent events in the corresponding COEX/memory network.

Note: For clinicians who are less transpersonally inclined, the processing of ancestral trauma can be conceptualised as working with introjected personality parts, passed down the generations in response to trauma.

When bridging somatically to abstract material that has no obvious reference point in a client's biographical history, the COEX framework combined with information from an AIP case conceptualisation can be used to work with this material creatively in the imaginal space. The imprint of ancestral trauma can also be reprocessed as a forth prong using the somatic graft technique whereby a more recent node in that network is activated, then this somatic response is implanted onto the scene of the transpersonal trauma, finally BLS is used to reprocess the emergent material. If using Grof's birth matrix model, the themes that emerge on psychedelics, combined with any biographical information, can be used to reconstruct a birth experience in the imaginal space. The feelings from the trip can be grafted onto the imagined birth experience in an attempt to activate any unprocessed material in the network. BLS can then be used to activate and reprocess anything that emerges.

For example, a client described how they were tormented about whether he had made the right decision during a break-up from a partner and was using words like 'it feels like I am impaled on the decision I have made' whilst holding onto the right-hand side of his chest. It was known from his history taking that he had had a collapsed lung on this side in his late teens where there remained a significant scar. He had also previously shared that in a past life regression with a hypnotherapist he discovered that he was stabbed in the chest and died. So, we activated the somatic feeling in response to the recent break-up along with the NC 'I can't trust my judgement' and grafted the somatic response onto a made-up scene of being impaled with a spear through his chest.

More detail emerged when BLS was added: he was stuck against a wall unable to move. He re-experienced the initial, desperate struggle and then submitted to the pain and his impending doom. During this reprocessing, he was making links to other events in his life where this pattern had manifested. When the perceived death was reprocessed, he shifted to a third-person perspective and SUDs reduced to 0 as in standard EMDR. When he re-evaluated the current relationship trigger, SUDs were now 0 and the PC 'I did the best I could' naturally emerged.

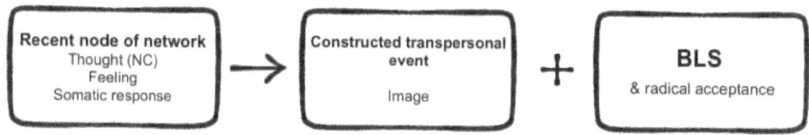

Figure 11.1 Diagram illustrating using the somatic graft technique to construct and reprocess a transpersonal experience.

Dreamwork

A client's subconscious often knows that an EMDR session is coming, and the night before the appointment dream content will often correspond with the touchstone memory that is then reprocessed. For example, the participant in the 'eMDMAdr' vignette in Chapter 6 had a dream the night before the treatment where a tidal wave swept her away. This represented the touchstone memory that emerged during the psycholytic session, where her mother threw her across the room when she was a toddler.

Dreams have been used as a source of information for millennia, and there is evidence of dream interpretation dating back to 3100 BC Mesopotamia (modern-day Iraq) (Black et al., 1998). Dreamwork is also a predominant part of Native American culture where it is believed to be a powerful tool for guidance and healing. It is central to entheogenic shamanic ritual in which dream incubation practices such as ritual drumming or singing prior to sleep are thought to enhance lucid dreaming (Winkelman, 2010). Dream analysis is also a core intervention in Freudian and Jungian analysis because it is deemed the 'royal road to a knowledge of the unconscious activities of the mind' (Freud, 1900, p. 769).

In a standard EMDR assessment, it is recommended that clients are asked about the content of their dreams, because disturbed sleep is associated with unprocessed trauma. Although recurrent nightmares are of particular interest when assessing for maladaptively encoded trauma, it is also useful to enquire about the general timbre of their dream life as well as their general quality of sleep. Do they wake up feeling rested? Is there a core theme that regularly pops up in their dreams? If so, what is the negative cognition and feeling that fits best with this?

It can be useful to bring dreams into their awareness early on in the work by explaining the AIP conceptualisation of nightmares using their content as an example and linking it to their memory network themes (if possible). Encouraging clients to bring information about dream content from the start of therapy so they get into the habit of noting them down, rather than forgetting them. Any information from dreams can be used to inform and update the AIP conceptualisation.

Tip – Integrating dreamwork into PsyA-EMDR

It can be insightful to incorporate dreamwork into PsyA-EMDR because it is another portal into the client's subconscious. During the **assessment phase,** it can be useful to enquire about dreams and in any recurrent dreams or nightmares that have been experienced *at any point in their lives.* From an AIP perspective, recurrent themes during dreamtime indicate that the brain is trying to process information but is unable to because it is partly dissociated from the main memory networks, and the recurrent nature of them indicates that the brain is repeatedly attempting to reconsolidate the information. Dream content also reflects the impact of external stressors on the subconscious, which can be useful information to guide the work.

The **somatic bridge** can be used to access the corresponding subconscious material by getting the client to bridge from the FEELING, SENSATION, THOUGHT and NC elicited by the dream. The standard protocol can then be used to re-process and integrate the material.

Encouraging clients to track their dreams throughout the process of PsyA-EMDR can inform the work. Often their perspective or age will change in response to successful integration of trauma in a similar way to the perception of memories during reprocessing as they shift from state-specific pathogenic memories (first person perspective with strong affect) to episodic encoding (third-person narrative with no somatic response).

Consciousness research

In 2022, the Noble Prize in Physics was awarded to three scientists responsible for a series of ingenious experiments which proved the theory of 'quantum entanglement' (Aspect et al., 2022). The idea that Einstein refused to accept – that two quantum systems can be entangled so they can interact with one another across any distance – was at odds with the core premise of his theory of relativity: that nothing can move faster than the speed of light. This ground breaking research demonstrated that when two or more particles are generated or interact, the quantum state of each particle cannot be described independently, even if the particles are separated by a large distance. Instead, the quantum state of each particle must be described as part of the whole system (Brody, 2020).

Quantum entanglement offers a conceptual framework for interconnectedness and challenges the false idea of separation. No matter how far apart two particles are, you affect one and you automatically effect the other faster than the speed of light. This does not prove action at a distance, only that distance is an illusion and there is no such thing as separation. Marks-Tarlow (2018) uses the concept of nonlocality from quantum entanglement theory to explain the phenomenon of clinician intuition and other extrasensory perception (ESP)-type phenomena experienced in the psychotherapeutic space. This type of phenomena is being actively researched in the field of psychedelic research and, interestingly, the CIA has been conducting research in this area since the 1950s. There is freely available evidence of CIA research into psychedelics and their impact on ESP, which was being developed for the military in the 'psychic arms race' with the Soviet Union (Puharich, 1959; Mitchell et al., 2017). More recently, this research has been taken to another level in DMT trials where participants are attempting to map the 'DMT hyperspace' for an hour while under the influence of intravenously administered DMT (Gallimore & Strassman, 2016). These extraordinary experiments have opened an avenue of consciousness research that has the potential to shed light on commonly reported phenomena such as 'entity experiences' or 'immersion into alternate realities' (Davis et al., 2020).

Consciousness researcher Jeffery Martin has spent 20 years cataloguing 'persistent non-symbolic states' (PNSE) in over 10,000 participants across many cultures. He has stripped out the dogma to reveal overarching themes in altered states of consciousness across cultures (ASC; Martin, 2020). Martin reframes 'mystical experience' or 'non-duality' as the re-organisation of the brain and calls the state 'fundamental wellbeing.' He is conducting research into the use of microdosing ketamine to facilitate the transition into a state of fundamental well-being through the mediation protocols he is developing (Quesada, 2023). The term 'non-symbolic' was derived from Cook-Greuter's (2000) research involving ego development and transcendence. As previously mentioned, the default mode network (DMN), which is now thought to be the neurobiological substrate of the ego, is the filter that edits our experience based on prior held beliefs (based on interpersonal experience in childhood). The DMN has been shown to support meta-cognitive processes activated during introspection and day dreaming and is crucial for self-representation and reflective self-awareness (Winkelman, 2017). Substances like DMT and 5MEO-DMT are compounds that reliably create the sense of separation from the sense of self, also called 'ego death.' In this moment we are no longer defined by our past experiences and are free to be fully in the moment, without being taken out of the present by triggered body reactions from unintegrated trauma.

A word of warning from Martin's research relates to the temptation for 'spiritual bypassing' to attain PSNE. Martin highlights the unnecessary trend in the field of psychedelics of using 'breakthrough doses' to attain transcendent experiences. He instead proposes that lower doses could be used as a tool to hone consciousness skills to be able to consistently transition to states of fundamental well-being. The somewhat misguided belief that taking a 'heroic' dose of magic mushrooms and conversing with your ancestors is sufficient to experience sustained positive change, when in fact this is just bypassing the need to address fundamental aspects of your psyche in a psychotherapeutic space. A core aim of PsyA-EMDR is to harness the power of psychedelics to facilitate deep integration work with traumatic body-based memories to enable the individual to become more present. Embodiment is required to release the trauma and ultimately become free of the somatic tyranny of the past. Psychedelics can facilitate this process.

Summary

Psychedelic research is challenging traditional concepts of reality and we are living in a period of profound changes in human awareness. The ephemeral nature of physical reality is being called into question by emerging theories in quantum physics, and we are rapidly shedding old ideas and embracing new concepts. The internal evolution of the human spirit and expansion of consciousness is making us realise that there are other ways to live and experience the world. It is hoped that these new perspectives will encourage a trauma-focussed approach to 'psychotic' presentations, where lifelong medication has previously been the only solution. This view is outdated and EMDR therapy offers a robust alternative, with comprehensive stabilisation interventions to work with even the most treatment-resistant client groups.

The field of consciousness research that is emerging from the psychedelic renaissance is encouraging a fresh look at the previously maligned transpersonal domains of experience. If we believe that everything is an expression of the self, then regardless of our personal view of transpersonal phenomenology radical acceptance of whatever emerges is key to helping people to heal. Every part of the psyche is welcome in the psychotherapeutic space and the AIP model can be adapted to work with the transpersonal material that regularly emerges in PAP. The framework can be used to develop EMDR based techniques to work with this material by expanding the AIP model outside of declarative, biographical memories into Grof's concept of COEXs. For those more transpersonally inclined, the fractal theory of consciousness, can be used to make sense of ESP-type phenomena, such as synchronicities that occur at the fractal seams.

A dramatic paradigm shift in the natural sciences is required to accommodate shifts in understanding about consciousness and the nature of reality gleaned from psychedelic research. The systemic and cultural ramifications of such shifts in science and consciousness are, like the counterculture movement in the 1960s, likely to produce lasting individual and cultural impacts. The integration of current thinking in quantum science with trauma modalities like EMDR can provide a transpersonal lens that is rooted in solid science. The flexibility of the AIP model means it is easily expanded to provide a forth prong to the past, present and future model, offering a more coherent framework to work with perinatal and transpersonal material.

References

Aspect, A., Clauser, J. F., & Zeilinger, A. (2022). Pioneering quantum information science. *Nature Computational Science 2,* 687–688. https://doi.org/10.1038/s43588-022-00368-0

Black, J., Green, A., & Rickards, T. (1998). *Gods, demons and symbols of ancient Mesopotamia: An illustrated dictionary.* London: British Museum Press.

Borjigin, J., Lee, U., Liu, T., Pal, D., Huff, S., Klarr, D., & Mashour, G. A. (2013). Surge of neurophysiological coherence and connectivity in the dying brain. *Proceedings of the National Academy of Sciences, 110*(35), 14432–14437. https://doi.org/10.1073/pnas.1308285110

Brody, J. (2020). *Quantum entanglement.* Cambridge, MA: MIT Press. https://doi.org/10.7551/mitpress/12403.001.0001

Cole, M. W., Bassett, D. S., Power, J. D., Braver, T. S., & Petersen, S. E. (2014). Intrinsic and task-evoked network architectures of the human brain. *Neuron, 83,* 238–251. https://doi.org/10.1016/j.neuron.2014.05.014

Cook-Greuter, S. R. (2000). Mature ego development: Gateway to ego transcendence? *Journal of Adult Development, 7*(4), 227–240. https://doi.org/10.1023/A:1009511411421

Cornil, L., & van Limbergen, O. (2024). Treating relational trauma with EMDR. Presentation at the EMDR UK conference on 16th March 2024. Watsonville, CA: EMDR UK.

Crews, D. (2008). Epigenetics and its implications for behavioral neuroendocrinology. *Frontiers in Neuroendocrinology, 29*(3), 344–357. https://doi.org/10.1016/j.yfrne.2008.01.003

Davis, A. K., Clifton, J. M., Weaver, E. G., Hurwitz, E. S., Johnson, M. W., & Griffiths, R. R. (2020). Survey of entity encounter experiences occasioned by inhaled N, N-dimethyltryptamine: Phenomenology, interpretation, and enduring effects. *Journal of Psychopharmacology, 34*(9), 1008–1020. https://doi.org/10.1177/0269881120916143

Evans, J., Robinson, O. C., Argyri, E. K., Suseelan, S., Murphy-Beiner, A., McAlpine, R., Luke, D., Michelle, K., & Prideaux, E. (2023). Extended difficulties following the use of psychedelic drugs: A mixed methods study. *PLoS One, 18*(10), e0293349. https://doi.org/10.1371/journal.pone.0293349

Freud, S. (1900). *The interpretation of dreams.* London: Penguin.

Greenewald, J. (2021). UFOs: The Central Intelligence Agency (CIA) collection. Found at https://www.theblackvault.com/documentarchive/ufos-the-central-intelligence-agency-cia-collection/. Accessed 08.01.2024

Grof, S. (1980). *LSD psychotherapy*. Pomona, CA: Hunter House.

Grof, S. (1998). Human nature and the nature of reality: Conceptual challenges from consciousness research. *Journal of Psychoactive Drugs, 30*(4), 343–357. https://doi.org/10.1080/02791072.1998.10399710

Grof, S. (2016). *Realms of the human unconscious: Observations from LSD research*. Chicago, IL: Souvenir Press.

Grof, C., & Grof, S. (2017). Spiritual emergency: The understanding and treatment of transpersonal crises. *International Journal of Transpersonal Studies, 36*(2), 5. https://doi.org/10.24972/ijts.2017.36.2.30

Grof, S., & Grof, C. (1989). *Spiritual emergency: When personal transformation becomes a crisis*. Los Angeles: J.P. Tarcher.

Heisenberg, W. (1930). *Physikalische prinzipien der quantentheorie, leipzig: Hirzel english translation the physical principles of quantum theory*. Chicago, IL: University of Chicago Press. Reprinted Dover 1940.

Jung, C. G. (1952). *Synchronicity: An acausal connecting principle published in 1993*. Bollingen, CH: Bollingen Foundation.

Jung, C. G. (1960). *A review of the complex theory. Collected works (Vol. 8)*. Bollingen Series XX. Princeton, NJ: Princeton University Press.

Kohut, H. (1971). *The analysis of the self*. New York: International Universities Press.

Logie, R. & De Jong A. (2014). The "Flashforward Procedure": Confronting the catastrophe. *Journal of EMDR Practice and Research, 8*(1), 25–32. https://doi.org/10.1891/1933-3196.8.1.25

Mandelbrot, B. (1977). *The fractal geometry of nature*. New York, NY: W. H. Freeman.

Manfield, P., Lovett, J., Engel, L., & Manfield, D. (2017). Use of the flash technique in EMDR therapy: Four case examples. *Journal of EMDR Practice and Research, 11*(4), 195. https://doi.org/10.1891/1933-3196.11.4.195

Marks-Tarlow, T. (1999). The self as a dynamical system. *Nonlinear Dynamics, Psychology, and Life Sciences, 3*, 311–345. https://doi.org/10.1023/A:1021958829905

Marks-Tarlow, T. (2018). Fractal entanglement between observer and observed. *International Journal of Semiotics and Visual Rhetoric (IJSVR), 2*(1), 1–14. https://doi.org/10.4018/IJSVR.2018010101

Marks Tarlow, T. (2020). A fractal epistemology for transpersonal psychology. *International Journal of Transpersonal Studies, 39*(1), 7. https://doi.org/10.24972/ijts.2020.39.1-2.55

Marks-Tarlow, T., & Shapiro, Y. (2021). Synchronicity, acausal connection, and the fractal dynamics of clinical practice. *Psychoanalytic Dialogues, 31*(4), 468–486. https://doi.org/10.1080/10481885.2021.1925283

Martin, J. A. (2020). Clusters of individuals experiences form a continuum of persistent non-symbolic experiences in adults. *CONSCIOUSNESS: Ideas and Research for the Twenty-First Century, 8*(8), 1.

Matheson, S. L., Shepherd, A. M., Pinchbeck, R. M., Laurens, K. R., & Carr, V. J. (2013). Childhood adversity in schizophrenia: A systematic meta-analysis. *Psychological Medicine, 43*(2), 225–238. https://doi.org/10.1017/S0033291712000785

Mitchell, E., Puthoff, H., Graff, D., Geller, U., & In, R. T. (2017). *Phenomena: The secret history of the US Government's investigations into extrasensory perception and psychokinesis*. New York: Little, Brown and Company

Movalled, K., Sani, A., Nikniaz, L., & Ghojazadeh, M. (2023). The impact of sound stimulations during pregnancy on fetal learning: A systematic review. *BMC Pediatrics, 23*(1), 1–15. https://doi.org/10.1186/s12887-023-03990-7

Murray, R. M., Paparelli, A., Morrison, P. D., Marconi, A., & Di Forti, M. (2013). What can we learn about schizophrenia from studying the human model, drug-induced psychosis? *American Journal of Medical Genetics Part B: Neuropsychiatric Genetics, 162*(7), 661–670. https://doi.org/10.1002/ajmg.b.32177

NICE. (2014). *Psychosis and schizophrenia in adults – treatment and management* (Clinical Guideline 136). London: National Collaborating Centre for Mental Health.

Paulsen, S. (2017). *When there are no words: Repairing early trauma and neglect from the attachment period with EMDR therapy*. Bainbridge Island, WA: Bainbridge Institute for Integrative Psychology.

Popkey, A. (2005). DeTUR, an urge reduction protocol for addictions and dysfunctional behaviours. In R. Shapiro (Ed.), *EMDR solutions: Pathways to healing* (pp. 167–188). New York: W.W. Norton & Company.

Puharich, A. (1959). *The sacred mushroom: Key to the door of eternity*. Garden City, NY: Doubleday & Company.

Quesada, D. (2023). Awaken interviews Dr.Jeffery Martin Pt 2 - Evolution of consciousness beyond the mind. Found at https://awaken.com/2023/02/awaken-interviews-dr-jeffery-martin-pt-2-evolution-of-consciousness-beyond-the-mind/. Accessed 29.01.2024

Shapiro, F. (2001). *Eye movement desensitization and reprocessing: Basic principles, protocols and procedures* (2nd ed.). New York, NY: Guilford Press.

Sin, J., & Spain, D. (2017). Psychological interventions for trauma in individuals who have psychosis: A systematic review and meta-analysis. *Psychosis, 9*(1), 67–81. https://doi.org/10.1080/17522439.2016.1167946

Strassman, R. (2000). *DMT: The spirit molecule: A doctor's revolutionary research into the biology of near-death and mystical experiences*. New York: Simon and Schuster.

Varese, F., Sellwood, W., Pulford, D., Awenat, Y., Bird, L., Bhutani, G., Carter, L.A., Davies, L., Aseem, S., Davis, C. & Hefferman-Clarke, R., (2023). Trauma-focused therapy in early psychosis: results of a feasibility randomized controlled trial of EMDR for psychosis (EMDRp) in early intervention settings. *Psychological Medicine*, pp.1–12. https://doi.org/10.1017/S0033291723002532

Varese, F., Smeets, F., Drukker, M., Lieverse, R., Lataster, T., Viechtbauer, W., & Bentall, R. P. (2012). Childhood adversities increase the risk of psychosis: A meta-analysis of patient-control, prospective- and cross-sectional cohort studies. *Schizophrenia Bulletin, 38*(4), 661–671. https://doi.org/10.1093/schbul/sbs050.0

Vollenweider, F. X., & Smallridge, J. W. (2022). Classic psychedelic drugs: Update on biological mechanisms. *Pharmacopsychiatry, 55*(3), 121–138. https://doi.org/10.1055/a-1721-2914

Winkelman, M. (2010). *Shamanism: A biopsychosocial paradigm of conscious-ness and healing.* Santa Barbara, CA: ABC-CLIO. https://doi.org/10.5040/9798216014133

Winkelman, M. J. (2017). The mechanisms of psychedelic visionary experiences: Hypotheses from evolutionary psychology. *Frontiers in Neuroscience, 11,* 539. https://doi.org/10.3389/fnins.2017.00539

12 The future of PsyA-EMDR therapy

Tropoflavin
7,8-Dihydroxyflavone ($C_{15}H_{10}O_4$)

DOI: 10.4324/9781003431718-12

A systematic review of 12 studies demonstrated that the intensity of a psychedelic mystical experience correlated with positive treatment outcomes (Ko et al., 2022). However, not everyone possesses the physical capacity or the psychological stability to withstand the intensity of such interventions. This creates an 'issue of accessibility' ethical dilemma. Non-hallucinogenic psychoplastogens represent a promising alternative to psychedelics when used as an adjunct to psychotherapy, offering many of the potential therapeutic benefits, without the intense psychoactive effects typically associated with traditional psychedelics. These substances may provide treatment options for those deemed unsuitable for classic psychedelic administration, widening the treatment pathways available.

Exercise (De Sousa Fernandes et al., 2020), omega 3 fatty acids (Crupi et al., 2013), some dietary supplements such as N-acetylcysteine (Tardiolo et al., 2018) and cannabinoids such as THC and CBD (Valeri & Mazzon, 2021) also appear to have neuroprotective and pro-neurogenic effects. Alongside these behavioural and nutritional factors, there are a growing number of pharmaceutical molecules that also produce measurable changes in neuroplasticity. This group of drugs produces rapid and sustained effects on neuronal structure and function. The pharmaceutical application of such molecules is still being assessed, but early indications indicate gentler and more sustained effects, manifesting therapeutic benefits after a single administration, without the psychological risks and legislative barriers associated with the application of classic psychedelics (Vargas et al., 2021).

Psychoplastogens appear to induce changes in neuronal structure by activating key proteins involved in cell growth, autophagy and synapse formation (Olson, 2018; Hoeffer & Klann, 2010). One illustrative example is 7,8-dihydroxyflavone, known as Tropoflavin. This non-psychedelic psychoplastogen has demonstrated therapeutic efficacy in animal models for a variety of psychiatric disorders (Chang, 2016). By promoting synaptic plasticity, such compounds have the potential to alleviate symptoms of various mental health conditions, including depression, anxiety and PTSD (Vargas et al., 2021). Research into psychoplastogens is still in its infancy, but early findings suggest they could revolutionise the field of mental health treatment by providing novel accessible pathways to healing and growth. Determining how to deploy psychoplastogenic medicines most effectively at scale will be an important consideration. What is certain is that more research is needed to firmly establish the risks and benefits associated with the application of these novel compounds.

When considering the future of PsyA-EMDR therapy, it is useful to address some of the challenges and opportunities arising in the evolving landscape of psychedelic treatments. In this chapter, we build on the foundations of the AIP framework, delving into the implications and future direction of PsyA-EMDR therapy and highlighting opportunities for further development, innovation, collaboration and enhanced care outcomes. Alongside this, if we are to assess the efficacy and impact of this (or any other) approach, an understanding of the core processes and mechanisms is also necessary. While much remains unknown, the AIP conceptualisation offers a valuable framework for exploring the therapeutic potential of psychedelics when used in conjunction with EMDR therapy.

Repeated exposure to trauma, especially when paired with insufficient mental hygiene practices, leads to an accumulation of dysfunctionally stored material. This reduces resilience, ultimately leading to an increased risk of PTSD and other secondary psychopathologies (Bremner, 2006). If early intervention was prioritised, there would be less need for psychedelics or any other psychotherapeutic intervention. Early diagnostic and therapeutic interventions, for example, the 'Right to Choose' pathway (NHS England, n.d.) or the 'Open Dialogue' model (Seikkula et al., 2006) act as preventative care, reducing the number of treatment sessions required, reducing patient risk and preventing symptoms from becoming chronic and/or systemic. Lengthy wait times for accessing treatments are also counterproductive to health outcomes. As we explore and navigate the intricacies of accessibility, there is an emerging need to move away from healthcare systems that operate within a two-tiered structure. In such systems, those with financial resources can access private treatments, and those unable to afford them, often individuals with a higher trauma load, cannot. Social inequality is emerging as a notable/significant risk factor, whereby limited accessibility leads to complications that affect the safety and efficacy of mental health provision (Kirkbride et al., 2024). Consequently, psychedelic therapy might pose an increased risk for marginalised communities and individuals lacking the financial resources to access treatments promptly. Prioritising inclusive treatment options that emphasise early intervention should be a key focus as we progress towards scalable psychedelic treatments. Such approaches may help to alleviate the impact of secondary compilations and foster long-term well-being outcomes for everyone.

Social exclusion is just one of several systemic and cultural factors that contribute to risk in psychedelic treatment provision. Making changes to the social and cultural environment could help to minimise the spectrum of risks associated with PAP delivery.

Wider systemic/cultural areas that contribute to risk in PAP delivery

Legislation

- The lack of evidence-based drug legislation continues to obstruct meaningful research opportunities.
- There is a lack of understanding and guidance by professional governing bodies about psychedelic therapies, which prevents practitioners and service users from making informed choices about psychedelic treatment options.

Education

- There is a lack of psychedelically informed inpatient care settings.
- There is insufficient breadth and depth of training for practitioners, resulting in professionals working outside their training competencies.
- There is a lack of psychoeducation, resources and training opportunities for practitioners.
- There are limited legitimate experiential training opportunities for practitioners to experience psychedelic treatments themselves.

Pharmacology

- Pharmaceutical protectionism can obstruct the rigours of scientific scrutiny.
- The potential for profiteering can bias the data available.
- Novel compounds are being developed, tested and patent-protected. Many traditional medicines, which cannot be patented, are under-researched.
- There is not enough evidence published about adverse drug effects, or disappointing experiences.
- Non-disclosure agreements in clinical research prevent practitioners from sharing their learning about clinical challenges.

Psychology

- There is a lack of trauma-informed practice across all levels of engagement in psychedelic provision.
- For those destabilised by psychedelics, adequate tools to work therapeutically with the emergent content have not yet been developed or scientifically verified. Further evidence is needed for efficacious methods when working with those experiencing adverse reactions such as HPPD.

Substance

- There continues to be social stigma associated with psychedelic drug use which impacts the mindset of those in receipt of psychedelic treatments.
- There is an insufficient evidence base to support appropriate dose, sequence or substance selection.
- There is a lack of awareness that high-dose experiences aren't necessarily conducive to enhanced therapeutic outcomes. Low-dose experiences can be supported and simultaneously enhanced using spiritual emergence practices already used by EMDR therapists to induce and enhance mystical-like experiences.
- Substance variants have not yet been specifically explored. For example, there are paradigmatic differences between ways of working therapeutically with fast-acting decontextualising psychedelics such as 5-MeO-DMT / N,N-DMT and trust-enhancing empathogens such as MDMA. Whilst helpful, therapeutic generalisations need to be carefully assessed against ideographic differences of the subjective drug effects. A rich spectrum of therapeutic interventions needs to reflect these phenomenological variants and individual needs.

Setting

- There is insufficient learning from recreational use, substance misuse, underground treatment settings and acute care service users' experiences.
- There is a growing popularity in illegal underground treatment settings where inexperienced practitioners can compromise patient safety and harm the reputation of PAP.
- There is a lack of emphasis on therapeutic outcomes in medicalised settings. For example, working therapeutically with those who have had Ketamine as an aesthetic or neuroprotective agent is often unexplored or overlooked.

Practitioner

- Therapists need adequate supervision by those suitably trained and highly experienced in this area of practice. There is a limited pool of practitioners who qualify, and opportunities that engender mistake-friendly environments to support practitioner development are still fewer.
- There is a lack of opportunity to work in interdisciplinary teams, where an expanded skill sets lead to a greater number of treatment options.
- Practitioners should be encouraged to have sufficient insight into their own personal material, which is currently not a mandatory requirement

for many mental health practitioners, for example psychiatrists and clinical psychologists.

Research

- Relying on data obtained from neuroimaging is insufficient to elucidate the underlying mechanisms of EMDR and other psychedelic therapies.
- The refinement of practical applications in conjunction with data collection is necessary to advance our understanding.

Clinical decision-making

Finding suitable support for the most vulnerable members of society requires the provision of treatments that align with a person's capacity to engage in therapy. For some, relational interventions are sufficient to lead to significant and lasting change and, for many, trauma-focused interventions such as EMDR therapy will facilitate positive change/healing. The most complex presentations are often described as 'treatment resistant' and are passed around between different services, running the risk of being retraumatised in the process. Social stigma and history both play a role in reinforcing this outcome, as many of society's most vulnerable people are deprioritised by political systems. Many people in this situation are left with no alternative than to self-medicate for their symptoms. In his book, In the Realm of Hungry Ghosts, Gabor Mate states that,

> There is no war on drugs because you can't war on inanimate objects. There's only a war on drug addicts, which means we are warring on the most abused and vulnerable segments of society
>
> (Mate, 2018).

Given the impact that social stigma has on provision, further exploration of the impact that these factors play on the availability of psychedelic treatments and clinical reasoning is warranted. What factors would justify traditional interventions? And when could psychedelic alternatives be offered?

And so, proponents of EMDR therapy justifiably question: why not stay with the evidence-based 8-phases of standard EMDR therapy? When is standard protocol EMDR therapy insufficient as a stand-alone? What justifies the need to incorporate psychedelics into a treatment plan? Answering these questions necessitates a detailed analysis of the phenomenological and practical variances between EMDR therapy and PsyA-EMDR therapy. Integrating the 8-phases of EMDR into the psychedelic medication session is at the forefront of applied practice. Current research is constrained by financial and legislative barriers, but valuable insights can be gleaned from practice-based evidence gained from therapists already working in the emerging field of PsyA-EMDR therapy. Widening access to either treatment will depend on a variety of factors.

Widening the treatment domain

In PAP, case conceptualisations and the resulting clinical formulations inform decisions about whom to treat, what treatment to administer, the appropriate dosage, substance and sequence and what therapy to provide, as well as the timing and location of these interventions. Such decisions typically stem from a nuanced clinical decision-making process, which combines the holistic needs of the individual, with patient empowerment, clinical judgement, contextual factors, legislative requirements and service availability.

The decision-making matrix diagram outlined below can be used as a formulation tool to assist clinicians when considering the suitability of PsyA-EMDR therapy. In terms of treatment participation, there are four stepped levels. The goal is to widen the treatment domain that resides between the inner most and outer most levels. This can be achieved by addressing the issues that reside at each level. Inspired by the model outlined in Kate Raworth's book, doughnut economics (Raworth, 2017), these levels include the individual personal foundations, standard protocol EMDR therapy, PsyA-EMDR therapy and the social global ceilings. Thus, the standard protocol EMDR therapy and PsyA-EMDR therapy levels are referred to as 'the treatment domain.' The diagram outlines the key issues that reside at each level, and what ceilings need to be tackled to enhance access to the treatment domain. Widening accessibility supports inclusion and can be achieved through political, social, economic, educational, therapeutic or medical input.

Widening the treatment domain can be achieved by:

1 Working to address the issues that reside in the inner most circle, the 'individual personal foundations.' The issues at this level represent a person's essential needs, the dimensions that are deemed to be necessary for ensuring a person's safety and well-being throughout the course of an intervention. These represent the minimum requirements for accessing treatments safely. For example, health issues may be prohibitive to participation, such as the use of benzodiazepine medications which are contraindicatory for EMDR. However, after therapeutic or medical input, there may be a reduced need for these medications. Once these individual personal foundations have been fulfilled, a person may

then be deemed suitable for the next level, the use of standard protocol EMDR therapy.

2 Standard protocol EMDR therapy is used before administering psychedelic medications. Indications that someone might be suitable for standard protocol EMDR, but not yet suitable for psychedelic administration, are outlined in the diagram at this level. These issues can be addressed using the 8-phases of EMDR standard protocol. For example, a prohibitive diagnosis such as bipolar disorder may be treated using conventional EMDR methods, and, once stabilised, these patients might then be deemed suitable for the psychedelic-assisted therapy component. It should also be noted that those who do respond well to EMDR therapy may no longer need psychedelic medications, as usually symptoms subside with EMDR therapy alone, reducing the need for psychedelics. This should be deemed an ideal outcome.

3 At the PsyA-EMDR level, clinical decision-making incorporates situational variants that may contribute towards individualised care planning. For example, EMDR techniques can be applied to previous psychedelic experiences without the need for any additional medications. For example, many people have already had recreational or medical psychedelic experiences that have been left unexplored and unintegrated. The therapeutic value of these existing cohorts merits further exploration. See Chapter 4, 'Ethics' demonstrating the value of working therapeutically with Ketamine that had been previously prescribed as a neuroprotective anaesthetic in the case material titled 'An underused stroke of insight.' Working with historic material such as this should be prioritised before giving any further psychedelic medications.

4 Once all the foundations are in place and access to PsyA-EMDR can be considered, subsequent limitations become cultural, political or systemic. These issues are described as the 'social global ceilings.' This level in the diagram represents the social and environmental limitations that cap or limit access to the treatment domain. These ceilings cannot be exceeded without political or social reform. For example, the lack of evidence to support psychedelic therapy practice will likely limit service availability in medical settings, until commissioners are able to fund treatments that stand on a (as yet non-existent) body of research evidence. The issues represented at this level highlight the key areas that need to be addressed to improve individual and societal access to psychedelic-assisted therapies.

To reiterate, the goal is to widen the treatment domain, ensuring that interventions occur within the safe and just parameters that are depicted in between the innermost and outermost rings. This diagram highlights the complex matrix of considerations that are necessary to inform the clinical decision-making process and improve accessibility.

To use metaphor to simplify the explanation, this diagram resembles a 2-dimensional 'exploded bagel.' The outer layers constitute the bagel itself, appearing as fragmented segments and representing the individual personal foundations and the social global ceilings. In between these layers lies the nourishing filling layer, symbolised by standard protocol EMDR, and could be seen as the meaty bit of the sandwich (or vegan equivalent). In addition, there is an optional extra in this sandwich-making extravaganza, depicted as the dressing. This dressing can be added to lubricate and enrich the experience of eating the sandwich. This dressing represents the psychedelic-assisted component of the therapy. The dressing isn't fundamental, but it does enhance the experience and make it more palatable. The aspects identified in each segment of this cut up bagel can be used to support the clinical decision-making processes at each layer. Metaphorically, the overall goal is to increase the portions of filling in this bagel so that it becomes more appetising and can feed more people, thus widening the treatment domain to enhance accessibility.

Warning

The potential impact of psychedelic medications on pre-existing psychotic and bipolar disorders is unclear. A history or family history of mania, psychosis (including drug-induced psychosis) can heighten the risks associated with psychedelic medications. EMDR therapy as a stand-alone could offer a safer and more suitable therapeutic alternative. Suitability needs to be assessed on a case-by-case basis and may depend upon several external factors. If symptoms of psychosis or mania are present and interfering with an individual's competency, safety and stabilisation need to be prioritised.

Therapist safety

Practitioner safety is paramount, and all aspects of psychedelic therapy need to be adequately risk-assessed. In many countries, working with classified substances is illegal outside of licenced clinical research settings. With legislative change on the horizon, therapists are strongly encouraged

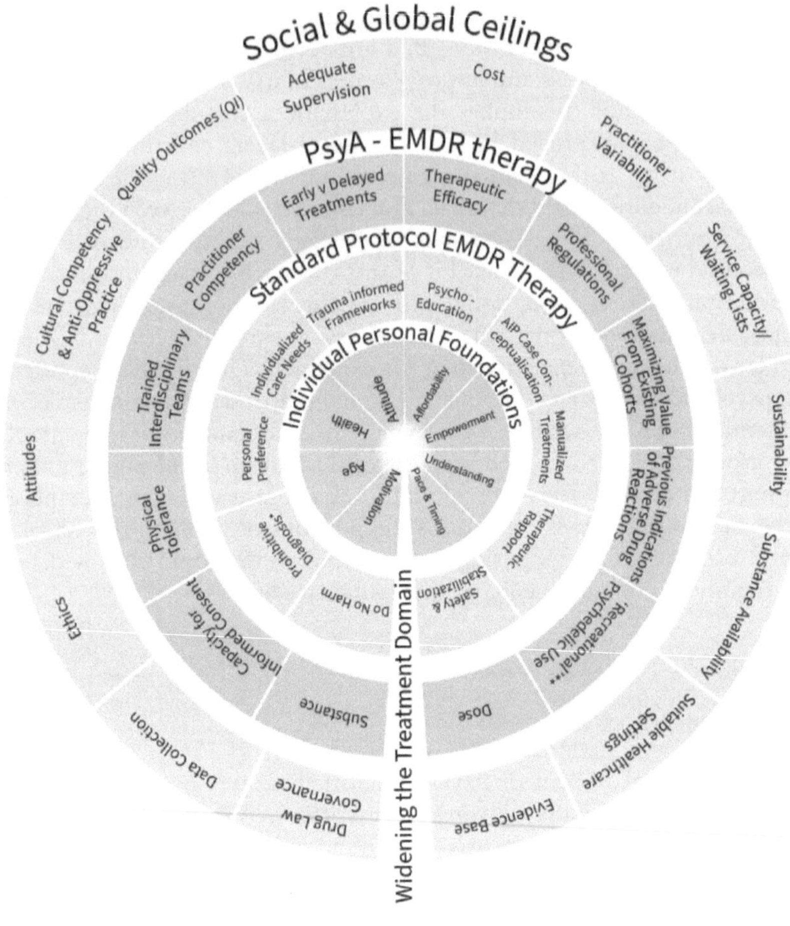

Figure 12.1 The decision-making matrix identifies various factors that support and guide the expansion on the treatment domain for PsyA-EMDR therapy, supporting patient-centred, inclusive treatment outcomes.

to stay within the law for all matters relating to their clinical practice and to seek guidance on local laws about what is permissible.

Working within one's own competency is paramount. Additional training and CPD are strongly recommended when working with psychedelic substances to support the safe navigation of the amplified content. The dose and substance selection should be matched to practitioner competency. Not all psychedelics are the same; having training in one substance does not necessarily indicate competency to work with all of them. As with any healthcare provision, it is good practice to periodically identify which areas require further development and seek out CPD to address any shortfalls. Practitioner experiential trainings are useful although there is a debate about whether first-hand experience of psychedelics is essential. Those working in the field should have opportunities to experience expanded states so that they are familiar with the terrain and get accustomed to sitting for other practitioners before working with the complexity of clinical cohorts. This includes breathwork, an alternative for those who have reservations about psychedelic substances.

Specialist supervision with those already working in the field is essential and supports a wider awareness of how to navigate the challenges that emerge. Cultivating mistake friendly environments whilst adopting a stance of not knowing supports reflective practice, as we continue to work towards an understanding of how to work with these substances and how to optimise their therapeutic value.

Compassion fatigue and practitioner burnout compromise practitioner and patient safety. Clinicians are encouraged to build in opportunities for self-care throughout their daily routines, such as practising meditation or engaging in other contemplative activities. Ethical pitfalls will emerge, even with the most well intending of practitioners when adequate self-care is compromised. Self-care needs to be prioritised during the session, within the team and at home (Rothschild, 2006).

Practitioners need to tend to their own self-development to know their growing edges, hot spots, blind spots and soft spots and to be aware of how these might get in the way of the therapeutic process. A minimal requirement for personal therapy might also be beneficial when training requirements are considered for accreditation as a psychedelic practitioner.

Vicarious traumatisation poses a significant risk to professionals working with complex cases. Developing focusing skills is useful in preventing the formation of mental images of client material. It can be useful to stay as fully engaged with the client in the present moment as is possible. Notice the way their lips move as they speak rather than deploying imaginative narratives of their descriptions. Employing left-brain mindfulness techniques can help keep such traumatic images at bay, reducing the risk of vicarious traumatisation of the therapist. Self-care and personal therapy may also be useful. Working as a team helps to reduce the impact of the work. For treatment cohorts with a high trauma load, a floating therapist model could be deployed, much like that seen in EMDR 2.0 protocols.

Posture, body language and dress code all need careful consideration. Close attention should be paid to power differentials because of the inability to provide informed consent which can compromise patient and practitioner safety. We recommend that the use of therapeutic touch is avoided which adheres to the guidelines of many of the counselling accrediting bodies. Contract and discuss in advance to minimise the need for safety touch.

See Chapter 4, 'Ethics.' Videotape the psychedelic medication sessions as a safeguarding precaution. Some people experience paranoid delusions of abuse by therapists that did not happen. It is easy to ensure practitioner safety and dispel delusional beliefs by sharing the footage at a later date, once the content has been sufficiently worked with.

Many psychedelics have aphrodisiac effects and expanded states magnify erotic material. Psychedelics can intensify erotic transference and therapists should be adept at addressing and challenging therapist idolisation and look out for signs of therapeutic narcissism. Practitioners should be encouraged to stay out of intimate or sexual relationships with any clients or colleagues. Instead, explore the emergent content in clinical supervision. Where intimate relationships between co-therapists are already established, seek additional guidance about working with the enhanced transferential content. Professional colleagues may need to be challenged if there are signs or symptoms of therapeutic abuse.

Therapist Safety Checklist

- Are you feeling resourced?
- Do you have adequate self-care?
- Do you have support from your supervisor(s) and professional peers?
- Are you working within your competency?
- What skills do you need to develop to address any shortfalls in competency?
- Could you benefit from engaging in personal therapy?
- Are you familiar with the phenomenology of expanded states?
- Can you work as a team with colleagues to reduce the psychological load?
- Do you have peers in the field you can share ideas or issues with?
- Are you managing to maintain a healthy emotional boundary with your client's content?
- Do you have adequate safeguarding precautions in place to protect yourself? e.g. recording sessions.
- Have you clearly contracted around safety touch, and explained the alternatives to therapeutic touch?
- Are you aware of the power differentials that exist in the psychedelic work you are undertaking?
- Are you maintaining professional boundaries with your clients and colleagues?

No one can accurately foresee how these treatment options may unfold. Several other factors may affect the future delivery of PsyA-EMDR, and a few of these factors would merit further exploration. Some of these emergent themes are unpacked herein:

Building an evidence base

Before a pharmaceutical company can bring a new medicine to market, an evidence base is required to demonstrate drug efficacy. The evidence base for psychedelic drugs will likely support the availability of these medicines for use in healthcare settings, long before the existence of an evidence base to demonstrate the therapeutic efficacy of the PAP approach. And demonstrating evidence-based efficacy of the various PAP approaches will need to happen before a comparison of the efficacy of these different PAP's can be conducted. Demonstrating therapeutic efficacy is notoriously arduous and problematic, and yet health service commissioners rely on evidence-based practice for funding service provision. This means that interventions already in use at scale such as ACT are the approaches that have been most readily adopted. Compiling an evidence base requires a systematic approach. Breaking down the testing of the PsyA-EMDR protocol into it constituent parts, preparation, dosing, post stabilisation and integration. Each of these four cornerstones needs to be rigorously assessed. The risks already posed to vulnerable individuals by recreational psychedelic drug use and in psychedelic clinical research trials mean that the cornerstone of post-dose stabilisation is likely to be the first evidence-based performance indicator for the value and efficacy of PsyA-EMDR therapy. As psychedelic medications are rolled out, training therapists to work with challenges associated with the delivery of PAP at scale is timely. We need effective therapeutic applications and suitably trained practitioners securely in place for when issues relating to scalability begin to emerge in mental health services. Government and institutional strategies need to support CPD opportunities, and practitioner experiential trainings prioritised, to prepare practitioners for working in the field.

Cost and effectiveness

When considering scalability, the cost and effectiveness of any intervention will determine how likely it is to be incorporated into health service provision. In health economics and outcomes research, Quality-Adjusted Life Year (QALY) is the measurement used to assess the value of medical interventions (Drummond, 2015). QALY combines both the quantity and quality of life lived as a result of a particular health intervention. QALYs allow researchers and policymakers to compare the effectiveness of different interventions across various health conditions and populations, providing a standardised metric for decision-making for resource allocation in healthcare. Trauma is widespread and highly correlated with poor mental health (Kessler et al., 1995). As models of mental distress move away from "what is wrong with you?" towards transdiagnostic trauma-informed frameworks that consider "what happened to you?" (Sweeney, 2018), there has been a movement towards trauma-informed approaches in mental health provision. Therapies designed to address trauma enhance quality of life and accelerate recovery (Herman, 2015). Consequently, the cost and efficacy ratings of trauma therapies may indicate the best outcomes in QALY measurements and are likely to indicate the future trajectory of this work. In non-psychedelic therapy settings, EMDR appears to be the most cost-effective intervention for adults with PTSD (with a probability of 0.34 amongst the 11 evaluated therapy options at a cost-effectiveness threshold of £20,000 per QALY (Mavranezouli et al., 2020). This is followed by combined somatic/cognitive therapies, self-help with support, psychoeducation, selective serotonin reuptake inhibitors (SSRIs), trauma-focused cognitive behavioural therapy (TF-CBT), self-help without support, non-TF-CBT and combined TF-CBT/SSRIs were ranked in descending order of cost-effectiveness. Notably, counselling was found to be less cost-effective than no treatment at all. Whilst QALY measurements are not yet known for psychedelic treatments delivered in healthcare settings, the existing QALY data may provide some indication of the likely outcomes for future decision-making in psychedelic healthcare resource allocation.

Neurodiversity

Neurological differences encompass a wide range of conditions, including autism spectrum disorder (ASD) and attention deficit hyperactivity disorder (ADHD). Such individuals often experience challenges in various domains of functioning, such as social interaction, communication and attention regulation. Emerging research suggests that psychedelic therapies may hold some promise in addressing some of the symptoms associated with these neurodevelopmental conditions (Orsini, 2020). Whilst the underlying mechanisms are not fully understood, potential benefits include an amelioration in some of the behavioural traits associated with ASD, such as improved emotional regulation, enhanced social connectedness and reduced symptoms of anxiety and depression (Markopoulos et al., 2022). The interactions of psychedelic medications in neurodivergent populations remain uncertain, highlighting the need for further investigation into their specific effects. Evidence indicates that the effect of medications can vary, for instance, non-psychedelic ADHD medications have been shown to elicit distinct effects in individuals with and without ADHD (Lakhan et al., 2012). Rigorous formulation practices are essential when treating neurodiverse populations so as to give the clinician the opportunity to better understand the client and their needs. During formulation, it can be helpful to decipher what traits were already there before the trauma and consider how to better manage working memory and relational factors if problems with processing do emerge. Despite preliminary findings, further research is needed to elucidate safety and efficacy and to explore any potential adjustments or adjunct treatments that might be deemed necessary. Those with neurodiverse conditions will likely require a comprehensive and individualised care approach. More evidence is needed to clarify exactly how psychedelic treatments might be finetuned for those with social-behavioural disorders.

Forensics and clinical psychopathy

Research indicates that lifetime psychedelic use is associated with an 18% decrease in the probability of being arrested for violent crime (Holoyda, 2020), significantly reduces the risk of arrest for intimate partner violence(Walsh et al., 2016) and reduces the probability of committing physical assault (Hendricks, 2018). This data suggests that psychedelics could hold therapeutic potential for those at risk of violent behaviours. Research into trauma-informed care for adults involved in the prison system demonstrates that EMDR significantly reduces recidivism (Brown et al., 2015), is an efficient and effective means of addressing those with adverse developmental experiences which contribute to offense pathways (Ronald et al., 2016) and may reduce an offender's justification for victimising others (Finlay, 2002). A comprehensive framework for integrating EMDR into psychedelic therapy in forensic populations does not yet exist in the literature. This gap prompts a theoretical illustration for the feasibility of one potential future application.

Fanatical extremists hold extreme political or religious views; exemplified by individuals affiliated with the far-right, Islamist extremists and proponents of the incel movement. Individuals prone to ideological extremism frequently harbour histories marked by betrayal trauma (Freyd, 1996). Preventing and countering violent extremism has become a ubiquitous feature of national strategies and early intervention is a key approach (Stephens et al., 2021). An individual's first encounter with the law, before they become desensitised to judicial processes, is key in terms of outcome impact (Silber, 2007), therefore facilitating early interventions is crucial to disrupt patterns before they become entrenched. EMDR is under investigation as a treatment for radicalised individuals (Ramaswamy, 2024), whereby dynamic risk factors are conceptualised through the AIP model as an expression of pathogenic memories, and where positive memories facilitate the mobilisation of protective factors (Dieu et al., 2019). Many of those affected by extremist ideologies have previously engaged in recreational psychedelic use, and PsyA-EMDR could be used to integrate these recreational experiences, without the need for further psychedelic administration. Furthermore, empathogens such as MDMA could be useful in assisting targeted preventative deradicalisation interventions. At the point of first arrest, MDMA-assisted EMDR therapy could be useful in supporting attachment formation and resourcing for trauma reprocessing. Numerous aetiological parallels exist between extremism and other forensic presentations. For example, many child sex offenders also exhibit features of betrayal trauma (Levenson et al., 2014) and may demonstrate comparable responses to trauma-focused psychedelic treatments (Tenenbaum, 1961). EMDR has successfully been used in forensic settings with child sex offenders in the US and the UK for over ten years (Ricci & Clayton, 2016), and the addition of psychedelic medications has the potential to enhance such treatments. Of course, much more research and a forensic analysis of the data sets would be necessary before introducing these treatments into forensic cohorts. Until a robust evidence base for psychedelic therapies exists, and until psychedelic treatments are fully supported and endorsed by regulatory processes, it is likely that these treatments would not be suitable for such cohorts, due to the inevitable emerging ethical considerations. Ultimately, strict adherence to evidence-based practice is essential when navigating the intricate terrain of any psychedelic-assisted therapy within forensic setting, and to date, research into this area is scarce (Holoyda, 2020).

The future of group work

Group therapy offers a unique therapeutic experience that can be used either as a stand-alone or to supplement individual therapy. Community integration initiatives such as psychedelic integration circles are already being used to enhance therapeutic value through horizontal models of community-centred care. Group therapy can be particularly beneficial to individuals seeking social support, diverse perspectives and opportunities for interpersonal growth, normalisation and experiential learning. Group work is also more cost-effective than individual therapy, so more accessible for people on low incomes.

The potential for group traumatic episode protocol (G-TEP) EMDR to be incorporated into community, retreat and medical settings for the integration of psychedelic-assisted therapy presents an intriguing avenue for therapeutic advancement. G-TEP is designed to address collective traumas experienced by groups such as war or natural disasters and holds promise in facilitating the processing and integration of psychedelic experiences within a supportive group context. In group settings, G-TEP PsyA-EMDR therapy could aid in navigating and integrating psychedelic experiences in a group setting with the option of sharing themes or experiences that emerge. This could offer a more structured approach to addressing collective traumas and societal challenges that may surface and foster a sense of cohesion, understanding and community among participants. G-TEP interventions are often EMDr, whereby the focus is on desensitisation (rather than reprocessing), whilst keeping a narrow focus on the identified target. This means that full integration of the corresponding memory network may not be possible in the way that it is in individual work. For G-TEP participants who have recently had psychedelics, it might be that EMDr is sufficient to facilitate more comprehensive integration, due to the increased neuroplasticity at the time of the group processing. Further individual work can then be used to get into the root node and complete the target. The group experience is likely to promote deeper insights, both within the individual and on a community level.

The importance of endings

At the outset of any psychedelic therapy intervention, it is crucial to consider its eventual conclusion. The ending will shape the overall therapeutic trajectory, ensuring a cohesive journey and allowing for intentional planning and preparation, whilst fostering a sense of safety and purpose throughout the whole process. As well as providing a sense of closure, a thoughtfully structured ending will provide a sense of resolution, facilitating integration, promoting lasting change and enhancing the overall therapeutic impact of the experience. The ending is especially important for those with attachment trauma where the potential for enactments and heightened projective identification can otherwise play out.

With every ending, there comes a new beginning and, as this book draws to its conclusion, it is perhaps useful to consider what new beginnings will emerge hereafter. In his book, *How to Change your Mind*, Michael Pollan describes the need to imagine new ceremonial paradigms to fit our times, whereby ingenuity and attunement to both the individual and the medicine will be required. There is a need for culturally appropriate frameworks for setting out how this work is offered, with embedded structures for appropriate meaning making. A greater thoughtfulness will be needed from guides or facilitators in western settings (Pollan, 2018). Such structures might be symbolised and held by the therapeutic frame, signifying the fundamental importance of the opening and the ending or completing of the process.

In closing

In closing, the practical applications outlined in this book will help to expose a more complete spectrum of understanding about the benefits, challenges and nuances of this treatment. Whilst EMDR therapy stands on a solid body of evidence, adding psychedelic medications to this integrative approach holds great promise but clearly requires further investigation. Additional adaptations and finetuning will then emerge from experience and changes will no doubt be made to the protocols outlined herein. It is hoped that this book will lay the foundations to build a more robust evidence base for EMDR as a PAP moving forward. Subsequent editions will likely support further developments, providing more detailed troubleshooting guidance and optimising safer and more consistent delivery of this novel treatment. This book sketches out an overview to illustrate a new way of working, but for now it is not yet possible to foresee or curate a more definitive guide. As practice-based evidence for PsyA-EMDR therapy expands, new insights will be generated from working in the field, which can then be incorporated into protocols and practice. This book marks just the start of a growing edge of pracademia that will no doubt continue to unfold.

Psychologist, educator, originator and developer of EMDR therapy, Francine Shapiro recognised the challenges of fitting a novel panacea into traditional therapeutic structures. Shapiro described, "As with any field, if something does not fit into the current understanding of how things work, it raises eyebrows, hackles or both" (Shapiro, 2012). Our own experiences of writing this book have highlighted the value of collaborative partnerships as a bedrock of validation, support, inspiration and growth. There is strength in relationship, where creativity, enthusiasm and passion get nurtured, encouraged and validated, with love. Our relationship has been integral to giving each of us the confidence to passionately share our ways of working with the wider community. We hope that our partnership inspires others to develop collaborations of their own. Practitioner communities offer a refreshing alternative to corporate interests and top-down institutional academia. Practitioner collaborations draw upon interdisciplinary skill sets through self-experimentation, reflective practice, reflexive practice and mutual respect. The authors encourage the readership to join special interest groups (SIGs) where other people with shared interests and expertise may continue to collaborate, encourage and inspire. Where no communities exist, the readership is encouraged to set up their own networks and working groups. These grass roots movements offer a bottom-up approach to clinical change. A refreshing alternative in the emerging field.

Like the sun, pinching out from the horizon, the new dawn of psychedelic therapy is beginning to unfold. This ground-breaking work requires that our field of understanding develops as fast as is possible, but as slow as is necessary. New methods will give rise to new understandings and further expose the fabric of what is possible. Over time, this will eventually lead to a firm body of evidence, for what looks set to be a promising new era in trauma-responsive healing.

References

American Psychiatric Association. (2013). *Diagnostic and statistical manual of mental disorders* (5th ed.). Arlington, VA: American Psychiatric Publishing

Berne, E. (1961). *Transactional analysis in psychotherapy: A systematic individual and social psychiatry.* New York: Grove Press.

Bremner, J. D. (2006). Traumatic stress: Effects on the brain. *Dialogues in Clinical Neuroscience, 8*(4), 445–461. https://doi.org/10.31887/dcns.2006.8.4/jbremner

Brown, S.H., Gilman, S.G., Goodman, E.G., Adler-Tapia, R., & Freng, S. (2015). Integrated trauma treatment in drug court: Combining EMDR therapy and seeking safety. *Journal of EMDR Practice and Research, 9*(3), 123–136. https://psycnet.apa.org/doi/10.1891/1933-3196.9.3.123

Chang, H. A., Wang, Y. H., Tung, C. S., Yeh, C. B., & Liu, Y. P. (2016). 7, 8–Dihydroxyflavone, a tropomyosin-kinase related receptor b agonist, produces fast-onset antidepressant-like effects in rats exposed to chronic mild stress. *Psychiatry Investigation, 13*(5), 531–540. https://doi.org/10.4306/pi.2016.13.5.531

Crupi, R., Marino, A., & Cuzzocrea, S. (2013). n-3 fatty acids: Role in neurogenesis and neuroplasticity. *Current Medical Chemistry, 20*(24), 2953–2963. https://doi.org/10.2174/09298673113209990140

De Sousa Fernandes, M. S., Ordônio, T. F., Santos, G. C. J., Santos, L. E. R., Calazans, C. T., Gomes, D. A., & Santos, T. M. (2020). Effects of physical exercise on neuroplasticity and brain function: A systematic review in human and animal studies. *Neural Plasticity, 2020*, 8856621. https://doi.org/10.1155/2020/8856621

Dieu, E., & Torte St Jammes, J. (2019). Interest of AIP and EMDR in a new conceptualization of "TIM-E Criminology": Example of radicalized offenders' treatment. Conference: EMDRIA conference 2019, Ontario, CA: Changing lives.

Drummond, M. F., Sculpher, M. J., Claxton, K., Stoddart, G. L., & Torrance, G. W. (2015). *Methods for the economic evaluation of health care programmes.* Oxford: Oxford University Press.

Finlay, P. (2002). Eye movement desensitization and reprocessing (EMDR) in the treatment of sex offenders. *Dissertation Abstracts International, 63*(10), 4899. Found at https://connect.springerpub.com/highwire_display/entity_view/node/69581/full. Accessed 16.04.2024

Freyd, J. J. (1996). *Betrayal trauma: The logic of forgetting childhood abuse.* Cambridge, MA: Harvard University Press.

Hendricks, P. S., Crawford, M. S., & Cropsey, K. L. (2018). The relationships of classic psychedelic use with criminal behavior in the United States adult population. *Journal of Psychopharmacology, 32*(1), 37–48. https://doi.org/10.1177/0269881117735685 10.1177/0269881117735685

Herman, J. (2015). Trauma and recovery: The aftermath of violence from domestic abuse to political terror. New York: Basic Books.

Hoeffer, C.A., & Klann, E. (2010). mTOR signalling: At the crossroads of plasticity, memory and disease. *Trends in Neurosciences, 33*(2), 67–75. https://doi.org/10.1016/j.tins.2009.11.003

Holoyda, B. (2020). The psychedelic renaissance and its forensic implications. *Journal of the American Academy of Psychiatry and the Law, 48*(1), 87–97. https://doi.org/10.29158/JAAPL.003917-20

Kessler, R. C., Sonnega, A., Bromet, E., Hughes, M., & Nelson, C. B. (1995). Posttraumatic stress disorder in the national comorbidity survey. *Archieves of General Psychiatry, 52*(12), 1048–1060. https://doi.org/10.1001/archpsyc.1995.03950240066012

Kirkbride, J. B., Anglin, D. M., Colman, I., Dykxhoorn, J., Jones, P. B., Patalay, P., Pitman, A., Soneson, E., Steare, T., Wright, T., & Griffiths, S. L. (2024). The social determinants of mental health and disorder: Evidence, prevention and recommendations. *World Psychiatry, 23*(1), 58–90. https://doi.org/10.1002/wps.21160

Knipe, J. (2016). Loving eyes protocol. Found at https://emdrtherapyvolusia.com/wp-content/uploads/2016/12/Loving_Eyes_Protocol.pdf. Accessed 15.04.2024

Ko, K., Knight, G., Rucker, J. J., & Cleare, A. J. (2022). Psychedelics, mystical experience, and therapeutic efficacy: A systematic review. *Frontiers in Psychiatry, 13*, 917199. https://doi.org/10.3389/fpsyt.2022.917199

Lakhan, S.E., & Kirchgessner, A. (2012). Prescription stimulants in individuals with and without attention deficit hyperactivity disorder: Misuse, cognitive impact, and adverse effects. *Brain and Behavior, 2*(5), 661–677. https://doi.org/10.1002/brb3.78

Levenson, J. S., Willis, G. M., & Prescott, D. S. (2014). Adverse Childhood Experiences in the Lives of Male Sex Offenders: Implications for trauma-informed care. *Association for the Prevention and Treatment and Prevention of Sexual Abuse, 28*(4), 340–359. https://doi.org/10.1177/1079063214535819

Markopoulos, A., Inserra, A., De Gregorio, D., & Gobbi, G. (2022). Evaluating the potential use of serotonergic psychedelics in autism spectrum disorder. *Frontiers in Pharmacology, 12*,749068. https://doi.org/10.3389/fphar.2021.749068

Mavranezouli, I., Megnin-Viggars, O., Grey, N., Bhutani, G., Leach, J., & Daly, C. (2020). Cost-effectiveness of psychological treatments for post-traumatic stress disorder in adults. *PLoS ONE, 15*(4), e0232245. https://doi.org/10.1371/journal.pone.0232245

Maté, G. (2008). *In the realm of hungry ghosts: Close encounters with addiction.* North Atlantic Books.

National Health Service (NHS) England. (n.d.). Personalised care and choice. Found at https://www.england.nhs.uk/personalisedcare/choice/#:~:text=The%20NHS%20Constitution%20for%20England,support%20to%20make%20these%20choices

Olson, D. E. (2018). Psychoplastogens: A promising class of plasticity-promoting neurotherapeutics. *Journal of Experimental Neuroscience, 12*, 1179069518800508. https://doi.org/10.1177/1179069518800508

Orsini, A. P. (2020). *Autism on acid. How LSD helped me understand, navigate, alter & appreciate my autistic perceptions.* Chicago, IL: Independently Published.

Pollan, M. (2018). *How to change your mind: What the new science of psychedelics teaches us about consciousness, dying, addiction, depression, and transcendence.* Westminster, London: Penguin Press.

Ramaswamy, R. (2024). Trauma, Identity & Extremism. Poster Presentation. EMDR UK Conference 2024, New York.

Raworth, K. (2017). *Doughnut economics: Seven ways to think like a 21st–century economist.* New York: Random House Business.

Ricci, R. J., & Clayton, C. A. (2016). EMDR with sex offenders: Using offense drivers to guide conceptualization and treatment. *Journal of EMDR Practice and Research, 10*(2), 104. https://doi.org/10.1891/1933-3196.10.2.104

Ronald R.J., & Clayton, C.A. (2016). EMDR with sex offenders: Using offense drivers to guide conceptualization and treatment. *Journal of EMDR Practice and Research, 10*(2), 104–118. https://doi.org/10.1891/1933-3196.10.2.104

Rothschild, B. (2006). *Help for the helper: The psychophysiology of compassion fatigue and vicarious trauma.* New York: Norton.

Seikkula, J., Aaltonen, J., Alakare, B., Haarakangas, K., Keränen, J., & Lehtinen, K. (2006). Five-year patience of first-episode nonaffective psychosis in open-dialogue approach: Treatment principles, follow-up outcomes, and two case studies. *Psychotherapy Research, 16*(2), 214–228. https://doi.org/10.1080/10503300500268490

Shapiro, F. (2012). *Getting past your past. Take control of your life with self-help techniques and EMDR therapy.* Emmaus, PA: Rodale Books.

Shapiro, F. (2017). *Eye Movement Desensitization and Reprocessing (EMDR) therapy: Basic principles, protocols, and procedures* (3rd ed.). New York: Guilford Press.

Silber, M. D., & Bhatt, A. (2007). *Radicalization in the West: The homegrown threat.* New York: NYPD Intelligence Division.

Stephens, W., Sieckelinck, S., & Boutellier, H. (2021). Preventing violent extremism: A review of the literature. *Studies in Conflict & Terrorism, 44*(4), 346–361. https://doi.org/10.1080/1057610X.2018.1543144

Sweeney, A., Filson, B., Kennedy, A., Collinson, L., & Gillard, S. (2018). A paradigm shift: Relationships in trauma-informed mental health services. *BJPsych Advances, 24*(5), 319–333. https://doi.org/10.1192/bja.2018.29.

Tardiolo, G., Bramanti, P., & Mazzon, E. (2018). Overview on the effects of *n*-acetylcysteine in neurodegenerative diseases. *Molecules, 23*(12), 3305. https://doi.org/10.3390/molecules23123305.

Tedeschi, R. G., & Calhoun, L. G. (2004). Posttraumatic growth: Conceptual foundations and empirical evidence. *Psychological Inquiry, 15*(1), 1–18. https://doi.org/10.1207/s15327965pli1501_01

Tenenbaum, B. (1961). Group therapy with LSD-25. A preliminary report. *Nervous System Diseases, 22*, 459–462.

Valeri, A., & Mazzon, E. (2021). Cannabinoids and neurogenesis: The promised solution for neurodegeneration? *Molecules, 26*(20), 6313. https://doi.org/10.3390/molecules26206313

Vargas, M., Meyer, R., Avanes, A., Rus, M., & Olson, D. (2021). Psychedelics and other psychoplastogens for treating mental illness. *Frontiers in Psychiatry, 12*, 727117. https://doi.org/10.3389/fpsyt.2021.727117

Wade, C. (2024). To test the feasibility of a research study design for a future RCT examining the efficacy of AI-EMDR vs Standard Protocol (SP) for clients with attachment-informed complexity, Poster Presentation. EMDR UK Conference 2024, New York.

Walsch, Z., Hendricks, P.S., & Smith, S. (2016). Hallucinogen use and intimate partner violence: Prospective evidence consistent with protective effects among men with histories of problematic substance use. *Journal of Psychopharmacology, 3*, 601–607. https://doi.org/10.1177/026988111664253

World Health Organization (WHO). (2018). *International classification of diseases for mortality and morbidity statistics* (11th ed.). Geneva: World Health Organization.

Index

Note: *Italic* page numbers refer to figures.